AF443421

# The Effective Management of
# Breast Cancer

## Second edition

# The Effective Management of Breast Cancer

## Second edition

*Edited by*

Robert Leonard BSc MB BS MD FRCP
*Professor of Medical Oncology
and Director, South West Wales Cancer Institute, Wales, UK*

Andreas Polychronis MB MRCP
*Clinical Research Fellow in Medical Oncology
and Assistant Editor, Journal of Evaluation in Clinical Practice,
Imperial College of Science, Technology and Medicine, London, UK*

Andrew Miles MSc MPhil PhD
*Professor of Public Health Sciences
& Editor-in-Chief, Journal of Evaluation in Clinical Practice
Barts and The London,
Queen Mary's School of Medicine and Dentistry
University of London, UK*

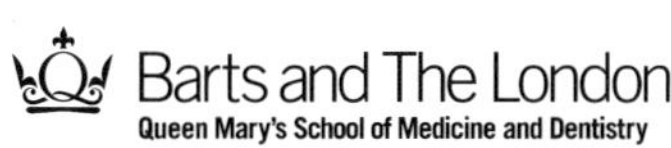
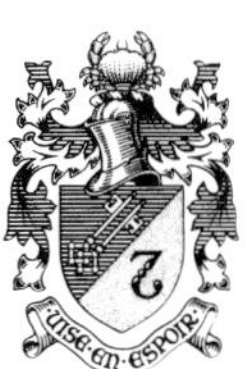
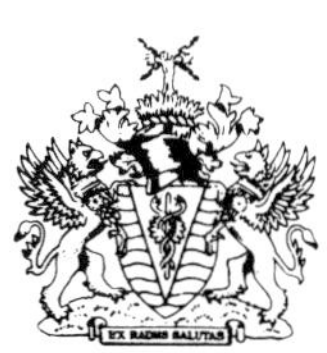
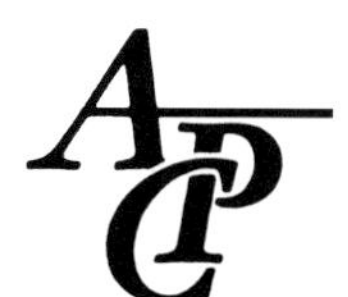

| British<br>Association of<br>Surgical Oncology | The Royal<br>College of<br>Radiologists | Association<br>of Cancer<br>Physicians |
| --- | --- | --- |

AESCULAPIUS MEDICAL PRESS
LONDON  SAN FRANCISCO  SYDNEY

Published by

Aesculapius Medical Press (London, San Francisco, Sydney)
PO Box LB48, Mount Pleasant Mail Centre, Farringdon Road, London EC1A 1LB, UK



**British Library Cataloguing in Publication Data**
A CIP catalogue record for this book is available from the British Library

ISBN 1 903044 41 3

While the advice and information in this book are believed to be true and accurate at the
time of going to press, neither the authors nor the publishers nor the sponsoring institutions
can accept any legal responsibility or liability for any errors or omissions that may be made.
In particular (but without limiting the generality of the preceding disclaimer) every effort
has been made to check drug usages; however, it is possible that errors have been missed.
Furthermore, dosage schedules are constantly being revised and new side effects recognised.
For these reasons, the reader is strongly urged to consult the drug companies' printed
instructions before administering any of the drugs recommended in this book.

*Further copies of this volume are available from:*

Claudio Melchiorri
Aesculapius Medical Press
PO Box LB48, Mount Pleasant Mail Centre, Farringdon Road, London EC1A 1LB, UK

Fax: 020 8525 8661
Email: claudio@keyadvances4.demon.co.uk
www.keyadvances.org.uk

Copy edited by The Clyvedon Press Ltd, Cardiff, UK

Typeset, printed and bound in Britain
Peter Powell Origination & Print Limited

# Contents

# Contributors

Richard Adams BMedSci BM BS MRCP(UK), Specialist Registrar and Research Fellow in Clinical Oncology, Velindre Hospital NHS Trust, Cardiff, UK

Andre Ahr MD, Department of Gynecology and Obstetrics, J.W. Goethe University, Frankfurt am Main, Germany

Timothy J. Archer FRCS, Consultant Surgeon, Ipswich Hospital, Ipswich

Peter Barrett-Lee MD FRCR FRCP(Edin) FRCP(Lond), Consultant Clinical Oncologist, Velindre Hospital NHS Trust, Cardiff, UK

Michael Baum FRCS, Professor of Surgery, Meyerstein Institute of Oncology, and Academic Department of Surgery, University College London Hospitals NHS Trust, London, UK

Nicolas Beechey-Newman FRCS, Consultant Surgeon, Department of Academic Oncology, Guy's Hospital, London, UK

Nigel J. Bundred MD FRCS, Professor in Surgical Oncology, South Manchester University Hospital, Manchester, UK

David A. Cameron MD FRCP, Consultant Medical Oncologist, Department of Oncology, University of Edinburgh, Edinburgh, UK

Sandra M. deCanha MB ChB MMed, Department of Clinical Oncology, Mount Vernon Hospital, Middlesex, UK

Andrew Champion BSc PhD, Centre Manager, National Collaborative Centre for Cancer, Cardiff, Wales, UK

Robert Coleman MD FRCP (Lond. and Edin.), Professor of Medical Oncology, Academic Unit of Clinical Oncology, Cancer Research Centre, Weston Park Hospital, Sheffield, UK

Isabel dos Santos Silva MD MSc PhD, Clinical Senior Lecturer in Epidemiology, Non-Communicable Disease Epidemiology Unit, London School of Hygiene and Tropical Medicine, London, UK

Diana M. Eccles MD FRCP, Consultant/Senior Lecturer in Cancer Genetics, Wessex Regional Genetics Service, Southampton University Hospitals Trust, Cancer Sciences Research Division, Wessex Clinical Genetics Service, Princess Anne Hospital, Southampton, UK

Ian O. Ellis FRCPath, Professor of Cancer Pathology, University of Nottingham, UK

Paul Ellis MD FRCP, Consultant Medical Oncologist, Guy's and St. Thomas's Hospital, London, UK

Christopher W. Elston MD FRCPath, Professor of Tumour Pathology, University of Nottingham, UK

Julie Evans BSc MSc, Senior Qualitative Researcher, Department of Primary Health Care, University of Oxford, UK

Andrew M. Hanby BM FRCPath, Professor of Breast Pathology, University of Leeds, UK

Jane Hanson BSc PhD, Programme Co-ordinator for Cancer Services Group, Wales, UK

Uwe Holtrich PhD, Department of Gynecology and Obstetrics, J.W. Goethe University, Frankfurt am Main, Germany

Peter J. Hoskin BSc MD FRCP FRCPath, Professor of Clinical Oncology, Mount Vernon Hospital, Middlesex

Stephen R. D. Johnston MA PhD FRCP, Consultant Medical Oncologist, Royal Marsden Hospital, London, UK

Thomas Karn PhD, Department of Gynecology and Obstetrics, J.W. Goethe University, Frankfurt am Main, Germany

Manfred Kaufman MD, Department of Gynecology and Obstetrics, J.W. Goethe University, Frankfurt am Main, Germany

Ashutosh Kothari MS DNB MNAMS, Senior Research Fellow, Department of Academic Oncology, Guy's Hospital, London, UK

Andrew H. S. Lee MRCP MRCPath, Consultant Histopathologist, Nottingham City Hospital, Nottingham, UK

Robert Leonard BSc MB BS MD FRCP, Professor of Medical Oncology & Director, South West Wales Cancer Institute, Swansea, Wales, UK

Ann McPherson CBE FRCGP FRCP DCH, General Practitioner, Lecturer, Department of Primary Health Care, University of Oxford, UK

Fergus Macbeth FRCR, Consultant Clinical Oncologist, Velindre Hospital, Wales

Robert Mansel MD FRCS, Professor of Surgery, University of Wales College of Medicine, Cardiff

David W. Miles MD BSc FRCP, Senior Lecturer in Medical Oncology, ICRF Breast Cancer Biology Group, Guy's Hospital, London, UK

Sarah E. Pinder FRCPath, Senior Lecturer and Consultant Histopathologist, University of Nottingham, UK

Andreas Polychronis MB MRCP, Clinical Research Fellow in Medical Oncology and Assistant Editor, *Journal of Evaluation in Clinical Practice*, Imperial College at the Hammersmith Hospital, London.

Suman Prinjha PhD, Senior Qualitative Researcher, Department of Primary Health Care, University of Oxford, UK

Richard M. Rainsbury MBBS BSc MS FRCS, Director, Oncoplastic Breast Unit, Royal Hampshire County Hospital, Winchester, Hampshire, UK

Carmel Sheppard RGN BSc MSc Dip. Counselling, Consultant Nurse – Breast Care, Portsmouth Hospitals NHS Trust / University of Southampton, UK

Valerie Speirs BSc PhD, Senior Lecturer and Team Leader, Molecular Medicine, University of Leeds, UK

C Michael Steel PhD DSc FRCP FRCPath FRCS FRSE, Professor in Medical Science, Bute Medical School, University of St Andrews, Fife, UK

Jeffrey S. Tobias, Professor of Clinical Oncology, Meyerstein Institute of Oncology, and Academic Department of Surgery, University College London Hospitals NHS Trust, London, UK

Lindsay W Turnbull BSc MB ChB DMRD FRCR MD, Postgraduate Medical Institute of the University of Hull, Centre for Magnetic Resonance Investigations, Hull Royal Infirmary, Hull, UK

Lorraine E Turner RGN BSc, Research Sister, South Manchester University Hospital, Manchester, UK

Jayant S. Vaidya MB BS MS DNB FRCS PhD, Meyerstein Institute of Oncology, and Academic Department of Surgery, University College London Hospitals NHS Trust, London, UK

John Yarnold BSc MRCP FRCR, Professor of Clinical Oncology, Royal Marsden Hospital, Sutton, Surrey, UK

Charlotte Westbury BSc MRCP FRCR, Clinical Research Fellow, Institute of Cancer Research, London, UK

# Preface

More than three decades of epidemiological studies have identified various adult risk factors for breast cancer. In recent years, however, research has raised the possibility that factors operating *in utero* and in early life may be as important in the aetiology of mammary carcinomas as those acting in adult life. Associations have been reported, although not always consistently across all studies, between breast cancer risk and various *in utero* exposures. In particular, the evidence points to a positive association between birth weight and breast cancer risk at pre-menopausal, but not postmenopausal, ages. Published data are also consistent with maternal pre-eclampsia or eclampsia being associated with a reduced risk of breast cancer. Being born a twin is associated with an increased risk. Rapid childhood growth, as indicated by the timing of menarche, leg length and adult height, has also been associated with an increase in the risk of breast cancer. Support for the role of pre- and postnatal growth rates in the aetiology of this cancer is also provided by evidence of a positive association between adult serum levels of insulin-like growth factors and subsequent risk of breast cancer. Although there are still many unanswered questions regarding the role of early life exposures on breast cancer risk, and how they may interact with the established adult risk factors, these findings imply the need for research and for efforts in prevention to shift from adult to early life. Indeed, it is precisely to such a detailed consideration that dos Santos Silva turns in the opening chapter of Part One of this volume, which we have dedicated, through Chapters 1–3, to a thorough overview of our current understanding of the aetiology, epidemiology and genetics of breast cancer.

In Chapter 2, we turn to a discussion of recent progress in studies of the molecular biology of breast cancer and the modifiers of penetrance. As Steel describes, breast cancer is thought to arise through the progressive accumulation of mutations in specific oncogenes and tumour suppressors. Germ-line mutations in some of these genes account for familial predisposition but, as this author discusses, there is a huge gap between epidemiology-based estimates of the total contribution of genetics to breast cancer (from 20 to 80%), and most genetic factors in breast cancer remain undetermined. BRCA1 and BRCA2 are, of course, the most intensively studied of the known "breast cancer genes", but despite the scale of investigation their functions remain inadequately characterized, although they both appear to participate, with many other gene products, in homologous recombination of DNA (in double-strand break repair and in meiotic interchange). They may, however, also act as transcription factors, and microarray analysis of gene expression in BRCA1 or BRCA2 mutation-bearing cancers does indeed demonstrate patterns that are distinct from those of sporadic breast cancers. For example, inactivation of p53 is very common and may contribute to the high pathological grade typical of BRCA1 mutant tumours in particular. Truncating mutations throughout either gene carry substantially increased risks of breast and ovarian cancer. BRCA2 mutations also confer risks of pancreatic, urothelial and other tumours. For both, mutation site influences the relative risks of breast and ovarian cancer but other factors, genetic and environmental, appear to be even more important in determining tumour-specific and overall penetrance.

Genetic counselling for breast cancer risk involves assessing all available evidence to determine the likelihood of a genetic predisposition to breast cancer, the mode of inheritance (if any), the likelihood of genetic testing being helpful and the interpretation of any test results. This information must then be translated into an assessment of cancer risks for families and individuals which will directly inform the discussion of options for risk management. Individuals at risk will come to a genetic assessment with variable background knowledge and very varied experiences of cancer that will affect the way that information is perceived and dealt with, and it is to a thorough description of these factors that Eccles turns in Chapter 3. Interpreting and estimating genetic and epidemiological risks is complex, and although many methods have been described, few have been widely validated prospectively. Genetic services have a regional base, usually in a teaching hospital with outreach clinic availability, but in general terms it is true to say that the availability of special interest cancer genetics clinics remains 'patchy', mainly due to the current shortage of clinical geneticists with oncology training and an interest in clinical cancer genetics. The use of skilled genetic counsellors is widespread in offering genetic counselling services throughout the UK and the management options for an individual at risk include prevention and early detection by screening. But choices will depend on level of risk and risk perception. For the patient diagnosed with hereditary breast cancer, management options may differ, and it is still unclear whether treatment strategies need to take into account the potential differential response to adjuvant therapies in hereditary breast cancer and whether these have a different prognosis to age-matched sporadic cancers.

We have dedicated Part Two of the text, through Chapters 4–7, to detailed discussion of the imaging, biopsy and endoscopy of breast cancer. Using gadolinium-based intravenous contrast agents, fast imaging techniques and dedicated receiver coils, dynamic contrast-enhanced magnetic resonance imaging (DCE-MRI) is becoming an invaluable tool in the diagnosis and treatment of breast disease. This technique has been termed 'dynamic' because it relies on rapid data acquisition before, during and after the bolus administration of an MR-specific contrast agent. Using this method of data acquisition, sensitivities for symptomatic cases are now in excess of 95% and specificities greater than 90% for invasive breast cancer. The high sensitivity and specificity of DCE-MRI relies on the use of intravenous gadolinium, which passes into the extravascular space and accumulates in tissues with high vascularity. The justification for using gadolinium, as Turnbull describes in Chapter 4, is that most cancers induce neo-vascularisation. A carcinoma larger than 3 mm in diameter secretes pro-angiogenic molecules which increase the vascularity of the region by recruiting new vessels. Other factors that encourage tissue enhancement are expansion of the extracellular space, increased interstitial pressure and increased capillary permeability due to an abnormal basement membrane or cytokine-mediated effects. These result in more rapid accumulation of gadolinium in cancers than in benign lesions. MRI therefore shows considerable promise for improved management of patients with primary breast malignancy. The comparative benefit and cost-effectiveness of this technique with respect to other imaging modalities is currently under evaluation, but interest will centre around alternation in surgical management, in particular reduction in the requirement for re-operation for positive resection margins, the role of MRI in assessment of microcalcification and assessment of the efficacy of neoadjuvant chemotherapy.

Despite the early work of Sartorius and colleagues in the late 1970's (which demonstrated that the breast consists of 15–20 radially arranged lobules, each opening at the nipple through a major duct), the breast, as Beechey-Newman and Kothari discuss in Chapter 5, still appears to remain overwhelmingly considered as a solid organ. The mammary gland is an unusual organ in that most of its development takes place at puberty and subsequent development is limited to pregnancy and lactation. Almost 90% of all breast cancers, as the authors remind us, are described histopathologically as invasive ductal or lobular carcinomas and it is now established that these histologically distinct breast epithelial tumour types originate from the epithelial lining of the intralobular ducts and terminal ducto-lobular units. Almost without exception, breast carcinomas express protein characteristics of ductal luminal epithelial cells. Studies into the natural history of breast cancer have revealed that the journey from the first signs of epithelial cell atypia to frank invasive malignancy may take several years. In this process of transformation, up to and including the stage of ductal carcinoma *in situ*, the problem is confined entirely to the breast duct. Once the invasive stage of cellular neoplasia is reached then the accepted paradigm is that it should be regarded as a systemic disease, rather than a loco-regional entity. The histological recognition and classification of these pre-invasive states has been advanced greatly over the past two decades. However, the most significant benefits from the application of these advances may still be to come. Beechey-Newman and Kothari are, of course, correct in their assertion that none of the imaging modalities available for the diagnosis of early breast cancer today give us direct access to the ductal epithelium, which is the point of origin of all breast carcinomas. Holland and associates, in 1990, demonstrated that only 50% of micropapillary or cribriform DCIS is associated with microcalcification, and it fails to show *in situ* malignancy in the region of the nipple in 70% of the cases. Other pre-malignant conditions such as atypical ductal hyperplasia are rarely, if ever, detected by any of the existing imaging modalities. It follows, therefore, that an imaging technique that offers direct visualization of the mammary ductal epithelia has the potential to provide greater accuracy in the diagnosis of benign and malignant pathology. It is for this reason that the authors advance the concept and technique of breast duct microendoscopy as a "revolutionary method" of breast imaging for 2005 and beyond, which will for the first time allow the assessment of the part of the breast that is of most importance to us – the ductal epithelium.

The aims of non-operative diagnosis are essentially threefold and namely that patients can undergo one therapeutic surgical procedure, facilitate counselling of patients and reduce the number of diagnostic surgical biopsies for benign disease. To achieve this the pathologist needs to be able reliably to diagnose malignancy, to distinguish between invasive and *in situ* carcinoma, to make definitive benign diagnoses and to explain clinical and imaging abnormalities, including calcification. The major difference between needle core biopsy (NCB) and fine needle aspiration cytology (FNAC) is the additional architectural information provided by NCB and it is to a detailed evaluation of the relative usefulness of these techniques that Lee and associates turn in Chapter 6. Both FNAC and NCB have well established roles in diagnosing malignancy in symptomatic patients, but the authors are clear that in screening patients, the absolute sensitivity for carcinoma and specificity are significantly higher for NCB and, indeed, the distinction between *in situ* and invasive carcinoma cannot be made with FNAC. With NCB the positive predictive value of a diagnosis of invasion is virtually 100% but about 20% of patients with a diagnosis of only DCIS on core will also have invasion in the subsequent surgical specimen. FNA cannot reliable distinguish normal breast tissue from benign lesions, whereas the architectural information provided by NCB often enables definitive diagnosis of benign lesions such as fibroadenomas and NCB is, additionally, better at assessing calcification. The authors discuss how a radiograph of the specimen can show whether the calcification has been sampled, and the histological changes associated with the calcification identified. Calcification is never seen in FNAC so there is less certainty that the correct area has been sampled. The advantages of NCB described by Lee and colleagues undoubtedly explain why many breast units to assess most lesions using NCB but it remains the case that in a small number of patients core biopsy is either contraindicated or may be difficult, so that either FNAC or surgical biopsy has to be performed. A problem with infrequent use of FNAC is maintenance of competence of both the aspirator and the pathologist. Neither FNAC or NCB is perfect and the authors are clear that it remains essential that the results of both FNAC and NCB are assessed in the light of the clinical and imaging findings, ideally in the context of multidisciplinary meetings.

As we move further into 21$^{st}$ century Medicine, the place of the histopathologist in the diagnosis, determination of treatment and as a pivotal player in the development of new therapies for breast cancer appears surprisingly secure. We say, with Hanby and Speirs, writing in Chapter 7, 'surprisingly secure', because with the characterization of the human genome, many colleagues have felt increasingly certain that knowledge of the genome alone may be enough to enable us to tackle the diagnosis and treatment of disease, arguably rendering histopathological analysis redundant. For Hanby and Speirs, such predictions remain quite premature, and many histopathological challenges remain ahead in the analysis of breast cancer. These become manifest as changes evolve in the spectrum and quality of material received, in the form of novel imaging techniques and the approaches taken to obtain a biopsy. They also include the reliable assessment of molecular markers of predictive value, such as HER2, the anticipation of new targets, and the problems we face in measuring these. Finally, there is the hope for a better breast cancer taxonomy and the ability to predict outcome and to inform and direct therapy with far more precision. The authors describe how the quest for new markers, and their analysis in large patient cohorts, has been considerably accelerated by cDNA arrays. Such arrays allow the analysis of large numbers of gene expression levels, potential targets then can be localized immunohistochemically or by *in situ* hybridization on tissue microarrays. These methods, the authors emphasise, will be further augmented by the increasing introduction of proteomic array technology. Whether these approaches will make conventional morphological analysis redundant therefore remains to be seen. However, these array methods have already demonstrated considerable prognostic power. The vast amount of data is subject to bioinformatics/AI analysis, which conceivably could include morphological data. In this way, distinct clusters with distinct morphologies and different drug response profiles might be defined, so allowing histopathological triage of tumours into different groups which then may be subject to more focused, though costly analysis. Against this, it is likely that better discrimination of risk and prediction of benefit will encourage a better targeted use of expensive and toxic therapy. This is, as Hanby and Speirs admit, exciting though at the time of writing, purely speculative, and the results of further studies which will specifically test such possibilities are awaited with great interest.

We have dedicated Part Three of this volume, through Chapters 8–12, to a detailed review of the current evidence and opinion base for surgical intervention in early and recurrent breast cancer. In the opening chapter of this Part, Mansel reminds us that the current status of sentinel node biopsy remains rather confused. Although there are several multi-centre randomised trials of the technique which have been funded in the USA and Europe, there are still no conclusive results available from completed trials. The literature consists of large numbers of small audit studies usually from single centres, largely showing that a success rate varying from around 70% to >95% can be achieved in locating the sentinel node and a false negative rate of between 0 and 25%. The standards set by the ALMANAC study in the UK, of which Mansel has been a principal investigator, are that a surgeon should achieve a 95% success rate and a false negative rate of around 5%. In the USA, as the author goes on to discuss, some surgeons have switched to using sentinel node biopsy as their standard of care for small tumours, although this change in practice is not always based on institutional audit data. A consensus meeting in Philadelphia in the USA decided that sentinel node biopsy is still not the standard of care for routine use and that the data from the randomised trials should be awaited before laying down new practice. Also, as the author describes, it was felt that institutions should validate surgeons' techniques by auditing a series of sentinel node biopsies compared against a gold standard axillary staging technique so that individual rates are known for both success and false negative values. In the UK, the ALMANAC study is the main randomised trial which is currently accruing patients and which has to date randomised many hundreds of patients. The target is 1300 and this will give sufficient power to examine the patient acceptability, psychosocial outcomes and health economic issues. It is likely that sentinel node biopsy will produce a saving in time in the operating theatre and a reduction in morbidity. However, the main question for patients is the issue of whether a sentinel node procedure alone is safe enough to accept a negative result indicating no requirement for further axillary surgery to provide accurate prognostication further treatment. The answer to this question awaits some long term data which currently do not exist.

Breast surgery is now an established subspecialty of general surgery in the UK, with the traditional model of the general surgeon with a subspecialty interest in breast surgery having changed, irrevocably, as Rainsbury describes in Chapter 9. On the one hand, shorter training programmes, the European Working Time Directive, better outcomes and mounting patient, provider and professional expectations are leading to greater specialization. On the other hand, today's trainees with a subspecialty interest in breast surgery are acquiring a new range of skills and competencies, with more than 80% prioritizing training in breast reconstruction. Heightened trainee expectations are generating innovative new initiatives that cross the traditional boundaries between breast and plastic surgery, encouraging the acquisition of hybrid skills. Growing collaboration between the British Association of Surgical Oncology, British Association of Breast Surgery and the British Association of Plastic Surgeons has, as Rainsbury describes, resulted in a new cross-specialty training programme in oncoplastic breast surgery with this new specialization being seen to combine the best principles of tumour resection (to achieve wide, tumour-free margins), with the best principles of breast reconstruction (to optimize cosmetic outcomes while minimising complications).

The use of systemic drug therapy before surgery for operable breast cancer became more common in the latter half of the 1980s, with three principal arguments being advanced in justification of this approach. Once it has been clearly established that breast conservation was a safe and appropriate way to manage smaller cancers, it was felt that the reduction in tumour size achieved with drug therapy might allow more women to have successful breast conservation. Laboratory studies predicted that that initiation of effective systemic therapy before removal of the primary tumour would result in improvements in metastasis-free survival for the patients. Additionally, by observing possible tumour response to the therapy, the most appropriate post-surgical adjuvant therapy could be chosen. Several studies have addressed these issues but not without controversy. One school of thought expresses concerns that delaying surgery, particularly in those patients whose tumours were not very responsive, might compromise operability, increase operative complications and possibly even long-term local control. In Chapter 10, Cameron elegantly reviews the accumulated literature and considers recent data. He concludes that pre-operative chemotherapy has clearly come of age and that published data are convincing that there is no survival detriment resulting from delayed surgery. He feels it is equally clear that those women whose tumours respond will live longer, and that it is the pathological rather than clinical response that best predicts for long-term outcome.

Can a 'low risk' subgroup be identified in whom radiotherapy can be safely omitted after breast conservation surgery? It is to this particular question that Westbury and Yarnold turn in Chapter 11. Readers will be aware of the systematic review published by the Early Breast Cancer Trial Collaborative Group (EBCTCG) which demonstrated that randomization to radiotherapy after mastectomy or breast preserving surgery prevents, on average, 20 isolated local recurrences per 100 women irradiated at 10 years. This achieves a 5% absolute reduction in breast cancer deaths at 20 years. The same benefit is seen after mastectomy or tumour excision, in pN- and pN+ patients and those treated with or without adjuvant chemotherapy or endocrine therapy. Although an excess cardiac mortality offset this benefit in early trials, the evidence suggests that modern radiotherapy techniques are less harmful. The prevention of 5 breast cancer deaths by the prevention of 20 local recurrences means that irradiation of a group with a 10% local recurrence risk avoids, on average, 2 breast cancer deaths. This represents the threshold of benefit at which adjuvant systemic therapy is commonly recommended. Current practice in the UK, as the authors discuss, is to select patients for radiotherapy with a local-regional recurrence risk in the region of 30% or more viz. pT3 or pN+(>4), in whom the chest wall recurrence risk is >40% after mastectomy. In fact, there is a strong case for recommending patients with pT2 disease and/or any lymph nodes positive for post-mastectomy radiotherapy, regardless of adjuvant systemic therapy. Where breast conserving surgery is concerned, it is currently impossible reliably to identify subgroups with a local recurrence risk <10% at 10 years. Current observational and randomized studies suggest that, even in small screen-detected lesions less than 10mm in diameter, the breast relapse rate is in the range 10–20% at 10 years. In spite of this, audits of patients with small-screen detected lesions in England treated in the 1990's, suggest that around 20% of patients treated by breast preserving surgery are not referred for radiotherapy. Regardless of what form of local surgery or systemic therapies are applied, the prevention of 4 local-regional recurrences by radiotherapy prevents 1 breast cancer death. For Westbury and Arnold, current thresholds for breast cancer radiotherapy in the UK are the legacy of a by-gone era and perpetuate unnecessary breast cancer mortality and they are clear that lower thresholds for treatment need to be adopted, together with routine techniques for excluding heart from the treatment volume.

The ability of prognostic criteria to predict individual disease progression and clinical outcome remains imperfect. This uncertainty in forecasting outcome means that some patients who need adjuvant treatment do not receive it, whereas others are unnecessarily treated and as a result are exposed to the risk of side effects without good reason. For Karn and associates, writing in Chapter 12, improved tools are therefore clearly needed for the assessment of prognosis in breast cancer and a major goal, therefore, is the development of an individual risk-profile system with high accuracy and reproducibility to estimate patients' prognosis and best treatment. The completion of the Human Genome Project and the development of new, high performance screening techniques have revolutionized the ways in which researchers can study the pathogenesis of disease and the analysis of the levels of expression of thousands of genes in parallel with the use of DNA or mRNA chips has shown distinct patterns in different types of tumour. Because the expression of the genes is measured, such analysis is mostly referred to as expression profiling. These patterns can classify histologically similar tumours into specific subtypes, a process that provides clinically relevant information. Several studies on mammary carcinomas have aimed to categorise several subtypes of breast cancer, but these studies have mostly lacked correlation with classic clinical variables and follow-up data. Global determination of cellular transcriptional activity is expected to identify gene expression signatures that predict clinical behaviour of tumours and Karn and his colleagues provide a stimulating overview of this new technology and how it may be employed in the identification of patients at high risk of tumour recurrence. They are clear that expression profiling, which has for some time been able to distinguish known subtypes of breast cancer, has now been able to identify novel subgroups, which differ in their clinical behaviour and which will have an impact on future treatment decisions. They conclude by anticipating that further studies will generate profiles that directly allow the individual prediction of response to a specific therapy.

We have dedicated Part Four of the volume, through Chapters 13–20, to a detailed review of radiation and medical therapy in breast cancer. In the opening chapter, Tobias, Vaidya and Baum discuss the concept of conformal intra-operative brachytherapy in reducing radiotherapy dose in early breast cancer, an interesting, novel approach to treatment that is attracting considerable interest in the field. They discuss the origins of this technique and the early experience of its use and results, describing their own studies in detail together with a very full discussion of the benefits of the technique in terms of rapid access to radiotherapy. We move, in Chapter 14, to de Canha and Hoskin's elegant review of current thinking on the role of radiotherapy in metastatic disease. Palliative radiotherapy, as these authors document, represents around 50% of any departmental workload and 30% of palliative patients will have breast cancer. Breast cancer palliation therefore takes up around 15% of all radiotherapy activity and represents a major workload. The main indications for palliative radiotherapy in breast cancer are bone pain, pathological fracture, spinal cord compression and brain metastasis, although other, less common, scenarios where palliative radiotherapy is of value include chest wall fungation, cranial nerve palsies, choroidal metastasis, symptoms from enlarged lymph nodes and soft tissue disease. In the multicentre randomised trials of bone metastasis listed by the authors, breast cancer represents around 40% of patients. These show that single doses of radiation are effective and equivalent to more protracted courses of treatment for both pain relief and acute toxicity. Where there are several sites of pain then wide field radiotherapy (hemibody radiotherapy) or radioisotope treatment with strontium or samarium are highly effective. Where bone metastases are complicated by inoperable pathological fracture local radiotherapy is also indicated and de Canha and Hoskin discuss how in the management of brain metastasis careful patient selection is required to obtain optimal results and avoid treatment for those patients who will not benefit. Survival is, as they discuss, closely related to performance status and the presence or absence of metastasis in other sites. Multiple metastasis in a patient with good performance status and disease control or absent metastasis elsewhere should, the authors recommend, receive whole brain radiotherapy and doses of 12Gy in 2 fractions, or 20 to 30Gy in 5 to 10 fractions are commonly given and considered equally effective. There is some evidence, as the authors conclude, that a slightly higher radiation dose has small benefits in patients with better performance status and in patients with solitary metastasis surgical excision should be considered with post-operative radiotherapy or where this is not surgically possible stereotactic radiotherapy.

During the past 15–20 years, it has become acceptable to use systemic therapy before surgery for operable breast cancer. The available literature clearly shows it to be a safe and feasible approach, with no survival detriment consequent upon surgery being delayed due to the pre-operative use of systemic therapy. The published series also suggest that there is a higher rate of breast conservation with this approach, although a few questions persist about the durability of some of this organ preservation. Prognostic factors have been derived; some are the same as for post-surgical adjuvant therapy, but the more informative ones relate to the extent of pathological tumour response. Although clinical response is associated with a better outcome, it is not as good a discriminator as the microscopic response. Current approaches are to use this setting as a test-bed for newer regimens/approaches, since it not only reflects the adjuvant setting better than patients with advanced malignancy, but has the added advantage of providing efficacy data (as seen in both clinical and pathological response rates) much quicker than adjuvant trials. Perhaps most interesting are the studies that try and use this setting further to understand tumour biology, but with the exception of one randomised trial with endocrine agents, they have not fulfilled their early promise. It is to the place of adjuvant systemic chemotherapy, by definition that therapy given after surgery in operable disease, that Adams, Barrett-Lee and Ellis turn in Chapter 15. As the authors discuss, systemic therapy in this setting has been shown to provide survival benefit to all groups of breast cancer patients regardless of menopausal, nodal, or hormonal receptor status, in the latest 2000 polychemotherapy overview by the Early Breast Cancer Trialists' Collaborative Group. In metastatic breast cancer resistant to anthracyclines, the taxoids paclitaxel and docetaxel have been shown to have useful activity with response rates of the order of 40–50%. It has therefore been postulated that sequential administration of these non-cross resistant agents in the adjuvant setting may lead to further gains. Initial results of this approach in the US were encouraging, with the CALGB 9344 study of 3170 patients randomised between four cycles of AC over 12 weeks vs. four cycles of AC followed by four cycles of paclitaxel over a total of 24 weeks, showing a reduction in the annual odds of recurrence by 22% and death by 26% at 30 months. However, a relatively recent update of this trial, and two subsequent trials of similar design, have cast doubts on the benefits of the paclitaxel arm. The NCRN/CRUK Taxotere as Adjuvant Chemotherapy Trial TACT) is therefore testing the hypothesis that the addition of four cycles of sequential docetaxel following 4 cycles of FEC will result in significant disease-free & overall survival benefit when compared with standard UK anthracycline-based chemotherapy of similar duration. Subsidiary studies will assess the QoL, health economic and cost-utility aspects of the treatments. This study already recruited over 1,500 patients in its first year, and is on course to complete recruitment ahead of schedule.

Having considered systemic therapy in the adjuvant setting, we move, in Chapter 16, to a listing and description of current chemotherapy trials in breast cancer. As Polychronis and Leonard discuss, a variety of cytotoxic and hormonal agents provide significant palliation for patients with metastatic breast cancer and the role of cytotoxic chemotherapy is well established for patients with life-threatening disease that requires rapid tumour control. Although polychemotherapy regimens produce higher response rates compared with single agent therapy, the survival impact is modest. Anthracycline plus taxane regimens are the most effective therapy, at the price of higher toxicity and should, the authors judge, be considered for patients with rapidly growing visceral metastases, lymphangitic spread or locally advanced breast cancer. For the majority of patients, then, the available data support the sequential use of single agent chemotherapy or the usual two to three drug combination regimens (eg, FAC, FEC, CMF). It must be remembered, they emphasize, that there is still a law of diminishing returns with successive lines of chemotherapy. Particularly as more complex adjuvant chemotherapy combinations are being used routinely, as Adams and colleagues discuss in Chapter 15, it is likely that well tolerated novel agents or combinations will replace anthracycline-based regimens in the palliation and management of relapsed disease.

Targeted therapies are not a new concept in the field of breast cancer. Strategies aimed at targeting the oestrogen receptor are, particularly, hardly new, but the identification and exploitation of other targets has taken longer than had been hoped. It is, as Miles discusses in Chapter 17, over 30 years since growth receptors were identified, but only in the past three years or so has a treatment targeting those receptors become available. Women whose tumours express HER2 at high levels have, as Miles documents, a relatively poor prognosis with a median survival of 3 years, compared with 6–7 years for HER2-negative cases, as Slamon first demonstrated in 1987. Many studies published subsequently, have demonstrated that HER2 overexpression is associated with other features of a poor prognosis, namely high tumour grade/s-phase fraction and oestrogen and progesterone receptor negativity. In many series, however, HER2 status remains an independent poor prognostic factor. Whether HER2 status is a predictor of poor response to other treatment modalities in breast cancer, namely hormonal and cytotoxic therapy, remains contentious. Conflicting data are presented in the literature regarding the ability of HER2 positivity to predict relative resistance to hormonal therapy and chemotherapy. The major difficulty in interpreting these studies are that they are retrospective analyses and in many instances there is no satisfactory 'control' arm against which to test attributable benefit of a treatment intervention in different HER2 subgroups. Although debate on this area is bound to continue, Miles feels it unlikely that prospective studies of adjuvant hormonal and/or chemotherapy will be stratified according to HER2 status. Such is the conflicting nature of the literature about HER2 as a predictive factor that a rational view would be that no active therapeutic option should be disregarded based solely on the HER2 status of a patient's tumour. Miles is clear that HER2 testing should be considered in patients with breast cancer, less perhaps because of its usefulness as a prognostic or predictive factor, but more to define whether the humanised monoclonal antibody to this growth factor receptor may be of use in patient management. Indeed, the use of trastuzumab in combination with chemotherapy has been demonstrated to prolong survival in women with metastatic breast cancer and the significance of this observation is perhaps implicit in the fact that few agents have shown such a benefit in this setting and certainly the additional toxicity associated with this benefit seems small. New combinations and schedules employing trastuzumab seem very promising but will need to be evaluated further.

A significant proportion of breast cancers are oestrogen dependent and are therefore amenable to endocrine therapy. While tamoxifen, a competitive non-steroidal anti-oestrogen, has been the mainstay of treatment for over 20 years, progress has been made with the development of third generation, potent oral aromatase inhibitors, including the non-steroidal inhibitors anastrazole and letrozole, together with the steroidal inhibitor exemestane, which are effective in reducing serum oestrogen levels in post-menopausal women. In Chapter 18, Johnston provides a particularly detailed review of these new generation aromatase inhibitors and their relative efficacy in the pre-operative, adjuvant and post-operative settings. In the metastatic setting, for example, Phase III trials in over 2000 post-menopausal women following failure of tamoxifen have demonstrated clinical superiority and improved tolerability over megestrol acetate, such that aromatase inhibitors may now be considered the standard of care as second line endocrine therapy. More recently, trials have asked whether these drugs should challenge tamoxifen as the first line agent of choice. In a US trials of 353 post-menopausal women, anastrozole, as Johnston describes, was associated with a significant improvement in time to disease progression compared with tamoxifen (5.6 to 11.1 months) although in a second larger European study the two drugs were equivalent. A large trial in 973 post-menopausal women showed a significant improvement both in response rate (30% vs 20%) and time to disease progression (9.2 vs 6.3 months), $p = 0.00001$) for patients treated with letrozole compared with tamoxifen. Interest has recently focussed, as this authors goes on the discuss, on the role of these drugs as pre-operative endocrine therapy for post-menopausal women with primary ER+ breast cancer. Results with letrozole have confirmed a higher response rate in terms of tumour shrinkage whether defined clinically, by ultrasound or mammography. In the adjuvant setting, clinical trials are addressing the potential role of aromatase inhibitors compared with tamoxifen, given either alone or in combination/sequence to tamoxifen. Early results are expected within the next few years, and if positive, may herald, Johnson is clear, a revolution in the endocrine treatment options for post-menopausal women with breast cancer.

Careful, or perhaps even simply an *outline* reading of the constituent chapter of the present volume so far, will have made clear to the specialist and non-specialist reader alike, the extraordinary progress made in recent years in the understanding of the aetiology and pathogenesis, natural history, and effective treatment of breast cancer. In Chapter 19, Johnston continues from his text in Chapter 18, by describing the current trends in ongoing research. Indeed, the most recent and significant advances have occurred, as he describes, in the development of systemic approaches for the treatment of advanced breast cancer. In particular, new endocrine therapies have challenged tamoxifen as the first-line therapy for oestrogen receptor (ER) positive breast cancer. Aromatase inhibitors have proved more effective with higher response rates and a better tolerability profile, significantly delaying progression of disease. In contrast, selective estrogen receptor modulators (SERMs) have proved disappointing in clinical trials, despite pre-clinical promise that their reduced agonist effects may improve upon the adverse effects of tamoxifen. A key problem in the clinic, as Johnston discusses, remains the development of endocrine resistance, either from the outset or as an acquired phenomenon after initial sensitivity to either tamoxifen or aromatase inhibitors. Experiments in the laboratory have shown that peptide growth factor pathways become up-regulated in cells exposed to long-term endocrine therapy, providing cells with an escape mechanism. Cross-talk occurs between these pathways to augment and amplify both oestrogen and growth factor signalling. Various signal transduction inhibitors (STIs) have been developed which block these pathways, including tyrosine kinase inhibitors, farnesyl transferase inhibitors, and cell cycle inhibitors, and experiments have shown that these drugs may be effective in hormone-resistant breast cancer, as Johnston discusses. In hormone-sensitive disease STIs, given in combination with endocrine therapy, may significantly prolong disease control by preventing the up-regulation of signalling pathways which leads to acquired resistance. Clinical trials of STIs, many or which are orally active and well tolerated, have started in patients with advanced breast cancer, including randomised studies in combination with tamoxifen or aromatase inhibitors. In concluding, Johnston is clear, as we agree, that these developments give hope that our new understanding of breast cancer molecular biology may at last translate into improved treatments for the disease.

No 'advanced disease' section of a volume on the effective management of breast cancer would be complete without a discussion of progress in the effective palliation of the late and often end-stage symptoms of disseminated disease, and it is to the role of bisphosphonate treatment for the management of bone metastases that Coleman turns in Chapter 20, the concluding chapter of Part Four. Advanced cancers frequently metastasise to bone and the resulting bone destruction is associated with a variety of skeletal complications, including pathological fractures, bone pain, impaired mobility, spinal cord compression and hypercalcaemia. The scale of these problems and their impact on human suffering is made clear by the commonly quoted statistic that some 1.5 Million cancer patients worldwide have bone metastases and experience their associated symptoms. While lacking in the ultimate goal of medical cure, there is a variety of treatments currently available for bone metastases and these include radiation therapy, surgery, bisphosphonates and analgesics, in addition to standard anti-cancer therapy. The primary goal of therapy is to minimise bone pain and morbidity and improve mobility and quality of life. Coleman is clear that bisphosphonates should now be considered part of standard management for breast cancer patients with symptomatic bone disease. Certainly, the available evidence, as this authors discusses, indicates that the aminobisphosphonates, and in particular zoledronic acid, are the most effective agents to prevent skeletal complications and relieve bone pain but he is clear that further work to define the optimal schedule of treatment, and when to start and stop treatment, is needed. Bone resoption markers may be useful in this regard. Current data suggest that oral clodronate may be useful in the adjuvant setting and that it reduces treatment-induced bone loss. However, larger, confirmatory trials are required before adjuvant bisphosphonates can be recommended for routine use.

We have dedicated Part Five, the penultimate Part of this volume, to discussion of key clinical considerations in the management of the menopausal patient, the ways in which an 'emotional adjustment' of the patient to her diagnosis and prognosis might be enhanced, and the role of the clinical nurse specialist in assisting breast surgeons, oncologists and palliative physicians in the provision of effective clinical care within the context of the multidisciplinary clinical team. Seventy percent of women who develop breast cancer are post-menopausal, with the remaining 30% often becoming prematurely menopausal following treatment for the disease. For breast cancer patients to make an informed decision about their transition through the menopause, Turner and Bundred believe it essential that their educational needs be met. Indeed, it is important that clinicians counsel women about the precipitation or exacerbation of hot flushes, especially if they are about to begin chemotherapy or tamoxifen. Worryingly, Schneider, some years ago now in 1997, identified that among pre- and post-menopausal women in the UK, between 40% and 60% had never discussed the menopause with their doctor. Only 4% of women aged 40–49 years in a study reported by Barlow and associates, consulted their general practitioner in relation to their menopausal symptoms. Within this context, Turner and Bundred recommend that clinicians and breast care specialists should therefore consider the development of protocols guiding appropriate menopausal management for women with a history of breast cancer as well as women going through the 'natural' menopause.

Modern medicine has been accurately characterised, perhaps, as being dominated and determined by the so-called 'biomedical paradigm' of disease pathogenesis and treatment. The last 20 years have seen a growing emphasis on what might be termed 'holistic' approaches to the treatment of disease in general and, latterly, to understanding – and treating – the psychological morbidity associated with disease: not only that experienced by the patient, but also that experienced by the immediate carers who are also directly affected by the 'catastrophe' that is a cancer diagnosis. In Chapter 22, McPherson and her colleagues, with direct reference to these considerations, describe the concept and application of a novel intervention aimed at increasing the 'emotional adjustment' of breast cancer patients. The authors invite the reader to consider the impact of 'bad news'. Indeed, "imagine", they suggest, "being told you have a life threatening illness….imagine that you are at home preparing supper for your family and the telephone rings and its your doctor (who says) unfortunately, the lump you found is indeed cancer". Or imagine being told that: "the cancer has spread and the treatment available will not necessarily be a cure, will cause your hair to fall out, make you sick, may cause diarrhoea and has other possible nasty side-effects". The authors are clear: such news will have to be given to the 36,000 or so women in the UK, each year, all of whom will have to deal with such unfamiliar and unexpected issues and feelings. Against this startling, but very real, scenario, McPherson and associates describe their novel intervention which they advance as a unique website that shows what the experience of illness is really like for patients – DIPEx – experiences of health and illness (www.dipex.org). The primary motivation leading to the creation of the intervention comes from Ann McPherson, a GP, the first author of this chapter, following her own diagnosis of breast cancer and her own wrestling with the diagnosis and support systems available to her. It is, we suggest, a salutary reminder as to the limitations of what we try to do, and make available for, breast cancer patients, and it functions, we suggest, as a so-called 'wake up call' as to the many aspects of 'holistic' breast cancer care that remain to be properly addressed as party of a more comprehensive approach to effective clinical care of the patient.

This theme of 'holistic care' continues in Chapter 23 with a discussion of the role of the clinical nurse specialist as an integral member of the multidisciplinary clinical team. Sheppard is, like McPherson and colleagues in the preceding chapter, clear that although we can never truly understand the unique personal experience of any woman following a diagnosis of breast cancer, a great deal of research over the last twenty years or so has enabled us to understand better and in more detail the complexities of the effects of the disease on quality of life and psychological health. Indeed, numerous studies have shown that the prevalence of anxiety and depression ranges between 25% and 50%. Despite this knowledge, there is evidence that psychological morbidity repeatedly goes unrecognised, with the primary focus of care remaining firmly fixed on the biomedical agenda. Sheppard shows the development of the role of the breast care nurse against this background and describes the *modus operandi* of the specialist nurse as it is current characterised.

We move in Part 6, the final Part, through Chapters 24–26, to a detailed consideration of issues of key importance to the clinical governance of breast cancer services. In the opening chapter of this Part, Archer reviews the history of political directives of direct relevance to breast cancer care and asks whether government targets are likely to make a significant difference to the health of patients with breast cancer or continue merely to function as political expedients. His chapter leads us on to a similarly 'political' issue: the processes and policies employed by the National Institute for Clinical Excellence (NICE) and specifically how these are impacting on treatment availability in Oncology generally, and breast cancer in particular. Ellis is clear that the regional inequality in cancer care across the UK and the increasing development of a two-tiered system whereby patients with wealth or health insurance have access to treatments that the rest of the world considered standard, whereas NHS patients do not, is nothing short of a national disgrace. He hopes, as do we, that NICE will address a range of issues that are in need of urgent consideration in order to ensure that patients are able to be offered state-of-the-art therapies. Indeed, many sceptical clinicians wait with interest to see if ring-fenced resources will automatically become available following so-called 'positive' NICE guidance. So far, this has not been remotely the case and Ellis is clear that NICE has much to address in cancer medicine throughout 2005. Indeed, many colleagues, and indeed many patients and their carers, consider that the failures of government in this regard should be considered as part of the discussions that are now beginning to take place as the General Election draws nearer.

The final chapter of the volume, Chapter 26, has been contributed by Macbeth and his co-workers and describes their early experience in monitoring the performance of breast cancer teams in Wales. The notion of 'clinical governance', though still poorly defined in intellectual terms, has made it explicit at least in outline concept that all health professionals are now accountable individually and collectively for the quality of the care that they give to patients. The quality and performance of cancer teams are increasingly questioned and failures are attracting unwelcome public attention. Ultimately, this need for more open scrutiny may be a good thing, but there are real problems in measuring how 'good' a clinician or a team is. Assessing quality is difficult. Firstly, how is quality defined and when parameters are delineated, how are they to be characterised and measured? If standards are to be implemented, on what evidence are they to be based? And what constitutes 'agreed clinical knowledge' that would then become appropriately implemented into practice? Macbeth and his colleagues duly consider many of these key questions of fundamental importance to anything which might be described as 'good' clinical care and their early experience, described within this closing chapter, has many lessons on which all colleagues working with cancer medicine might reflect.

It has been our aim in this text to provide an authoritative update on current science and opinion in the understanding and management of breast cancer that is as succinct as possible but as comprehensive as necessary. Consultants in surgical, clinical and medical oncology and their trainees will find it of immediate significance as part of continuing professional development and specialist training, respectively, and we advance it specifically as an excellent tool for these purposes. We anticipate, however, that this volume will prove of considerable value to nurse specialists and oncology pharmacists and to the planners and commissioners of cancer services and we similarly commend the book to these colleagues as part of their own continuing professional education. In conclusion, we thank Pfizer Ltd, and the former company Pharmacia Ltd, for the grants of unrestricted educational sponsorship that helped organise national symposia on the effective management of breast cancer in collaboration with the Association of Cancer Physicians, The Royal College of Radiologists and the British Association of Surgical Oncology, at which synopses of the constituent chapters of this volume were presented, and some of which grants have additionally assisted in the production and national dissemination of this text.

*Robert Leonard* BSc MB BS MD FRCP
*Andreas Polychronis* MB MRCP
*Andrew Miles* MSc MPhil PhD

London, May 2005

PART 1

# Aetiology, epidemiology and genetics

# Chapter 1

# Breast cancer aetiology: shifting the emphasis from adult to early life risk factors

*Isabel dos Santos Silva*

## Introduction

Epidemiological research into the aetiology of breast cancer has mainly focused on reproductive and other adult-life risk factors. However, the established risk factors seem to account for only half of all breast cancers (Madigan *et al.* 1995). In recent years, epidemiological research has raised the possibility that factors operating *in utero* and in early life may also be important in the aetiology of this tumour. In this chapter, we begin by reviewing briefly the established adult-life risk factors for breast cancer followed by a more detailed evaluation of the recent evidence linking breast cancer with pre-natal and early life exposures.

## Adult-life risk factors

Several risk factors for breast cancer have been established, most of which relate to reproductive events. Risk is increased by an early onset of menarche, nulliparity, late age at first birth and late natural menopause. These known risk factors for breast cancer can be understood as measures of cumulative exposure of the breast tissue to endogenous oestrogens and, possibly, progesterone. A recent re-analysis of data from nine prospective studies showed that in post-menopausal women high levels of serum oestrogens were strongly associated with an increased risk of breast cancer (EHBCC 2002). The evidence in pre-menopausal women is less consistent (Thomas *et al.* 1997), perhaps because it is difficult to measure accurately the impact of oestrogen due to menstrual fluctuation. There is also evidence that high plasma levels of prolactin (Hankinson *et al.* 1999) and of androgens (EHBCC 2002) may be important in post-menopausal women.

Prolonged breastfeeding delays the re-establishment of ovulation after a complete pregnancy and could therefore protect against breast cancer. The evidence in support of this hypothesis has been largely inconsistent partly because most studies have been conducted in populations where the lifetime duration of breastfeeding of most women is rather short. But a recent pooled re-analysis of individual data from 47 epidemiological studies conducted in 30 countries showed that lactation for long periods protects against breast cancer (CGHFBC 2002).

Recent pooled re-analyses of individual data from more than 50 epidemiological studies have provided evidence that the use of exogenous hormones may affect the risk of breast cancer (CGHFBC 1996, 1997). Post-menopausal hormone replacement therapy seems to be associated with an excess risk of breast cancer in current and recent users (CGHFBC 1997). Oral contraceptive use has only a small effect on risk of breast cancer, which is to increase the risk in current and recent users (CGHFBC 1996).

The effect of adiposity, as measured by body mass index (BMI), can also be seen within the oestrogen hypothesis. Most studies showed a positive association between BMI and post-menopausal risk of breast cancer, although the relative risks found in cohort studies (van den Brandt *et al.* 2000) are much closer to the null value than those found in case–control studies (Hunter & Willett 1996). In post-menopausal women, the extra-glandular conversion of androstenedione to oestrone and then oestradiol in adipose tissue accounts for 90% of circulating oestradiol (Grodin *et al.* 1973). Moreover, increased weight is not only associated with higher post-menopausal oestrogen levels but also with reduced levels of SHBG and, therefore, with greater tissue availability of oestrogens (Siiteri *et al.* 1981). For pre-menopausal breast cancer, however, the relation of obesity with breast cancer is inverted. A recent meta-analysis (Ursin *et al.* 1995) concluded that there was an inverse association of BMI with pre-menopausal breast cancer, which was stronger in cohort than case–control studies. This protective effect of obesity in younger women could not be adequately explained by difficulties in detection of tumours in heavy women. It could, however, be due to the association of pre-menopausal obesity with anovulation and progesterone deficiency. Recent research (based on recall data) seems to suggest that weight gain may also be an important risk factor for post-menopausal breast cancer (Le Marchand *et al.* 1988a; Ballard-Barbash *et al.* 1990; Brinton & Swanson 1992; Trentham-Dietz *et al.* 1997), and in some studies this effect was shown to be independent of BMI (Ballard-Barbash *et al.* 1990; Trentham-Dietz *et al.* 1997).

## Adolescent and childhood risk factors

Both early age at menarche and tall adult height are positively associated with an increased risk of breast cancer thus raising the hypothesis that factors operating in childhood and adolescence may also be important in the aetiology of this tumour (de Waard & Trichopoulos 1988). This is further supported by studies showing that high pre-menopausal plasma levels of insulin-like growth factor-I (IGF-I), a hormone that promotes growth, are associated with an increased risk of breast cancer (Hankison *et al.* 1998; Toniolo *et al.* 2000).

It is unclear by what mechanism adult height is a predictor of risk of breast cancer, particularly in affluent populations in which the prevalence of malnourishment during growth is unlikely to be large. Genetic and environmental factors, including diet, may influence the hormones that regulate epiphysial closure and thus adult height

(Ballard-Barbash 1994). These hormones may also affect subsequent risk of breast cancer. Thus, adult height is probably not a risk factor in itself, but it may be a marker of exposure to nutritional factors during puberty. Alternatively, adult height may be just an indirect marker for mammary gland size and, by inference, a rough indicator of the number of ductal stem cells at risk of malignant transformation (Trichopoulos & Lipman 1992).

Few investigations (Brinton & Swanson 1992; Li *et al.* 1997; Berkey *et al.* 1999) have attempted to examine changes in height and weight during childhood and adolescence and risk of breast cancer later in life. Overall, they seem to indicate that risk is increased in women who were taller and leaner in the pre-pubertal period and, thus, had a relatively early growth spurt and an earlier age at menarche. Most of these studies relied on the women's ability to recall their height in the distant past.

Although age at menarche and growth during childhood and adolescence are known to be influenced by nutritional status early in life, the few breast cancer studies (Hislop *et al.* 1986; Pryor *et al.* 1989; Potischman *et al.* 1998) that have assessed adolescent diet retrospectively from adults have been inconclusive. Hypotheses relating to childhood and adolescence diet are difficult to test directly in humans because recorded measures of dietary intake at young ages are scarce and reports by adults of their dietary intake in the distant past are unlikely to be sufficiently valid.

## Pre-natal influences on risk of breast cancer

In 1990, Thrichopoulos suggested that *in utero* exposure to high levels of oestrogens might increase the risk of breast cancer later in life on the basis of four assumptions: (1) endogenous oestrogens are important risk factors for breast cancer; (2) exposures that act post-natally can also act pre-natally; (3) levels of endogenous oestrogens are at least 10 times higher during pregnancy than during other periods of adult life; and (4) there is wide inter-individual variation in the levels of pregnancy oestrogens and this variability is probably related to exogenous factors (Thrichopoulos 1990).

This hypothesis, which has since evolved to include other endocrine factors, was a useful starting point which has sparked a considerable amount of work into the pre- and perinatal origins of breast cancer. As it is not currently possible to test this hypothesis using biological data on oestrogen levels experienced by women while *in utero* many decades ago, epidemiological research has so far relied on indirect markers of exposure to high or low levels of pregnancy oestrogens. Such indirect measures include, among others, size at birth, gestational age, preeclampsia/ eclampsia and twinship.

### Size at birth

Several studies have used birth weight as a marker of the *in utero* environment. Their characteristics and main findings are summarised in Table 1.1. These studies differed in terms of their design (cohorts, population-based case-control studies and case-

**Table 1.1** Birth weight and breast cancer risk

| Reference | Study design, country | Number of breast cancer cases/controls (or women in the cohort) | Birth weight (g) | RR* | Comments |
|---|---|---|---|---|---|
| Le Marchand et al. 1988 | Population-based case-control study, Hawaii, USA | 153 cases 461 controls | All ages 1162–2948 2949–3340 3341–4451 $p = 0.41$‡ | 1.00† 0.65 0.76 | Birth weight data obtained from birth records. No adjustment was made for maternal factors, other birth characteristics or adult risk factors. |
| Ekbom et al. 1992 | Population-based case-control study Sweden | 458 cases 1197 controls | All ages < 2500 2500–2999 3000–3499 3500–3999 ≥ 4000 $p = 0.25$‡ | 1.18 1.00† 1.29 1.47 1.23 | Birth weight data obtained from birth records. Relative risks adjusted for maternal characteristics but not for gestational age or adult risk factors. |
| Sanderson et al. 1996 | 2 population-based case-control studies, USA | 746 cases 960 controls | Ages 21–45 yrs < 2500 2500–2999 3000–3499 3500–3999 ≥ 4000 $p = 0.06$‡ | 1.3 1.0† 1.3 1.2 1.7 | Self-reported birth weight. Relative risks adjusted for subject's age, menopausal status and maternal smoking. Further adjustment for other perinatal and adult life risk factors did not affect the results. |
| | | 401 cases 439 controls | Ages 50–64 yrs. < 2500 2500–2999 3000–3499 3500–3999 ≥ 4000 $p = 0.06$‡ | 0.9 1.0† 1.1 0.8 0.6 | |

*Relative risk (RR) as estimated by odds ratios in case–control studies and rate ratios in cohort studies.
†Taken as the baseline category.
‡$p$-value for linear trend across the various birth weight categories.

contd

**Table 1.1** contd

| Reference | Study design, country | Number of breast cancer cases/controls (or women in the cohort) | Birth weight (g) | RR* | Comments |
|---|---|---|---|---|---|
| Michels *et al.* 1996 | Case-control study nested within the Nurses' Health Study, USA | 582 cases 1569 controls | *All ages* < 2500 2500–2999 3000–3499 3500–3999 ≥ 4000 $p = 0.008‡$ | 0.55 0.66 0.68 0.86 1.00† | Birth weight reported by mothers. Relative risks not adjusted for maternal factors or other perinatal characteristics but adjusted for adult risk factors. The relation between breast cancer and birth weight was more marked at ages under 45 ($p$ for trend = 0.05) and 45–50 years ($p$ = 0.03) than at older ages ($p$ = 0.18). |
| | | | *Ages < 45 yrs.* < 2500 2500–2999 3000–3499 3500–3999 ≥ 4000 $p = 0.05‡$ | 0.51 0.62 0.61 0.89 1.00† | |
| Ekbom *et al.* 1997 | Enlargement of the initial study by Ekbom *et al.* (1992), Sweden | 1068 cases 2727 controls | *All ages* < 2500 2500–2999 3000–3499 3500–3999 ≥ 4000 $p = 0.56‡$ | 0.80 1.00† 1.00 0.99 1.04 | Birth weight data obtained from birth records. Relative risks adjusted for maternal factors and for some perinatal characteristics but not for gestational age. No adjustment for adult risk factors. No evidence of interaction with age at diagnosis or menopausal status. |

*Relative risk (RR) as estimated by odds ratios in case–control studies and rate ratios in cohort studies.
†Taken as the baseline category.
‡$p$-value for linear trend across the various birth weight categories.

contd

**Table 1.1** contd

| Reference | Study design, country | Number of breast cancer cases/controls (or women in the cohort) | Birth weight (g) | RR* | Comments |
|---|---|---|---|---|---|
| Sanderson et al. 1998 | Two population-based case-control studies among women under the age of 45 years, USA | 510 case mothers<br>436 control mothers | *Age under 45 yrs.*<br>< 2500<br>2500–2999<br>3000–3499<br>3500–3999<br>≥ 4000<br>$p$ = n/a‡ | 1.2<br>1.0†<br>1.0<br>1.0<br>1.3 | Birth weight data reported by mothers.<br><br>Further adjustment for maternal factors, other perinatal characteristics and adult risk factors did not affect the results. |
| De Stavola et al. 2000 | National representative cohort of women born in 1946, Britain | 37 cases<br>2221 women in the cohort | *All ages*<br>< 3000<br>3000–3499<br>3500–3999<br>≥ 4000<br>$p$ = 0.09‡<br><br>*Premenopausal*<br>< 3000<br>3000–3499<br>3500–3999<br>≥ 4000<br>$p$ = 0.03‡ | 1.00†<br>1.05<br>1.76<br>2.02<br><br><br>1.00†<br>1.99<br>3.26<br>5.65 | Birth weight data obtained from birth records.<br><br>Relative risks adjusted for age only but further adjustment for birth characteristics and childhood and adulthood risk factors did not affect the results.<br><br>Data on gestational age not available in this study.<br><br>Women were still too young to allow separate examination of the association at postmenopausal ages. |

*Relative risk (RR) as estimated by odds ratios in case–control studies and rate ratios in cohort studies.
†Taken as the baseline category.
‡$p$-value for linear trend across the various birth weight categories.
n/a, Not given in the paper.

contd

**Table 1.1** contd

| Reference | Study design, country | Number of breast cancer cases/controls (or women in the cohort) | Birth weight (g) | RR* | Comments |
|---|---|---|---|---|---|
| Innes *et al.* 2000 | Population-based case-control study, USA | 484 cases 2870 controls | *Ages 14–37 years*<br>< 1500<br>1500–2499<br>2500–3499<br>3500–3999<br>≥ 4500<br>*p* = n/a‡ | 3.00<br>1.54<br>1.00†<br>1.08<br>3.10 | Birth weight data obtained from birth records.<br><br>Relative risks adjusted for gestational age, maternal and paternal age, preeclampsia, abruptio placentae, multifoetal gestation, birth order, race/ethnicity. |
| Andersson *et al.* 2001 | Cohort study, Sweden | 62 cases 1080 women in the cohort | *All ages*<br>1600–3000<br>3010–3349<br>3350–3590<br>3600–3960<br>4000–5500<br>*p* = 0.223‡ | 1.00†<br>1.14<br>1.64<br>1.56<br>1.57 | Birth weight data obtained from birth records.<br><br>Relative risks adjusted for cohort membership, gestational age, maternal; proteinuria, birth order and own parity. Further adjustment for age at menarche did not affect the results. |
| Hilakivi-Clarke *et al.* 2001 | Cohort study, Finland | 177 cases 3447 women in the cohort | *All ages (76% aged ≥ 50 at the time of diagnosis)*<br>≤2500<br>3000–<br>3500–<br>4000–<br>> 4000<br>*p* = NS‡ | 1.0†<br>1.4<br>1.9<br>1.5<br>1.9 | Birth weight data obtained from birth records.<br><br>Adjustment for gestational age did not affect the results. No adjustment was made for maternal factors or adult risk factors. |

*Relative risk (RR) as estimated by odds ratios in case–control studies and rate ratios in cohort studies.
†Taken as the baseline category.
‡*p*-value for linear trend across the various birth weight categories.
n/a, Not given in the paper.
NS, Not statistically significant (the actual *p*-value was not given in the paper).

contd

**Table 1.1** contd

| Reference | Study design, country | Number of breast cancer cases/controls (or women in the cohort) | Birth weight (g) | RR* | Comments |
|---|---|---|---|---|---|
| Hübinette *et al.* 2001 | Population-based case-control study of like-sexed twins, Sweden. <br><br> Two control groups: <br><br> (i) *Within pair comparison*: breast cancer-free female co-twins; <br> (ii) *Between pair comparison*: one twin randomly selected from a twin pair matched to the case on year of birth | (i) *Within pair comparison*: 96 cases and 96 co-twin controls; <br> (ii) *Between pair comparison*: 87 cases and 87 controls | (i) *Within pair comparison*: <br> < 1999 <br> 2000–2499 <br> 2500–2999 <br> ≥ 3000 <br> $p$ = <br><br> (ii) *Between pair comparison*: <br> < 1999 <br> 2000–2499 <br> 2500–2999 <br> ≥ 3000 <br> $p$ = | 1.0† <br> 2.3 <br> 2.8 <br> 3.5 <br> n/a‡ <br><br> 1.0† <br> 1.6 <br> 2.4 <br> 1.6 <br> n/a‡ | Birth weight data obtained from birth records. <br><br> No adjustment for adult life risk factors. |
| Kaijser *et al.* 2001 | Population-based case-control study of opposite sexed twins, Sweden | 90 cases <br> 90 controls | *All ages* <br> 1310–2000 <br> 2001–2500 <br> 2501–3000 <br> 3001–3500 <br> 3501–3980 <br> $p$ = 0.03‡ | 1.0† <br> 3.3 <br> 3.1 <br> 5.6 <br> 11.8 | Birth weight data obtained from birth records. <br><br> Relative risks adjusted for duration of gestation and male co-twin birth weight. |

*Relative risk (RR) as estimated by odds ratios in case–control studies and rate ratios in cohort studies.
†Taken as the baseline category.
‡$p$-value for linear trend across the various birth weight categories.
n/a, Not given in the paper.

contd

**Table 1.1** contd

| Reference | Study design, country | Number of breast cancer cases/controls (or women in the cohort) | Birth weight (g) | RR* | Comments |
|---|---|---|---|---|---|
| Sanderson et al. 2002 | Population-based case-control study, China | 288 cases 350 controls | *Ages 45 yrs and younger*<br>< 2500<br>2500–2999<br>3000–3499<br>3500–3999<br>≥ 4000<br>*p* = 0.32‡ | 0.9<br>1.0†<br>1.1<br>0.8<br>0.7 | Birth weight reported by mothers.<br><br>Relative risks adjusted for age, income, family history of breast cancer in first-degree relatives, history of fibroadenoma, age at menarche, parity, and age at first live birth. |
| Vatten et al. 2002 | Population-based study, Norway | 373 cases 1150 controls | *All ages*<br>< 3090<br>3090–3410<br>3420–3720<br>> 3730<br>*p* = 0.02‡ | 1.0†<br>1.1<br>1.2<br>1.4 | Birth weight data obtained from birth records.<br><br>Relative risks adjusted for year of birth, age at first birth and parity. |
| Titus-Ernstoff et al. 2002 | Population-based case-control study, USA | 1716 cases 1886 controls | *Postmenopausal ages*<br>< 2500<br>2500–2999<br>3000–3499<br>3500–3999<br>4000–4499<br>≥ 4500<br>*p* = 0.81‡ | 1.10<br>0.90<br>1.00†<br>1.07<br>0.89<br>1.18 | Self-reported birth weight.<br><br>Relative risks adjusted for age and state of residence. Further adjustment for other perinatal factors and known breast cancer risk factors did not affect these results. |

*Relative risk (RR) as estimated by odds ratios in case–control studies and rate ratios in cohort studies.
†Taken as the baseline category.
‡*p*-value for linear trend across the various birth weight categories.

contd

**Table 1.1** contd

| Reference | Study design, country | Number of breast cancer cases/controls (or women in the cohort) | Birth weight (g) | RR* | Comments |
|---|---|---|---|---|---|
| McCormack et al. 2003 | Cohort study, Sweden | 359 cases 5,358 women in the cohort | Ages < 50 years<br>< 3000<br>3000–3499<br>3500–3999<br>≥ 4000<br>$p = 0.006‡$ | 1.00†<br>1.61<br>2.43<br>3.48 | Birth weight data obtained from birth records<br><br>Relative risks adjusted for gestational age, marital status, age at first marriage, children in the home, educational level, occupational level and car ownership. |
| | | | Ages ≥ 50 years<br>< 3000<br>3000–3499<br>3500–3999<br>≥ 4000<br>$p = 0.87‡$ | 1.00†<br>0.75<br>0.97<br>0.87 | |

*Relative risk (RR) as estimated by odds ratios in case–control studies and rate ratios in cohort studies.
†Taken as the baseline category.
‡$p$-value for linear trend across the various birth weight categories.

control studies nested within cohorts), source of birth weight data (birth records, self-recall, or maternal recall) and ability to control for other maternal, perinatal and adult life risk factors.

Most studies that have examined the relation between birth weight and subsequent risk of breast cancer had a case–control design (Table 1.1). Two of these studies relied on self-reported birth weight (Sanderson *et al.* 1996; Titus-Ernstoff *et al.* 2002). The first one (Sanderson *et al.* 1996), a pooled analyses of data from two population-based case–control studies in the USA, revealed a J-shaped association at pre-menopausal ages (Table 1.1), with small (less than 2500 g) and heavy babies (greater than 4000 g) being at an increased risk of developing breast cancer later in life relative to babies who were average (2500–2999 g). At post-menopausal ages, however, risk of breast cancer decreased with increasing birth weight although the test for trend was only borderline significant. The second study (Titus-Ernstoff *et al.* 2002), a large population-based case-control study conducted in the USA, revealed a J-shaped association between birth weight and risk of breast cancer at post-menopausal ages.

Three case–control studies relied on maternal reports (Michels *et al.* 1996; Sanderson *et al.* 1998; Sanderson *et al.* 2002) (Table1.1). One of these, a large case–control study nested within the US Nurses' Health Study, showed a strong relation between birth weight and risk of breast cancer later in life. Women who weighed less than 2500 g at birth had about half the risk of those who weighed 4000 g or more, after adjusting for age at diagnosis, parity, age at first birth, age at menarche, adult BMI and family history of breast cancer. The pooled analysis of data from two USA population-based case–controls studies (Sanderson *et al.* 1996) described above also collected information from the mothers of young women. As with the results based on self-reported data, there was evidence of a J-shaped relation between birth weight and risk of breast cancer at ages under 45 years. Further adjustment for maternal factors, other perinatal characteristics and adult risk factors did not affect the results. In contrast, there was no association between birth weight, as reported by the mothers, and risk of breast cancer in a study conducted among pre-menopausal women in a low-risk Chinese population, but few women had birth weights over 4000 g (Sanderson *et al.* 2002).

Birth weight information for the other remaining seven case-control studies were obtained from birth records and are therefore likely to be more valid. The findings from these studies were not consistent, however. Some reported a positive linear relation (Vatten *et al.* 2002) or a J-shaped association (Ekbom *et al.* 1992; Innes *et al.* 2000) between birth weight and subsequent risk of breast cancer, but two (Le Marchand *et al.* 1988b; Ekbom *et al.* 1997) found no association.

Two additional case–control studies (Hubinette *et al.* 2001; Kaijser *et al.* 2001) examined the relation between birth weight and risk of breast cancer among twins (Table 1.1). Both showed a 3.5- to 6-fold increased risk for higher (greater than 3000 g) compared with lower (less than 2000 g) birth weight twins. Compared with singletons, twins generally have shorter gestational ages and lower birth weights but potentially high exposure to hormonal factors. Although the birth weight thresholds for risk cannot be applied to singleton births, these studies provide additional evidence for a link between growth *in utero* and risk of breast cancer.

Only four cohort studies have assessed the relation between birth weight and risk of breast cancer and all of them relied on birth records (Table 1.1). Two showed a positive linear association between risk of breast cancer and birth weight, particularly strong at pre-menopausal ages. The first one (De Stavola *et al.* 2000) was conducted within a nationally representative cohort of British women born immediately after World War II who have been followed up since then. This association was not affected by other perinatal and later-life factors, but was strengthened by tallness in childhood. The second cohort study was a Swedish cohort of about 6,000 women born in the Uppsala Academic Hospital between 1915 and 1929 (McCormack *et al.* 2003). There was a positive and strong association with birth weight, with women who weighed at least 4 kg at birth being almost three times more likely to develop breast cancer at pre-menopausal ages (taken as being ages under 50 years). No association was found between birth weight and risk of breast cancer at post-menopausal ages. The other two cohort studies (Andersson *et al.* 2001; Hilakivi-Clarke *et al.* 2001) also reported positive linear associations between birth weight and all-ages risk of breast cancer but none was statistically significant.

In short, six studies, including two twins studies, found positive linear relations with birth weight (Michels *et al.* 1996; De Stavola *et al.* 2000; Hubinette *et al.* 2001; Kaijser *et al.* 2001; Vatten *et al.* 2002a; McCormack *et al.* 2003), and in some (Michels *et al.* 1996; De Stavola *et al.* 2000; McCormack *et al.* 2003) the association was particularly strong at pre-menopausal ages. In addition, two other studies (Andersson *et al.* 2001; Hilakivi-Clarke *et al.* 2001) reported non-significant positive linear associations with birth weight. J-shaped associations, with small and heavy babies being at an increased risk of developing breast cancer later in life relative to babies who were average, were reported by four others (Ekbom *et al.* 1992; Sanderson *et al.* 1996; Innes *et al.* 2000; Titus-Ernstoff *et al.* 2002). The remaining four studies (Le Marchand *et al.* 1988b; Ekbom *et al.* 1997; Sanderson *et al.* 1998, 2002) showed no relation between birth weight and risk of breast cancer. Possible reasons for the lack of consistency of the findings include differences in the accuracy of the birth weight data, lack of adjustment for known risk factors of breast cancer and other maternal and perinatal factors, and lack of stratification by menopausal status.

Birth weight depends on linear growth (as determined by birth length) and degree of obesity; it is not clear whether birth weight is a risk factor for breast cancer because it is a measure of linear growth or a measure of obesity. This issue was recently examined in the Swedish cohort of about 6,000 women born in the Uppsala Academic Hospital between 1915 and 1929 (McCormack *et al.* 2003) described above. There were positive and statistically significant associations of birth weight, birth length and head circumference with risk of breast cancer at pre-menopausal ages, which became stronger after adjustment for gestational age. Ponderal index (as a measure of fatness) was not associated with risk of breast cancer. Simultaneous modelling of these birth size measures with gestational age showed that for the same ponderal index and gestational age, a 2 cm increase (equal to one standard deviation (SD)) in birth length was associated with a 31% (95% confidence interval (CI): 2% to 67%) increase in risk of breast cancer at pre-menopausal ages. In contrast, for the same birth length and gestational age, an increase in ponderal index at birth of 2 kg/m$^3$ (equal to one SD) was associated with a small, but not significant, increase of 11% (−12% to 38%) in pre-menopausal risk of breast cancer. The effect of birth weight disappeared after adjustment for birth length or head circumference, whereas the effect of the latter measures remained statistically significant after adjustment for birth weight. The results were not affected by further adjustment for maternal characteristics and adult-life risk factors for breast cancer. Six other studies (Ekbom et al. 1992, 1997; Hilakivi-Clarke *et al.* 2001; Andersson *et al.* 2001; Hübinette *et al.* 2001; Vatten *et al.* 2002a) examined the relation between birth length and subsequent risk of breast cancer. Although their findings are consistent with an increase in the risk of breast cancer with increasing birth length, only in one (Vatten *et al.* 2002a) was the trend statistically significant.

The findings from the Uppsala study (McCormack *et al.* 2003) would point towards linear growth, as measured by birth length rather than fatness, being the critical factor in determining risk of breast cancer perhaps as a result of *in utero* exposure to high levels of oestrogens, insulin-like growth factors (IGFs) and other growth factors. Alternatively, or additionally, foetal growth could be associated with breast cancer through its association with post-natal growth rates. Foetal growth is a predictor of a woman's growth and development during childhood and early adult life (Sørensen *et al.* 1999; Tuvemo *et al.* 1999; dos Santos Silva *et al.* 2002). This was recently examined within a nationally representative cohort of British women born in 1946 who have since been followed up, and for whom height and weight measurements were obtained throughout childhood. In this cohort, the effect of birth weight on pre-menopausal risk of breast cancer did not change after simultaneous adjustment for height and BMI at age 2 years and yearly height and BMI velocity rates throughout childhood and adolescence, suggesting that the biological mechanism(s) underlying the association of birth weight with early breast cancer are independent of those underlying the effect of childhood and adolescence growth (dos Santos Silva *et al.* 2004).

## Gestational age

Two main hypotheses have been put forward about the possible effect of gestational age on breast cancer aetiology. One states that short gestational ages would be protective against breast cancer later in life because gestational age represents the duration of exposure of the breast to maternal pregnancy oestrogens and, possibly, to other growth factors, whereas the other predicts that short gestational ages would have an adverse effect because oestrogen secretion is enhanced in pregnancies destined to deliver prematurely (Ekbom et al. 2000).

The relation between gestational age and risk of breast cancer was examined in ten studies. Their findings have been largely inconsistent. Statistically significant negative associations were found in three (Ekbom *et al.* 1997, 2000; McCormack *et al.* 2003). The large Swedish cohort (McCormack *et al.* 2003) described above found a negative trend between gestational age and risk of breast cancer at pre-menopausal ages, which was statistically significant only after adjustment for birth size. For a given birth size, women born before 38 weeks of gestation were twice (relative risk (RR) = 2.10; 95% confidence interval (CI) =1.05, 4.21) more likely to develop breast cancer at pre-menopausal ages than those born after 40 weeks. This finding seems to indicate that for a given birth size a short gestational age, and hence a higher rate of foetal growth, is associated with a raised risk of pre-menopausal breast cancer. There was no association between gestational age and risk of breast cancer at post-menopausal ages. Further adjustment for other perinatal and adult-life risk factors did not affect the results.

A similar negative association was observed in a large Swedish population-based study (Ekbom *et al.* 1997), with women who were severely premature at birth (i.e. born before 33 weeks of gestation) being 3.96 (95% CI = 1.45, 10.81) more likely to develop breast cancer after adjustment for other perinatal factors. This finding was replicated in a cohort of 237 prematurely born women (before the 35th gestational week) identified among all (around 60,000) deliveries that occurred in the city of Stockholm from 1925 to 1934 (Ekbom *et al.* 2000). In women born before the 31st gestational week, the risk for breast cancer was increased 6.7 times (95% CI = 1.4, 19.5), and the risk before the age of 50 years was increased 12.2 times (95% CI = 1.5–45.1). A two- to fourfold increase was observed among women born in the 31st or 32nd gestational week. With longer gestational time, the relative risk of breast cancer declined.

In contrast, a linked registry study conducted in the USA showed a positive association, with women born before 33 weeks of gestation having a much lower risk of developing breast cancer later in life than those born at 37 or more weeks (odds ratio (OR) = 0.11; 95% CI=0.16, 0.79) after adjustment for other perinatal factors (Innes *et al.* 2000). Two twin studies have also shown strong positive associations between gestational age and risk of breast cancer (Hübinette *et al.* 2001; Kaijser *et al.* 2001). Other studies (Le Marchand *et al.* 1988; Sanderson *et al.* 1996; Michels *et al.* 1996; Hilakivi-Clarke *et al.* 2001) reported no association, but some (Sanderson *et al.* 1996; Michels *et al.* 1996) relied on very crude measures of gestational age as recalled by the women or their mothers. Difficulties in obtaining accurate measures of gestational age and lack of adjustment for birth size may have limited the interpretation of findings from these studies.

## Pre-eclampsia/eclampsia

Pre-eclampsia, a condition associated with reduced maternal urinary excretion, has been hypothesized to reduce risk of breast cancer in women born of these pregnancies. The earliest study to address this issue reported a non-significant increase in the risk of breast cancer with maternal pre-eclampsia (RR = 3.46; 95% CI = 0.86, 13.90), based on only four exposed cases (Le Marchand *et al.* 1988b). In contrast, a population-based Swedish study (Ekbom *et al.* 1992) described in Table 1.1 found a protective effect (OR = 0.41; 95% CI=0.22, 0.79) after adjustment for other perinatal variables. Data were unavailable, however, to allow evaluation of confounding or effect modification by the daughter's adult breast cancer risk factors. Additional evidence in favour of a protective effect of pre-eclamptic pregnancies was provided by data from two other case-control studies (Sanderson *et al.* 1998; Innes *et al.* 2000).

Although urinary oestrogen levels are clearly reduced in women presenting with pre-eclampsia during pregnancy, it is unclear whether concentrations also are reduced in blood (Stamilio *et al.* 2000). Other biological factors that are potentially altered in pre-eclampsia may also play a role. Cord levels of alpha-fetoprotein (AFP) may be higher in pre-eclampsia than in normotensive pregnancies (Vatten *et al.* 2002b), and two studies have shown that high AFP levels in the circulation of pregnant women are associated with reduced subsequent risk for breast cancer in these women (Melbye *et al.* 2000; Richardson *et al.* 1998). Similarly, cord levels of IGF-I appear to be low in pre-eclampsia (Vatten *et al.* 2002c) and, as mentioned before, some studies (Hankinson *et al.* 1998; Toniolo *et al.* 2000) have shown that low circulating levels of IGF-I in pre-menopausal women are associated with reduced risk of breast cancer.

Further studies are required to confirm the association between maternal pre-eclampsia and reduced risk of breast cancer in daughters born of these pregnancies and to clarify the biological mechanisms underlying this association. These studies should take into account the severity of the disease as well as differences in birth weight and gestational age.

## Twins

Twin pregnancies are associated with higher maternal serum or urinary oestrogen levels relative to singletons (Duff *et al.* 1974). There is also some evidence that dizygotic (DZ) twinning might be associated with particularly high concentrations of maternal oestrogen levels because of the production of these hormones by two, rather than one, placentas.

Most (Hsieh *et al.* 1992; Braun *et al.* 1995; Ekbom *et al.* 1997), but not all (Sanderson *et al.* 1996), epidemiological studies have found an elevated risk of breast cancer in twin daughters compared with singletons. Studies comparing risk in DZ versus monozygotic (MZ) twins have produced less consistent results, partly because of difficulties in establishing zygosity. Some studies (Hsieh *et al.* 1992; Weiss *et al.* 1997) compared the risk for having a twin brother, as a proxy for being DZ, or having a twin sister, which is a mixture of MZ and DZ twins. But it is conceivable that having a male co-twin may have an effect beyond that of zygosity.

In general, studies based on twin registries (e.g. Ahlbom *et al.* 1997) do not seem to support the hypothesis that DZ twins are at a higher risk of breast cancer; these studies, however, are likely to have been affected by ascertainment and follow-up biases. Other epidemiological studies (e.g. Hsieh *et al.* 1992; Ekbom *et al.* 1997; Swerdlow *et al.* 1997) are more consistent with the hypothesis of a higher risk among DZ twins but they tend to be based on relatively smaller numbers. There is also some evidence that the effect of DZ twinning may be restricted to young women (Swerdlow *et al.* 1997).

## Other factors

Other perinatal factors have been investigated in a few studies as potential indicators of subsequent risk of breast cancer. Positive associations between maternal age and risk of breast cancer in daughters were reported in some studies (Rothman *et al.* 1980; Le Marchand *et al.* 1988b; Innes *et al.* 2000; Titus-Ernstoff *et al.* 2002; Ekbom *et al.* 1997), but not in others (Sanderson *et al.* 1996; McCormack *et al.* 2003). As total blood concentrations of oestrogens in pregnancy were found to be significantly lower in young (under 20 years) than in older women (20–29 years) in one study (Petridou *et al.* 1990), the relation between maternal age and breast cancer was interpreted as suggesting an aetiological role for oestrogen levels during pregnancy (although this hypothesis did not explain why a slightly smaller independent effect in the same direction was found in relation to paternal age). Interpretation of the findings is difficult because many studies did not adjust for the mother's number of previous pregnancies or for birth weight of the daughter.

One study (Titus-Ernstoff *et al.* 2002) found an inverse association between a woman's birth rank, adjusting for mother's age at the time of the birth, and subsequent risk of breast cancer, but this finding was not replicated in others (Le Marchand *et al.* 1988b; Sanderson *et al.* 1996; Ekbom *et al.* 1992, 1997; Innes *et al.* 2000; Vatten *et al.* 2002a; McCormack *et al.* 2003).

In a pooled analysis of data from two population-based case–control studies on maternal factors (as recalled by the mothers) and risk of breast cancer at young ages (under 45 years) (Sanderson *et al.* 1998), a pregnancy weight gain of 25–34 pounds was associated with a slight increase in the risk of breast cancer (OR = 1.5; 95% CI = 1.1, 2.0); however, there was no increase in risk with weight gains higher than this. This study (Sanderson *et al.* 1998) also reported positive associations of risk of breast cancer at young ages with maternal use of anti-emetic medication (OR = 2.9; 95% CI = 1.1, 8.1) and diethylstilboestrol (DES) (OR = 2.3; 95% CI = 0.8, 6.4). There were no associations with pre-pregnancy BMI, use of oral contraceptives or other hormones.

The possible role of parental smoking has been investigated in a few studies (e.g. Sanderson *et al.* 1996; Titus-Ernstoff *et al.* 2002), but no association was found.

Similarly, no association has been found between placental weight and risk of breast cancer (Ekbom *et al.* 1992; 1997; Hilakivi-Clarke *et al.* 2001; Vatten *et al.* 2002a).

Neonatal jaundice was found to be associated with a significantly increased risk of breast cancer later in life in a Swedish population-based case–control study (OR = 2.16; 95% CI = 1.25, 3.67) (Ekbom *et al.* 1997). The authors speculated that neonatal jaundice may be associated with high oestrogen levels as a result of impaired metabolism in the liver.

Various studies have examined the relation between having been breastfed and subsequent risk of breast cancer, but the results have been largely inconsistent (Ekbom *et al.* 1993; Titus-Ernstoff *et al.* 1998; Michels *et al.* 2001).

## Conclusions

More than three decades of epidemiological studies have identified various adult risk factors for breast cancer. In recent years, however, epidemiological research has raised the possibility that factors operating *in utero* and in early life may be as important in the aetiology of this tumour as those acting in adult life. Associations have been reported, although not always consistently across all studies, between risk of breast cancer and various *in utero* exposures. In particular, the evidence points to a positive association between birth size and risk of breast cancer, particularly strong at pre-menopausal ages. Rapid childhood growth, early menarche and adult height have also been associated with an increase in the risk of breast cancer. Published data are also consistent with maternal preeclampsia/eclampsia being associated with a reduced risk of breast cancer and being born a twin being associated with an increased risk. Preeclampsia and twinship are presumably indirect markers of *in utero* exposures. There are still many unanswered questions about the role of early-life exposures on risk of breast cancer, and how they may interact with the established adult risk factors, but these findings imply the need for research and preventive efforts to shift from adult to early life.

*References*

Ahlbom, A., Lichenstein, P., Malstrom, H., Feychting, M., Hemminki, K. & Pederson, N. L. (1997). Cancer in twins: genetic and nongenetic familial risk factors. *Journal of the National Cancer Institute* **89**, 287–293.

Andersson SW, Bengtsson C, Hallberg L, Lapidus L, Niklasson A, Wallgren A, Hukthén L (2001). Cancer risk in Swedish women: the relation to size at birth. *British Journal of Cancer* **84**, 1193–1198.

Ballard-Barbash, R., Schatzkin, A., Taylor, P. R. & Kahle, L. L. (1990). Association of change in body mass with breast cancer. *Cancer Research* **50**, 2152–2155.

Ballard-Barbash, R. (1994). Anthropometry and breast cancer. Body size – a moving target. *Cancer* **74**, 1090–1100.

Berkey, C. S., Frazier, A. L., Gardner, J. D. & Colditz, G. A. (1999). Adolescence and breast carcinoma risk. *Cancer* **85**, 2400–2409.

Braun, M. M., Ahlbom, A., Floderus, B., Brinton, L. & Hoover, R. N. (1995). Effect of twinship on incidence of cancer of the testis, breast and other sites (Sweden). *Cancer Causes and Control* **6**, 519–524.

Brinton, L. A., Swanson, C. A. (1992). Height and weight at various ages and risk of breast cancer. *Annals of Epidemiology* **2**, 597–609.

Collaborative Group on Hormonal Factors in Breast Cancer (CGHFBC) (1996). Breast cancer and hormonal contraceptives: collaborative reanalysis of individual data on 53297 women with breast cancer and 100239 women without breast cancer from 54 epidemiological studies. *The Lancet* **347**, 1713–1727.

Collaborative Group on Hormonal Factors in Breast Cancer (CGHFBC) (1997). Breast cancer and hormonal replacement therapy: collaborative reanalysis of data from 51 epidemiological studies of 52 705 women with breast cancer and 108 411 women without breast cancer. *The Lancet* **350**, 1047–1059.

Collaborative Group on Hormonal Factors in Breast Cancer (CGHFBC) (2002). Breast cancer and breastfeeding: collaborative reanalysis of individual data from 47 epidemiological studies in 30 countries, including 50302 women with breast cancer and 96973 women without the disease. *The Lancet* **360**, 187–195.

De Stavola, B. L., Hardy, R., Kuh, D., dos Santos Silva, I., Wadsworth, M. & Swerdlow, A. J. (2000). Birth weight, childhood growth and risk of breast cancer in a British birth cohort. *British Journal of Cancer* **83**, 964–968.

de Waard, F. & Trichopoulos, D. (1988). A unifying concept of the aetiology of breast cancer. *International Journal of Cancer* **41**, 666–669.

dos Santos Silva, I., De Stavola, B. L., Mann, V., Kuh, D., Hardy, R. & Wadsworth, M. E. J. (2002). Prenatal factors, childhood growth trajectories and age at menarche. *International Journal of Epidemiology* **31**, 405–412.

dos Santos Silva, I., De Stavola, B. L., Mann, V., Kuh, D., Hardy, R. & Wadsworth, M. E. J. (2004). Is the effect of birth weight on premenopausal breast cancer mediated by childhood growth? *British Journal of Cancer.* (In the press.)

Duff, G. B., Brown, J. B. (1974). Urinary oestriol excretion in twin pregnancies. *Journal of Obstetrics and Gynaecology* **81**, 695–700.

Ekbom, A., Trichopoulos, D., Adami, H.-O., Hsieh, C.-C. & Lan, S.-J. (1992). Evidence of prenatal influences on breast cancer risk. *The Lancet* **340**, 1015–1018.

Ekbom, A., Hsieh, C.-C., Trichopoulos, D., Yen, Y.-Y., Petridou, E. & Adami, H.-O. (1993). Breast-feeding and breast cancer in the offspring. *British Journal of Cancer* **67**, 842–845.

Ekbom, A., Hsieh, C.-C., Lipworth, L., Adami, H.-O. & Trichopoulos, D. (1997). Intrauterine environment and breast cancer risk in women: a population-based study. *Journal of the National Cancer Institute* **88**, 71–76.

Ekbom, A., Erlandsson, G., Hsieh, C.-C., Trichopoulos, D., Adami, H.-O., Cnattingius, S. (2000). Risk of breast cancer in prematurely born women. *Journal of the National Cancer Institute* **92**, 840–841.

Endogenous Hormones and Breast Cancer Collaborative Group (2002). Endogenous sex hormones and breast cancer in postmenopausal women: reanalysis of nine prospective studies. *Journal of the National Cancer Institute* **94**, 606–616.

Grodin, J. M., Siiteri, P. K. & MacDonald, P. C. (1973). Source of estrogen production in postmenopausal women. *Journal of Clinical Endocrinology and Metabolism* **36**, 207–214.

Hankinson, S. E., Willett, W. C., Colditz, G. A., Hunter, D. J., Michaud, D. S., Deroo, B., Rosner, B., Speizer, F. E. & Pollak, M. (1998). Circulating concentrations of insulin-like growth factor-I and risk of breast cancer. *The Lancet* **351**, 1393–1396.

Hankinson, S. E., Willett, W. C., Michaud, D. S., Manson, J. E., Colditz, G. A., Longcope, C., Rosner, B. & Speizer, F. E. (1999). Plasma prolactin levels and subsequent risk of breast cancer in postmenopausal women. *Journal of the National Cancer Institute* **91**, 629–634.

Hilakivi-Clarke, L., Forsén, T., Eriksson, J. G., Luoto, R., Tuomilehto, J., Osmond, C., Barker, D. J. P. (2001). Tallness and overweight during childhood have opposing effects on breast cancer risk. *British Journal of Cancer* **85**, 1680–1684.

Hislop, T., Coldman, A., Elwood, J., Brauer, G. & Kan, L. (1986). Childhood and recent eating patterns and risk of breast cancer. *Cancer Detection and Prevention* **9**, 47–58.

Hsieh, C.-C., Lan, S.-J., Ekbom, A., Petridou, E., Adami, H.-O. & Trichopoulos, D. (1992). Twin membership and breast cancer risk. *American Journal of Epidemiology* **136**, 1321–1326.

Hunter, D. J. & Willett, W. C. (1996). Nutrition and breast cancer. *Cancer Causes and Control* **7**, 56–68.

Hübinette, A., Lichtenstein, P., Ekbom, A. & Cnattingius, S. (2001). Birth characteristics and breast cancer risk: a study among like-sexed twins. *International Journal of Cancer* **91**, 248–251.

Innes, K., Byers, T., Schymura, M. (2000). Birth characteristics and subsequent risk for breast cancer in very young women. *American Journal of Epidemiology* **152**, 1121–1128.

Kaijser, M., Litchtenstein, P., Granath, F., Erlandsson, G., Cnattingius, S. & Ekbom, A. (2001). In utero exposures and breast cancer: a study of opposite-sexed twins. *Journal of the National Cancer Institute* **93**, 60–62.

Le Marchand, L., Kolonel, L. N., Earle, M. E. & Mi, M.-P. (1988a). Body size at different periods of life and breast cancer risk. *American Journal of Epidemiology* **128**, 137–152.

Le Marchand, L., Kolonel, L. N., Myers, B. C. & Mi, M.-P. (1988b). Birth characteristics of pre-menopausal women with breast cancer. *British Journal of Cancer* **57**, 437–439.

Li, C. I., Malone, K. E., White, E. & Daling, J. R. (1997). Age when maximum height is reached as a risk factor for breast cancer among young U.S. women. *Epidemiology* **8**, 559–565.

Madigan, M. P., Ziegler, R. G., Benichou, J., Byrne, C. & Hoover, R. N. (1995). Proportion of breast cancer cases in the United States explained by well-established risk factors. *Journal of the National Cancer Institute* **87**, 1681–1685.

McCormack, V. A., dos Santos Silva, I., De Stavola, B. L., Moshen, R., Leon, D. & Lithell, H. O. (2003). Foetal growth and subsequent risk of breast cancer: results from a long-term follow-up of a Swedish cohort of over 5000 women. *British Medical Journal* **326**, 248–251.

Melbye, M., Wohlfahrt, J., Lei, U., Norgaard-Pedersen, B., Mouridsen, H. T., Lambe, M. & Michels, K. B. (2000). Alpha-fetoprotein levels in maternal serum during pregnancy and maternal breast cancer incidence. *Journal of the National Cancer Institute* **92**, 1001–1005.

Michels, K. B., Trichopoulos, D., Robins, J. M., Rosner, B. A., Manson, J. E., Hunter, D. J., Colditz, G. A., Hankinson, S. E., Speizer, F. E. & Willett, W. C. (1996). Birth weight as a risk factor for breast cancer. *The Lancet* **348**, 1542–1546.

Michels, K. B., Trichopoulos, D., Rosner, B. A., Hunter, D. J., Colditz, G. A., Hankinson, S. E., Speizer, F. E. & Willett, W. C. (2001). Being breastfed in infancy and breast cancer incidence in adult life: results from the two Nurses' Health Studies. *American Journal of Epidemiology* **153**, 275–283.

Petridou, E., Panagiotopoulou, K., Katsouyanni, K., Spanos, E. & Trichopoulos, D. (1990). Tobacco smoking, pregnancy oestrogens and birth weight. *Epidemiology* **1**, 247–250.

Potischman, N., Weiss, H. A., Swanson, C. A., Coates, R. J., Gammon, M. D., Malone, K. E., Brogan, D., Stanford, J. L., Hoover, R. N. & Brinton, L. A. (1998). Diet during adolescence and risk of breast cancer among young women. *Journal of the National Cancer Institute* **90**, 226–233.

Pryor, M., Slattery, M., Robison, L. & Egger, M. (1989). Adolescent diet and breast cancer in Utah. *Cancer Research* **49**, 2161–2167.

Richardson, B. E., Hulka, B. S., Peck, J. L., Hughes, C. L., van den Berg, B. J., Christianson, R. E. & Calvin, J. A. (1998). Levels of maternal serum alpha-fetoprotein (AFP) in pregnant women and subsequent breast cancer risk. *American Journal of Epidemiology* **148**, 719–727.

Rothman, K. J., MacMahon, B., Lin, T. M., Lowe, C. R., Mirra, A. P., Ravnihar, B., Salber, E. J., Trichopoulos, D. & Yuasa, S. (1980). Maternal age and birth rank of women with breast cancer. *Journal of the National Cancer Institute* **65**, 719–722.

Sanderson, M., Williams, M. A., Malone, K. E., Stanford, J. L., Emanuel, I., White, E. & Daling, J. R. (1996). Perinatal factors and the risk of breast cancer. *Epidemiology* **7**, 34–37.

Sanderson, M., Williams, M. A., Daling, J. R., Holt, V. L., Malone, K. E., Self, S. G. & Moore, D. E. (1998). Maternal factors and breast cancer risk among young women. *Pediatric and Perinatal Epidemiology* **12**, 397–407.

Sanderson, M., Shu, X., Jin, F., Dai, Q., Ruan, Z., Gao, T.-Y. & Zheng, W. (2002). Weight at birth and adolescence and premenopausal breast cancer risk in a low-risk population. *British Journal of Cancer* **86**, 84–88.

Siiteri, P. K., Hanmmond, G. L. & Nisker, J. A. (1981). Increased availability of serum estrogens in breast cancer: a new hypothesis. In *Hormones and Breast Cancer* (Banbury Report 8) (ed. M. C. Pike, P. K. Siiteri, & C. W. Welsch), p. 87. Cold Spring Harbor, New York: Cold Spring Harbor Laboratory.

Sørensen, H. T., Sabroe, S., Rothman, K. J., Gillman, M., Steffensen, F. H., Fischer, P. & Sørensen, T. I. (1999). Birth weight and length as predictors for adult height. *American Journal of Epidemiology* **149**, 726–729.

Stamilio, D. M., Sehdev, H. M., Morgan, M. A., Propert, K. & Macones, G. A. (2000). Can antenatal clinical and biochemical markers predict the development of severe preeclampsia? *American Journal of Obstetrics and Gynaecology* **152**, 1121–1128.

Swerdlow, A. J., De Stavola, B. L., Swanwick, M. A. & Maconochie, N. E. S. (1997). Risks of breast and testicular cancers in young adult twins in England and Wales: evidence on prenatal and genetic aetiology. *The Lancet* **350**, 1723–1728.

Thomas, H. V., Key, T. J., Allen, D. S., Moore, J. W., Dowset M, Fentiman, I. S. & Wang, D. Y. (1997). A prospective study of endogenous hormone concentrations and breast cancer risk in premenopausal women. *British Journal of Cancer* **75**, 1075–1079.

Titus-Ernstoff, L., Egan, K. M., Newcomb, P. A., Baron, J. A., Stampfer, M., Greenberg, E. R., Cole, B. F., Ding, J., Willett, W. C. & Trichopoulos, D. (1998). Exposure to breast milk in infancy and adult breast cancer risk. *Journal of the National Cancer Institute* **90**, 921–294.

Titus-Ernstoff, L., Egan, K. M., Newcomb, P. A., Ding, J., Trentham-Dieta, A., Greenberg, E. R., Baron, J. A., Trichopoulos, D. & Willett, W. C. (2002). Early life factors in relation to breast cancer risk in postmenopausal women. *Cancer Epidemiology, Biomarkers and Prevention* 11, 207–210.

Toniolo, P., Brunning, P. F., Akhmedkhanov, A., Bonfrer, J. M., Koenig, K. L., Lukanova, A., Shore, R. E. & Zeleniuch-Jacquotte, A. (2000). Serum insulin-like growth factor-I and breast cancer. *International Journal of Cancer* **88**, 828–832.

Trentham-Dietz, A., Newcomb, P. A., Storer, B. E., Longnecker, M. P., Baron, J., Greenberg, E. R. & Willett, W. C. (1997). Body size and risk of breast cancer. *American Journal of Epidemiology* **145**, 1011–1119.

Trichopoulos, D. (1990). Hypothesis: does breast cancer originate in utero? *The Lancet* **335**, 939–940.

Trichopoulos, D. & Lipman R. D. (1992). Mammary gland mass and breast cancer risk. *Epidemiology* **3**, 523–526.

Tuvemo, T., Cnattingius, S. & Jonsson, B. (1999). Prediction of male adult stature using anthropometric data at birth: a nationwide population-based study. *Pediatric Research* **46**, 491–495.

Ursin, G., Longnecker, M. P., Haile, R. W., Greenland, S. (1995). A meta-analysis of body mass index and risk of premenopausal breast cancer. *Epidemiology* **6**, 137–141.

van den Brandt, P. A., Spiegelman, D., Yaun, S.-S., Adami, H.-O., Beeson, L., Folsom, A. R., Fraser, G., Goldbohm, R. A., Graham, S., Kushi L. *et al.* (2000). Pooled analysis of prospective cohort studies on height, weight, and breast cancer risk. *American Journal of Epidemiology* **152**, 514–527.

Vatten, L. J., Mæhle, Lund Nilsen, T. I., Tretli, S., Hsieh, C.-C., Trichopoulos, D. & Stuver, S. O. (2002a). Birth weight as a predictor of breast cancer: a case-control study in Norway. *British Journal of Cancer* **86**, 89–91.

Vatten, L. J., Romundstad, P. R., Odegard, R. A., Nilsen, S. T., Trichopoulos, D. & Austgulen, R. (2002b). Alpha-fetoprotein in umbilical cord in relation to severe pre-eclampsia, birth weight and future breast cancer risk. *British Journal of Cancer* **86**, 728–731.

Vatten, L. J., Nilsen, S. T., Odegard, R. A., Romundstad, P. R. & Austgulen, R. (2002c). Insulin-like growth factor I and leptin in umbilical cord plasma and infant birth size at term. *Pediatrics* **109**, 1131–1135.

Weiss, H. A., Potischman, N. A., Brinton, L. A., Brogan, D., Coates, R. J., Gammon, M. D., Malone, K. E. & Schoenberg, J. B. (1997). Prenatal and perinatal risk factors for breast cancer in young women. *Epidemiology* **8**, 181–187.

# Chapter 2

# The genetics of breast cancer – I: progress in molecular biology and modifiers of penetrance

*C. Michael Steel*

## Introduction

Little more than 20 years ago, it was customary to down-play the role of inheritance in breast cancer. Concerned patients were habitually reassured that familial clustering simply represented the chance aggregation of sporadic cases. More recently, the pendulum has swung towards the opposite extreme. Publicity surrounding the discovery of 'high penetrance breast cancer genes' (*BRCA1*, *BRCA2* and *p53*) has led to a dramatic shift in clinical genetics practice, with half or more of all referrals in several UK centres now attributable to concerns about familial breast cancer (Wonderling *et al.* 2001). Where cancer family services are not readily available, symptomatic breast clinics are in danger of being overwhelmed by demand for genetic counselling, so much so that doubts have been cast on the wisdom of GPs raising the issue of breast cancer family history with their patients (Women's Concerns Study Group 2001).

## The contribution of genetic factors to breast cancer

Striking examples of multi-case breast cancer families have been documented for over a century and it is surprising that, for so long, they made so little impact on the collective clinical psyche. However, it is becoming increasingly clear that these form only a minor component of the overall genetic contribution to breast cancer. Several very large surveys, documenting the prevalence of the disease among relatives of women with breast cancer, provide measures of its heritability (reviewed by Steel *et al.* 1991). The figures are not precise for two main reasons. First, ascertainment and confirmation of cases among relatives is an extremely difficult exercise and in some studies, including the very large 'Nurses Health' programme from the USA, only the maternal side of the family tree has been assessed, so that possible inheritance of risk through a male is not considered (Colditz *et al.* 1993). Second, members of the same family are likely to share a common 'lifestyle', so that it becomes difficult to separate genetic from environmental risk factors. Nevertheless, most commentators agree that heritable factors account for at least 30% of breast cancer risk and some would put that estimate considerably higher (Peto *et al.* 1999; Pharoah *et al.* 2002).

Germline mutations in *BRCA1*, *BRCA2*, *p53* and *PTEN*, in aggregate, probably account for fewer than 5% of breast cancers in most populations (Easton 1999). Hence there is a huge gap between the 'epidemiological' estimates of heritability and the frequency of recognised breast cancer genes. It seems likely that the shortfall is made up of a few 'high penetrance' genes, in which germline mutations are rare, and a larger number of rather common genetic variants, each conferring a modest increase in lifetime risk of breast cancer, possibly operating interactively with each other and with environmental factors. Many candidates have been proposed for such 'low penetrance' genes. Some of the strongest are listed in Table 2.1, but they also include components of the pathways of sex hormone production, response and elimination (Thomson & Ambrosone 2000), enzymes involved in the activation and detoxification of carcinogens (Dunning *et al.* 1999) and members of the complexes that determine fidelity of DNA replication and repair (Berwick & Vineis 2000). *ATM*, *CHK1* and *CHK2* may belong to this last category but their roles in familial breast cancer have still to be clarified (Inskip *et al.* 1999; Ingvarsson *et al.* 2002, Yarden *et al.* 2002; Meijers-Heijboer *et al.* 2002).

**Table 2.1** Single genes known (or strongly suspected) to confer heritable breast cancer risk

| Gene | Chromosomal location | Associated cancers | Other features |
|---|---|---|---|
| *BRCA1* | 17q | Ovary; possibly prostate, bowel and cervix | ER negative, high-grade 'atypical medullary' breast cancers. |
| *BRCA2* | 13q | Ovary; pancreas, biliary tract; possibly bladder and others | Variable pathological features of breast cancers. |
| *P53* | 17p | Childhood sarcomas (Li-Fraumeni syndrome) | Aggressive breast cancers. |
| *PTEN* | 10q | Thyroid and bowel (Cowden syndrome) | Hamartomas. Cephalomegaly. |
| *STK11* | 19p | Bowel (Peutz-Jegher's syndrome) | Pigmented macules on skin and mucosal surfaces |
| *PTCH* | 9q | Naevoid basal cell carcinomas; medulloblastoma (Gorlin syndrome) | Bifid ribs, odontogenic keratocysts. Agenesis of corpus callosum. |
| *CHK2* | 22q | Breast cancer risk increased in carriers of 1100delC | Does not alter penetrance of *BRCA1/2*. |
| *ATM* | 11q | Certain mutations may account for some breast cancer families | Heterozygote has no ataxia symptoms. |

See Lynch *et al.* (1997), Varley *et al.* (1997), de Jong *et al.* (2002) and other references cited in text.

Our own studies in St Andrews and Dundee have concentrated on the phenomenon of chromosomal sensitivity to irradiation in the G2 phase of the cell cycle, which is known to vary within the population (some 10% showing 'high G2 sensitivity'). It appears to be inherited as a single gene autosomal co-dominant trait, though different genes may be implicated in different families, and it has been associated, in many studies, with susceptibility to cancers, notably to breast cancer (reviewed by Bryant *et al.* 2002). In our series, the most striking finding was that breast cancers from women with high G2 sensitivity formed a distinct pathological subgroup, with highly favourable prognostic scores (Riches *et al.* 2001). The same pathological profile has been recorded for familial breast cancers not attributable to *BRCA1* or *BRCA2* mutations (Lakhani *et al.* 2000). However, the identity of the gene(s) involved in these families and their relation (if any) to G2 radiation sensitivity, remains unknown.

## The 'high penetrance' genes, *BRCA1/BRCA2* and their functions

*BRCA1* and *BRCA2* have been studied intensively since their discovery in 1994 and 1995, respectively (reviewed by Welcsh *et al.* 2000). Despite the similarity in their names and their shared involvement in breast cancer, structurally they are almost completely unrelated. Homology with genes in lower species is restricted to mammals and is not close. Few clues to their function emerge from sequence analysis. They have nuclear localisation domains and features that would support either protein–protein or protein–DNA interactions, or both. Yeast two-hybrid, co-precipitation and fluorescence co-localisation studies have identified several interacting proteins, including Rad51, p53, BARD1, p21 and ATM. They also interact with each other, though it is not certain how direct or indirect some of these interactions may be. In short, beyond suggesting that they may act as transcription factors, structural studies provide few clues to the underlying function(s) of either gene.

In the mouse, both genes are expressed widely during embryonic development (e.g. forebrain, thymus, gut, ovary, testis and adrenal) particularly in rapidly growing tissues. This also seems to be true in humans. The distribution and timing of expression are very similar for *BRCA1* and *BRCA2*. Both appear to be essential for normal development because homozygous knockout animals are non-viable. Simultaneous inactivation of *p53* mitigates the effect to some degree (see Scully and Livingston 2000). Conditional knockout in mice, targeted to mammary tissue, causes marked abnormalities of glandular development but no cancers and even with the addition of *p53* inactivation, only a few animals develop breast tumours (Xu *et al.* 1999). What does appear to be common to tissues with non-functional *BRCA1* or *BRCA2* is accumulation of DNA damage (specifically, increased sensitivity to radiation and other agents that induce double-stranded breaks) and gross chromosomal aberrations, both structural and numerical. The role of both genes in double-strand break repair by homologous recombination and in the related mechanism of DNA crossing-over in the meiotic synaptenemal complex is now well documented and tentative schemata explain their functional relationships with Rad51, ATM, FANCD, Chek1, Chek2, p53, p21 and DNA polymerase II in terms of these molecular processes. It is also becoming clear that they participate in chromatin remodelling, probably by influencing histone acetylation (Kote-Jarai and Eeles 1999; Chen *et al.* 1999; Li *et al.* 2000; Grompe & D'Andrea 2001; Yarden *et al.* 2002; Baldeyron *et al.* 2002). Despite the importance of these roles in the life of the cell and the organism, they may not describe the full range of *BRCA1* and *BRCA2* functions. They certainly do not provide an obvious explanation for their specific involvement in hereditary breast and ovarian cancer in humans. However, they are entirely consistent with the finding that breast tumours arising on a background of *BRCA1* or *BRCA2* mutations commonly show multiple aberrations and rearrangements at chromosomal and sub-chromosomal level (Tirkkonen *et al.* 1997; Crook *et al.* 1997). *BRCA1* tumours, in particular, tend to be of high pathological grade and are almost invariably oestrogen-receptor negative (Lakhani *et al.* 1998). Inactivation of *p53* is also present in most cases, all of these being adverse prognostic features. Recent developments in microarray gene expression analysis tend to support the view that that breast cancers attributable to *BRCA1* or *BRCA2* germline mutations show distinctive patterns of molecular evolution, but information on the identity of specific 'downstream' genetic alterations is still very limited (Hedenfalk *et al.* 2001; van't Veer *et al.* 2002).

## *BRCA1/2* mutations and breast/ovarian cancer risks

Germline frame-shift and other truncating mutations (though rarely missense mutations) at almost any point in either gene carry a substantial risk of breast cancer, often at an early age (more so for *BRCA1*). The actual level of this risk is controversial. There is little doubt that selection of extreme families by the Breast Cancer Linkage Consortium led to very high estimates of penetrance, which have not been confirmed in more recent population-based studies (reviewed by Narod 2002). On the other hand, as discussed below, the past history of a particular family may well be a better guide to risk for other mutation-carriers in that family than any estimate based on knowledge of the precise mutation or 'global' penetrance figures. Data from Scotland and Northern Ireland, based on over 100 consecutive mutation-bearing families, illustrate some of the relationships between molecular and clinical findings (Scottish/Northern Irish Consortium 2003). Breast cancer risks are broadly similar for *BRCA1* and *BRCA2* mutations but ovarian cancer is more than twice as common in *BRCA1* as in *BRCA2* families. We have confirmed that *BRCA1* mutations 3' of exon 11 carry a substantially reduced risk of ovarian cancer (and a slightly higher risk of breast cancer) than those in the 5' two thirds of the gene. For *BRCA2*, mutations in the central portion (termed by some the 'Ovarian Cancer Cluster Region', OCCR) are almost twice as likely to give rise to ovarian cancer as those outside this region. Nevertheless, individual families seem to refute these generalisations and, as has previously been noted for the Icelandic *BRCA2* 999 del5 founder mutation (Thorlacius *et al.* 1996), the pattern of associated cancers may differ widely among families with the same mutation. A particular case in point in our own series is *BRCA1* 4184 del4. Of three carrier families, one included both breast and ovarian cancers, one breast cancers only and the third had seven cases of ovarian cancer over four generations but no recorded breast cancers.

## Genetic modifiers of penetrance in *BRCA1/2* mutation-carriers

This specific observation suggests that some additional influence, modifying the effect of the *BRCA1* mutation, acted upon all affected members of the last family. Given its persistence over several generations, this is more likely to be a genetic than a shared environmental factor. Furthermore, its apparent co-inheritance with the mutation suggests that it may be a variant close to, or within, the *BRCA1* gene itself. Both *BRCA1* and *BRCA2* include several polymorphic regions and it is possible that one or more of these variants has an effect on breast cancer susceptibility though, in most cases, the evidence is, at best, equivocal (Dunning *et al.* 1997; Healey *et al.* 2000). The extent of promoter methylation has also been proposed as a molecular variable that may modify expression of *BRCA1* and hence affect penetrance of the cancer trait (Esteller *et al.* 2000) but, again, the hypothesis remains to be proved.

Unlinked genes considered as candidates for modifiers of *BRCA1/2* penetrance fall into three main categories (reviewed by Dunning *et al.* (1999) and Narod (2002)). First are those that affect the synthesis, function or elimination of sex hormones (oestrogen and androgen receptors, CYP19 aromatase, CYP17 17α steroid hydroxylase and nuclear receptor coactivator 3 NCO3—also known as AIB1), all of which are polymorphic and for each of which there is evidence for interaction with *BRCA1* or *BRCA2* in at least a few cases. Second are the genes whose products influence genome stability (Chen *et al.* 1999; Kote-Jarai & Eeles 1999; Scully & Livingston 2000; Welcsh *et al.* 2000; Li *et al.* 2000; Grompe & D'Andrea 2001; Yarden *et al.* 2002), such as *FANCD, ATM, Chek1, Chek2* and *Rad 51* which appear either to activate *BRCA1* and/or *BRCA2* by phosphorylation, or direct binding, in response to DNA damage (*ATM, FANCD, Chek2*) or co-operate with *BRCA1* and *BRCA2* in cell cycle arrest and DNA repair (*RAD51, Chek1*). A very strong effect of one *RAD51* variant (135C), present in around 7% of the population, has been demonstrated among carriers of the Ashkenazi Jewish *BRCA2* founder mutation (6174 delT). Penetrance was increased fourfold for women with the *RAD51* variant (Levy-Lahad *et al.* 2001). The finding has been confirmed in a second study but no effect was found for carriers of *BRCA1* mutations (Wang *et al.* 2001). The role of

*ATM* and *Chek2* polymorphisms or mutations, both as breast cancer risk factors in their own right and as possible modifiers of penetrance for *BRCA1/2* mutations, is currently eliciting a great deal of interest (see, for example, Chenevix-Trench *et al.* (2002) and Concannon (2002)) and, given the complexity of the field of DNA repair and cell cycle control, it seems very likely that further important discoveries, with implications for counselling and clinical management of women at increased genetic risk of breast cancer, will emerge in the course of the next few years. The third group of putative genetic modifiers includes all those genes that contribute to metabolism and excretion of potential carcinogens (*NAT1, GSTM1, GSTM3, GSTT, CYP1A1,* etc.). In most cases, only a modest effect would be expected from polymorphic variation at any of these loci and studies in familial breast cancer have not yet been conducted on a scale sufficient to prove or disprove any association.

## Environmental modifiers of penetrance

Environmental modifiers of genetic risk (Table 2.2) are generally of even greater concern to members of 'breast cancer' families because they present opportunities to reduce individual risks. Perhaps surprisingly, because of the almost invariable absence of oestrogen receptors from *BRCA1* mutant tumours, all the proven environmental modifiers involve the sex hormones (Narod 2002). Pregnancy appears to offer no protection, in contrast to its influence on sporadic breast cancer (Colditz *et al.* 1996; Jernstrom *et al.* 1999). Smoking, in at least one study, significantly reduced breast cancer risk in carriers of *BRCA1* or *BRCA2* mutations and this may be a consequence of its anti-oestrogenic effect (Brunet *et al.* 1998), though the effects of hormonal contraception and hormone replacement therapy on breast cancer risk in this setting are still uncertain (Narod, 2002). In relation to ovarian cancer, use of the combined oral contraceptive pill (which arrests ovulation) greatly reduces the incidence (or delays onset) of tumours in carriers of *BRCA1* mutations (Narod *et al.* 1998). Prophylactic oophorectomy also reduces the risk of breast cancer by around 50% in mutation carriers and this effect is not abrogated by giving exogenous oestrogen to control menopausal symptoms (Rebbeck *et al.* 2002; Kauff *et al.* 2002). Many centres advocate oophorectomy at around age 40 for known carriers of *BRCA1* or *BRCA2* mutations and there is substantial evidence that, as anticipated, this provides almost complete protection against ovarian and primary peritoneal cancer of ovarian type. The implication is that primary peritoneal cancers in this setting are, in their earliest (?pre-cancerous) stages, hormone dependent. Some of these are believed to arise from the fallopian tube epithelium, and excision of the tubes is advised at the time of oophorectomy. Even tubal ligation has been found to reduce the risk of ovarian cancer in *BRCA1* mutation carriers, though the mechanism is unclear (Narod *et al.* 2001). Very few ovarian cancers present before age 40 and many gynaecologists are reluctant to undertake oophorectomy before this age. However, the reduction of breast cancer risk is an important consideration and a significant number of *BRCA1* mutation carriers will develop breast cancer in their 30s, or even their 20s. The question then arises, can anti-oestrogens offer protection for young women who wish to retain fertility? The completed and ongoing tamoxifen trials do not give an unequivocal answer. Tamoxifen does appear to provide secondary protection in *BRCA1* carriers (i.e. it reduces the risk of a second primary breast cancer in those already affected) but longer follow-up is required before the primary prevention trials can be interpreted with confidence (Cuzick *et al.* 2003).

**Table 2.2** Inheritance of breast cancer risk: some proven and putative environmental modifiers

| Environmental factor | Observations |
| --- | --- |
| Prophylactic mastectomy | Major, specialised procedure but offers high level of protection. |
| Oophorectomy | Reduces risk of breast cancer. Protection not abrogated by HRT. |
| Anti-oestrogens | Still some controversy over effectiveness in *BRCA1/2* mutation carriers. |
| Pregnancies | May increase risks in *BRCA1/2* mutation carriers. |
| HRT | Probably increases risks of familial breast cancer but unproven. |
| Oral contraceptives | Probably increase breast cancer risk but clearly reduces ovarian cancer risk in *BRCA1/2* mutation carriers. |
| Diet: phytoestrogens | Linked to overall breast cancer risk. Supplements reduce breast mammographic density but not formally shown to reduce familial cancer risk. |
| Diet: selenium | Commonly deficient in Western diets. Links with breast cancer uncertain. |
| Smoking | Claimed to be protective in *BRCA2* carriers but associated factors complicate analysis. |
| Radiation | Theoretically increased risk for p53 mutation-carriers and possibly also for *BRCA1*, *BRCA2* and others. No formal confirmation. |
| Alcohol | Associated with increased overall risk of breast cancer. No data specific to familial cases. |

Data from Colditz *et al.* (1996), Narod (2002) and other references cited in text.

Prophylactic bilateral mastectomy is an option taken up by some young women at very high risk and, in skilled hands, it has been shown to reduce subsequent breast cancer risk by at least 90% (Hartmann *et al.* 2001; Meijers-Heijboer *et al.* 2001). However, the operation is highly specialised, both to ensure as near complete removal of breast epithelium as possible and to achieve cosmetically satisfactory reconstruction, where this is requested.

Intensive surveillance, usually implying annual clinical examination and mammography from age 35, is available in many centres for women at substantial familial risk. The results so far seem promising, though the subset of women with *BRCA1* mutations fares less well, even when breast cancers are detected at an apparently early stage (Moller *et al.* 2002). Magnetic resonance imaging may offer the promise of more effective screening (Stoutjesdijk *et al.* 2001) but much longer follow-up of larger numbers will be required to evaluate these approaches fully. Similarly, dietary modification, for example supplements of phyto-oestrogens or selenium, are still at the trial stage.

## Conclusion

Familial breast cancer is a real and, for many, a potentially devastating clinical problem. Overall, however, there are grounds for optimism that, as more is learned about its fundamental biology, this knowledge will be translated into effective and acceptable forms of management that will transform the lives of many women now at high risk.

## *References*

Baldeyron, C., Jacquemin, E., Smith, J. *et al.* (2002). A single mutated BRCA1 allele leads to impaired fidelity of double strand break end-joining. *Oncogene* **21**, 1401–1410.

Berwick, M. & Vineis, P. (2000). Markers of DNA repair and susceptibility to cancer in humans: an epidemiologic review. *Journal of the National Cancer Institute* **92**, 874–897.

Brunet, J.-S., Ghadirian, P., Rebbeck, T. *et al.* (1998). Effect of smoking on breast cancer in carriers of mutant BRCA1 or BRCA2 genes. *Journal of the National Cancer Institute* **90**, 761–766.

Bryant, P. E., Gray, L., Riches, A. C., Steel, C. M. *et al.* (2002). Technical report: the G2 chromosomal radiosensitivity assay. *International Journal of Radiation Biology* **78**, 863–866.

Chen, J.-J., Silver, D., Cantor, S., Livingston, D. M. & Scully, R. (1999). BRCA1, BRCA2 and Rad51 operate in a common DNA damage response pathway. *Cancer Research* (Suppl.) **59**, 1752s–1756s.

Chenevix-Trench, G., Spurdle, A.B. Gatei, M. *et al.* (2002). Dominant negative ATM mutations in breast cancer families. *Journal of the National Cancer Institute* **94**, 205–215.

Colditz, G. A., Willett, W. C. & Hunter, D. J. (1993). Family history, age and risk of breast cancer. *Journal of the American Medical Association* **270**, 338–343.

Colditz, G. A., Rosner, B. & Speizer, F. E. (1996). Risk factors for breast cancer according to family history of breast cancer. *Journal of the National Cancer Institute* **88**, 365–371.

Concannon, P. (2002). ATM heterozygosity and cancer risk. *Nature Genetics* **32**, 89–90.

Crook, T., Crossland, S., Crompton, M., Osin, P. & Gusterson, B. A. (1997). Molecular changes in BRCA1-associated breast cancer. *The Lancet* **350**, 638–639.

Cuzick, J., Powles, T., Veronesi, U. *et al.* (2003). Overview of the main outcomes in breast-cancer prevention trials. *The Lancet* **361**, 296–300.

De Jong, M. M., Nolte, I. M., te Meerman, G. J. *et al.* (2002). Genes other than BRCA1 and BRCA2 involved in breast cancer susceptibility. *Journal of Medical Genetics* **39**, 225–242.

Dunning, A. M., Healey, C. S., Pharoah, P. D. P., Teare, M. D., Ponder, B. A. J. & Easton, D. F. (1999). A systematic review of genetic polymorphisms and breast cancer risk. *Cancer Epidemiology, Biomarkers and Prevention* **8**, 843–854.

Dunning, A. M., Chiano, C. S., Smith, N. R. *et al.* (1997). Common BRCA1 variants and susceptibility to breast and ovarian cancer in the general population. *Human Molecular Genetics* **6**, 285–289.

Easton, D. F. (1999). How many more breast cancer predisposition genes are there? *Breast Cancer Research* **1**, 14–17.

Esteller, M., Silva, J. M., Dominguez, G. *et al.* (2000). Promoter hypermethylation and BRCA1 inactivation in sporadic breast and ovarian tumours. *Journal of the National Cancer Institute* **92**, 564–569.

Grompe, M. & D'Andrea, A. (2001). Fanconi anaemia and DNA repair. *Human Molecular Genetics* **10**, 2253–2259.

Hartmann, L. C., Sellers, T. A., Schaid, D. T. *et al.* (2001). Efficacy of bilateral prophylactic mastectomy in BRCA1 and BRCA2 gene mutation carriers. *Journal of the National Cancer Institute* **93**, 1633–1637.

Healey, C. S., Dunning, A. M., Teare, M. D. *et al.* (2000). A common variant in BRCA2 is associated with both breast cancer risk and prenatal viability. *Nature Genetics* **26**, 362–364.

Hedenfalk, I., Duggan, D., Chen, Y. *et al.* (2001). Gene-expression profiles in hereditary breast cancer. *New England Journal of Medicine* **344**, 539–548.

Ingvarsson, S., Sigbjornsdottir, B. I., Huiping, C., Hafsteinsdottir, S. H., Ragnarsson, G. *et al.* (2002). Mutation analysis of the CHK2 gene in breast carcinoma and other cancers. *Breast Cancer Research* **4**, R4.

Inskip, H. M., Kinlen, L. J., Taylor, A. M. R., Woods, C. G. & Arlett, C. F. (1999). Risk of breast cancer and other cancers in heterozygotes for ataxia–telangiectasia. *British Journal of Cancer* **79**, 1304–1307.

Jernstrom, H., Lerman, C., Ghadirian, P. *et al.* (1999). Pregnancy and risk of early breast cancer in carriers of BRCA1 and BRCA2. *The Lancet* **354**, 1846–1850.

Kauff, N. D., Satagopan, J. M., Robson, M. E. *et al.* (2002). Risk-reducing salpingo-oophorectomy in women with a BRCA1 or BRCA2 mutation. *New England Journal of Medicine* **346**, 1609–1615.

Kote-Jarai, Z. & Eeles, R. (1999). BRCA1, BRCA2 and their possible functions in DNA damage response. *British Journal of Cancer* **81**, 1099–1102.

Lakhani, S. R., Jacquemeier, J., Sloane, J. P. *et al.* (1998). Multifactorial analysis of differences between sporadic breast cancers and cancers involving BRCA1 and BRCA2 mutations. *Journal of the National Cancer Institute* **90**, 1138–1145.

Lakhani, S. R., Gusterson, B. A., Jacquemeier, J. *et al.* (2000). The pathology of familial breast cancer: histological features of cancers in families not due to mutations in BRCA1 or BRCA2. *Clinical Cancer Research* **6**, 782–789.

Levy-Lahad, E., Lahad, A., Eisenberg, S. *et al.* (2001). A single nucleotide polymorphism in the RAD51 gene modifies cancer risk in BRCA2 but not BRCA1 carriers. *Proceedings of the National Academy of Sciences of the United States of America* **98**, 3232–3236.

Li, S, Ting, N. S. Y., Zheng, L. *et al.* (2000). Functional link of BRCA1 and ataxia telangiectasia gene product in DNA damage response. *Nature* **406**, 210–215.

Lynch, E. D., Ostermeyer, E. A., Lee, M. K. *et al.* (1997). Inherited mutations in PTEN that are associated with breast cancer, Cowden disease and juvenile polyposis. *American Journal of Human Genetics* **61**, 1254–1260.

Meijers-Heijboer, H., van Geel, B., van Putten, W. L. *et al.* (2001). Breast cancer after prophylactic bilateral mastectomy in women with a BRCA1 or BRCA2 mutation. *New England Journal of Medicine* **345**, 159–164.

Meijers-Heijboer, H., van den Ouwenland, A., Klijn, J. *et al.* (2002). Low-penetrance susceptibility to breast cancer due to CHEK2 1100delC in non-carriers of BRCA1 or BRCA2 mutations. *Nature Genetics* **31**, 55–59.

Moller, P., Borg, A., Evans, G. *et al.* (2002). Survival in prospectively ascertained familial breast cancer: analysis of a series stratified by tumour characteristics, BRCA mutations and oophorectomy. *International Journal of Cancer* **101**, 555–559.

Narod, S. A., Risch, H., Moslehi, R. *et al.* (1998). Oral contraceptives and the risk of hereditary ovarian cancer. *New England Journal of Medicine* **339**, 424–428.

Narod, S. A., Sun, P., Ghadirian, P. *et al.* (2001). Tubal ligation and risk of ovarian cancer in carriers of BRCA1 or BRCA2 mutations. *The Lancet* **357**, 1467–1470.

Narod, S. A. (2002). Modifiers of risk in hereditary breast and ovarian cancer syndromes. *Nature Reviews Cancer* **2**, 113–123.

Peto, J., Collins, N., Barfoot, R. *et al.* (1999). Prevalence of BRCA1 and BRCA2 gene mutations in patients with early onset breast cancer. *Journal of the National Cancer Institute* **91**, 943–949.

Pharoah, P. D. P., Antoniou, A., Bobrow, M., Zimmern, R. L., Easton, D. F. & Ponder, B. A. J. (2002). Polygeneic susceptibility to breast cancer and implications for prevention. *Nature Genetics* **31**, 33–36.

Rebbeck, T. R., Lynch, H., Neuhausen, S. L. *et al.* (2002). Prophylactic oophorectomy in carriers of BRCA1 or BRCA2 mutations. *New England Journal of Medicine* **346**, 1616–1622.

Riches, A. C., Bryant, P. E., Steel, C. M., Gleig, A. *et al.* (2001). Chromosomal radiosensitivity in G2-phase lymphocytes identifies breast cancer patients with distinctive tumour characteristics. *British Journal of Cancer* **85**, 1157–1161.

Scottish/Northern Irish BRCA1/BRCA2 Consortium (2003). BRCA1 and BRCA2 mutations in Scotland and Northern Ireland. *British Journal of Cancer* **88**, 1256–1262.

Scully, R. & Livingston, D. M. (2000). In search of the tumour-suppressor functions of BRCA1 and BRCA2. *Nature* **408**, 429–432.

Stoutjesdijk, M. J., Boetes, C., Jager, G. J., *et al.* (2001). Magnetic resonance imaging and mammography in women with a hereditary risk of breast cancer. *Journal of the National Cancer Institute* **93**, 1095–1102.

Steel, C.M., Thompson, A. & Clayton, J. (1991). Genetic aspects of breast cancer. *British Medical Bulletin* **47**, 504–518.

Thompson, P.A. & Ambrosone, C. (2000). Molecular epidemiology of genetic polymorphisms in estrogen metabolising enzymes in human breast cancer. *Journal of the National Cancer Institute Monographs* **27**, 125–133.

Thorlacius, S., Olafsdottir, G., Trygvadottir, L. *et al.* (1996). A single BRCA2 mutation in male and female breast cancer families from Iceland with varied cancer phenotypes. *Nature Genetics* **13**, 117–119.

Tirkkonen, M., Johannsson, O., Agnarsson, B. A. *et al.* (1997). Distinct somatic genetic changes associated with tumour progression in carriers of BRCA1 and BRCA2 germline mutations. *Cancer Research* **57**, 1222–1227.

Van't Veer, L. J., Dai, H., van de Vijver, M. J. *et al.* (2002). Gene expression profiling predicts clinical outcome of breast cancer. *Nature* **415**, 530–536.

Varley, J. M., Evans, D. G. R. & Birch, J. M. (1997). Li-Fraumeni syndrome: a molecular and clinical review. *British Journal of Cancer* **76**, 1–14.

Wang, W. W., Spurdle, A. B., Kolachanaa, P. *et al.* (2001). A single nucleotide polymorphism in the 5' untranslated region of RAD51 and risk of cancer among BRCA1/2 mutation carriers. *Cancer Epidemiology, Biomarkers and Prevention* **10**, 955–960.

Welcsh, P. L., Owens, K. N. & King, M.-C. (2000). Insights into the functions of BRCA1 and BRCA2. *Trends in Genetics* **16**, 69–74.

Women's Concerns Study Group. (2001). Raising concerns about family history of breast cancer in primary care consultations: prospective, population based study. *British Medical Journal* **322**, 27–28.

Wonderling, D., Hopwood, P., Cull, A., Douglas, F., Watson, M., Burn, J. & McPherson, K. (2001). A descriptive study of UK cancer genetics services: an emerging clinical response to the new genetics. *British Journal of Cancer* **85**, 166–170.

Xu, X., Wagner, K.-U., Larson, D. *et al.* (1999). Conditional mutation of BRCA1 in mammary epithelial cells results in blunted ductal morphogenesis and tumour formation. *Nature Genetics* **22**, 37–43.

Yarden, R. I., Pardo-Reoyo, S., Sgagias, M., Cowan, K. H. & Brody, L. C. (2002). BRCA1 regulates the G2/M checkpoint by activating Chk1 kinase upon DNA damage. *Nature Genetics* **30**, 285–289.

# Chapter 3

# The genetics of breast cancer–II: progress in genetic counselling and clinical decision making

*Diana M. Eccles*

## Introduction

Genetic counselling for risk of breast cancer involves a stepwise process of gathering and assessing all the available evidence from an individual to determine the likelihood of a genetic predisposition to breast cancer being present in that individual's family.

Individuals at risk will come to a genetic assessment with variable background knowledge and very varied experiences of cancer, which will affect the way that information is perceived and dealt with. Interpreting and estimating genetic and epidemiological risks is complex, and although many methods have been described, few have been widely validated prospectively.

Cancer genetic services usually operate out of the regional genetics services. In the UK these services are usually based in teaching hospitals. Most services offer outreach specialist clinics and liaise closely with regional and district cancer services for the provision of cancer genetics. The use of skilled genetic counsellors with either a nursing or science background is helpful in offering services throughout the UK.

Clinical management options for an individual at risk include prevention and early detection by screening, but choices will depend on the estimated level of risk and the individual's perception of their own risk. For the patient diagnosed with hereditary breast cancer, management options offered may differ. However, it is still unclear whether treatment strategies need to take into account the potential differential response to adjuvant therapies in hereditary breast cancer.

## Genetic risk assessment and counselling

Genetic counselling is a process by which patients or relatives at risk of a disorder that may be inherited are advised of the consequences of the disorder, the probability of developing or transmitting it, and ways in which this may be prevented, avoided or ameliorated (Harper 1993).

This broad definition of genetic counselling applies to many situations dealt with in the genetics clinic. An individual with a family history of breast cancer can obtain an assessment of the likelihood that the breast cancer in her family is likely to be due to a highly penetrant dominant genetic predisposition (e.g. a mutation in the *BRCA1* gene), a familial susceptibility (perhaps because of a single low-penetrance gene or a combination of susceptibilities both genetic and environmental), or is more likely to have arisen by chance without necessarily any significant genetic susceptibility. From the likely inheritance pattern the usefulness of any molecular genetic tests can be determined, and from there the possibility that breast cancer might develop can be estimated. Based on this risk estimate, various management strategies may be offered (Eccles *et al.* 2000). These may be accepted or rejected, depending on the perception of the risk of breast cancer and the efficacy of the proffered interventions.

The main steps in the genetic assessment process are listed below.

1. Completion of a detailed three-generation family pedigree with confirmation of key diagnoses from medical records or death certificates. This can be very time consuming and is a considerable administrative burden for genetics services; in practice this is most often done by genetic nurse specialists or genetic associates.
2. Using the family history and other information to assess the likely mode of inheritance (if any). A variety of computations can be used in different situations.
3. Using all the available evidence to assess the likelihood of genetic testing being helpful.
4. Interpreting any molecular genetic test results (discussed in chapter 2).
5. Translating all available evidence into an assessment of cancer risk for a family member.
6. Communicating the risk in an accessible form.
7. Discussing options for risk management.

## Risk assessment: general principles

Breast cancer is a common disease, diagnosed in around 38,000 women annually in the UK (CRC 2001). Conventional epidemiological studies indicate that a major risk factor for breast cancer is increasing age. Other risk factors include early age at menarche, late menopause, hormone replacement therapy (all factors that prolong exposure to oestrogen) and family history of the disease.

Segregation analysis is a means of examining pedigree information from populations where the disease of interest is found, and determining what pattern of inheritance is likely from the available family history data. The parameters defined by segregation analysis include a measure of how common the putative gene or genes are in the population (frequency), and the chance of developing the disease if an individual inherits the disease gene (penetrance). Breast cancer segregation analyses have consistently shown that breast cancer can be inherited as a dominant predisposition with high penetrance, and that these high-risk genes are relatively infrequent in the population (Claus *et al.* 1994; Eccles *et al.* 1994). Segregation analysis cannot determine how many genes might determine the same pattern and expression of disease (several genes expressing the same disease phenotype is known as genetic heterogeneity). Thus it turns out, as highly penetrant breast cancer genes are discovered, that there are several genes that can cause dominantly inherited predisposition to breast cancer, but that these probably account for less than 5% of all breast cancer cases. The remainder could perhaps be explained by several lower-penetrance genes combined with environmental risk factors, or even other modes of inheritance including autosomal recessive inheritance (Antoniou *et al.* 2001).

There are undoubtedly many genes of lower penetrance than those that can readily be discovered using genetic linkage approaches. Candidate genes are, for example, those that determine endogenous oestrogen levels and enzymes that detoxify carcinogens (de Jong *et al.* 2002). They also possibly include genes that are involved in DNA repair, which are increasingly implicated in cancer predisposition (Meijers-Heijboer *et al.* 2002).

There are several computer programmes available that approach risk estimation either from a genetic perspective (Chang-Claude *et al.* 1999) or from an epidemiological perspective where family history is factored in with other known risk factors (Spiegelman *et al.* 1994). None of the available methods has been well validated in a range of clinical circumstances, and results for individuals need to be interpreted very carefully and not used in isolation (MacKarem *et al.* 2001). Where the family history is unlikely to represent a strong genetic predisposition, molecular genetic testing is unlikely to be helpful (Langston *et al.* 1996; Eccles *et al.* 1998; Janezic *et al.* 1999; Chang-Claude *et al.* 1999).

Where there is no family history of breast cancer, a combination of adverse epidemiological risk factors may confer a lifetime risk equivalent to that for a woman with one or two older relatives affected with breast cancer. Certain risk-reducing strategies may be equally valid in women at increased risk for other reasons than genetic predisposition (Rockhill *et al.* 2001).

## *Molecular testing*

If a suitable sample is available from a fully informed and consenting family member who has had a cancer likely to be associated with a high-risk gene mutation, a search for the causative mutation can be initiated on behalf of affected and at-risk family members. Such a search may reveal a disease-causing mutation where the protein product will clearly be abnormal and non-functional, a mutation or variant of uncertain significance (which in the main are of no clinical benefit), or it will reveal no mutation. No laboratory can currently detect all possible mutations, even with a variety of techniques, for reasons discussed elsewhere including genetic heterogeneity and the sensitivity of mutation searching for different classes of mutation. Mutation analysis is costly and a negative result is of no value in this context. It is important therefore to select carefully if limited resources are to be used responsibly, and to interpret the results correctly.

If a specific gene mutation is identified in an affected family member, more specific risk information can be given to family members, and the option of a predictive genetic test can be considered by each individual. A predictive genetic test will tell an individual categorically whether they have inherited the identified familial mutation. However, it will not clarify the precise cancer risk as this will still depend on other factors (genetic and environmental) that will influence the likelihood of the gene manifesting phenotypically as a cancer (gene penetrance and expression) (Begg 2002).

## Risk communication

### Clinical interpretation of risk

An estimation of the chance of an individual developing breast cancer, using any available computational method and family history data, will necessarily be associated with a degree of uncertainty relating to the appropriateness of the model used, and the common problem of missing or incorrect data. For example, in a family with two close relatives with breast cancer at 50–55 years, a wrong assignation of diagnosis, perhaps a colon cancer mistakenly believed to be ovarian cancer, would lead to an overestimate of the likelihood of a given family history to be due to a high-risk gene. A range of likely risk may be a more honest representation. Sometimes the actual risk estimate is only helpful in that it allows categorisation of the individual. The UK Cancer Genetics Group (associated with the British Society of Human Genetics) have agreed published guidelines, which may help to categorise patients into high risk, moderately increased risk or a risk similar to that in the general population. Moderate risk here was defined as over three times the age-related risk on the basis that this level of risk is achieved with risk factors other than family history where additional screening is not usually advocated (Eccles *et al.* 2000).

### Setting the scene

It is helpful in explaining risk to an individual to clarify the level of understanding they have already, any unexpected health beliefs, and any experiences of cancer and cancer diagnosis and treatment. To use a consultation most effectively it is sensible to establish what information that person and the referring doctor need, and what the individual wants to know. It is also important to take into account an indication of the level of perceived risk for that individual. Communicating the background risk of breast cancer can be important because this is often incorrectly perceived (Lloyd *et al.* 1996; Evans *et al.* 1993).

### Presentation of risks

The actual presentation of estimated risk might be as a lifetime risk (risk of developing breast cancer to age 80 years), a heterozygous risk (risk of being a gene carrier on the basis of family history data and age of the individual), and cumulative risk to a specified age (for example, the chance of being diagnosed with breast cancer before entering the National Breast Screening Programme at age 50 years), or a risk relative to an individual of the same age drawn at random from the general population. Often a risk category is all that is required along with a recommendation for management (Eccles *et al.* 2000).

### Risk perception

Perceived risk relates as much to previous experience and health beliefs as to estimated risk of breast cancer (Figure 3.1). A consultation to explain risk and offer management options does seem to allay anxieties, at least in the short term. However, because this is often coupled with screening interventions, it is still unclear what component of the consultation really allays fears, and the effect seems to be temporary. Further research in this area is needed to ensure appropriate service development and more effective risk communication (Hopwood 2000).

---

**Risk assessment**

- Likely mode of inheritance (if any)?

- Risk of cancer?

- Communication of risk

**Clinical decision making**

- Early detection (screening)

- Cancer prevention

- Cancer treatment

---

**Figure 3.1**  Clinical cancer genetics

## Cancer genetics services

Further to the Calman–Hine report on Cancer Services in the UK, a working party was commissioned by The Royal College of Physicians to examine the delivery of Cancer Genetics Services (Harper 1998). Services across the UK are developing roughly along the lines recommended in this report. Guidelines have been published for use in primary care (available from Cancer Research UK (CRUK); Primary Care Guidelines 2001), for use at breast unit level (Eccles *et al.* 2000), with higher-risk families being selected for formal genetic counselling by the specialist cancer genetics service; some of these families may be suitable for molecular genetic analysis. Across the UK, however, local research interests and funding issues still strongly influence referral patterns and available services (Wonderling *et al.* 2001). Similar provision exists across many other European countries but often, as in the USA, provision is through cancer services rather than genetics services (Hodgson *et al.* 1999).

# Clinical management issues

## Risk management

### Prevention

The two main approaches to cancer prevention are either medical or surgical measures. Such options might be offered depending on the estimated level of risk (by the health professional), and might be accepted depending on the perceived risk (of the individual expressing concern) and the perception of that individual of the efficacy of screening and treatment if cancer were to be diagnosed (Figure 3.2).

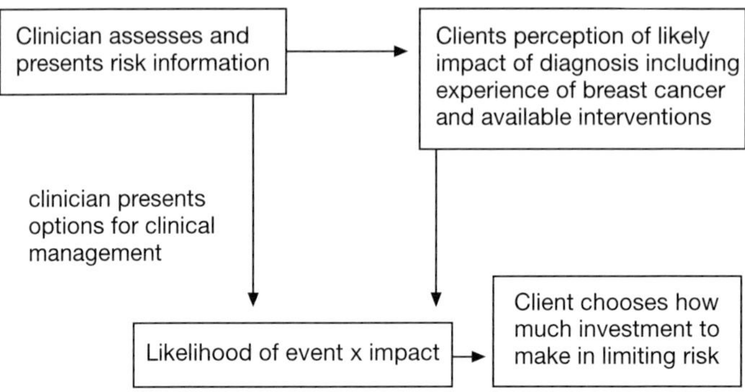


**Figure 3.2** Risk perception

### Medical approaches

Oestrogen exposure is a key risk factor in breast carcinogenesis. Many of the well-recognised epidemiological risk factors for breast cancer relate to those that increase oestrogen exposure (either endogenous or exogenous). For some years now there has been considerable interest in the use of selective oestrogen receptor modulators (notably tamoxifen; Powles *et al*. 1990; Fisher *et al*. 1998) to reduce risk of breast cancer, with up to 50% fewer oestrogen receptor (ER)-positive breast tumours being reported from the USA (NSABP1 trial; Fisher *et al*. 1998). More recently, 30% fewer ER-positive tumours were reported in the treatment arm for a fourth randomised intervention study investigating tamoxifen as a chemopreventive agent (IBIS investigators 2002). Side effects for tamoxifen are an issue, and any possible benefits in reduction in breast cancer mortality may be outweighed by the risks (increased thrombo-embolism and endometrial cancer risk).

More recently, attention has turned to GnRH antagonists like Zoladex (goserelin acetate), which switch off the pituitary–ovarian axis rendering the individual temporarily post-menopausal. Pilot studies in women at high risk of being a gene carrier have proven difficult to recruit to, but once patients are recruited compliance seems to be good (Evans 2001, 2002).

**Surgical approaches**

Risk-reducing mastectomy is offered in many centres for women at high risk of developing breast cancer. There is evidence that this does reduce risk of breast cancer effectively although not entirely (Hartmann *et al* 1999; Meijers-Heijboer *et al*. 2000; McDonnell *et al*. 2001). The acceptability of this measure will vary greatly according to cultural and social factors (Julian-Reynier *et al*. 2001).

Recent evidence confirming oophorectomy reduces the subsequent risk of breast cancer by up to 50% in premenopausal *BRCA1* gene carriers will perhaps lead to a different weighting in decisions about risk management (Rebbeck 2004; Armstrong 2004).

*Early detection*

Mammography is the most frequently used imaging modality for early detection of breast cancer. There is considerable controversy about the magnitude of mortality reduction attributable to mammography in screening trials (Davies *et al* 1995; Boddy & Ratain 1997; Black *et al*. 2002). This controversy is considerable for the age group under 50 years (Lucassen *et al*. 2001). Although there are several studies demonstrating that cancers can be detected in women under 50 years of age being screened for a family history of breast cancer, data on mortality are not available or are derived from surrogate end-points (Kollias *et al*. 1998; Kerlikowske *et al*. 2000). In addition, there are data that suggest for high-risk *BRCA1* gene carriers (where cancers tend to be high grade) mammography is relatively insensitive and that higher resolution modalities such as magnetic resonance imaging and possibly more frequent screening than annual may be more effective (Brekelmans *et al*. 2001). It is clear, however, that it will be important to evaluate screening modalities and regimens with good prospective studies taking actual cancer mortality into account (Armstrong & Weber 2001).

Ovarian screening using a combination of serum tumour markers (principally CA125) and pelvic ultrasound scanning has not been demonstrated to be effective in reducing cancer mortality in population-based studies. However, a current UK randomised trial of population screening in the over-50 year age group may clarify the role and efficacy of these modalities (Hogg & Friedlander 2004). Two UK studies may clarify the role of these modalities: a large population-based study in post-menopausal population risk women (Jacobs *et al*. 1999), and a CRUK study for women who may carry a genetic predisposition to ovarian cancer (UKFOCSS: www.ncrn.org.uk/portfolio/Data.asp). Both these studies are likely to take several years to reach any conclusions. Until definitive evidence of benefit is available, ovarian cancer screening should not be offered as a routine clinical service. Thus there is more likelihood that women will undergo prophylactic oophorectomy if they are thought to be at high risk for developing ovarian cancer (Emery *et al.* 1999), and this may in turn affect the likelihood of breast cancer developing in these women as outlined above.

## Cancer treatment

There are several areas of important clinical uncertainty about the management of hereditary breast cancer. One surrounds the prognosis for *BRCA1*-related breast cancers, for which the literature suggests that the overall survival is better, the same or much worse than sporadic cancers (Porter *et al.* 1994; Eccles *et al.* 2001; Verhoog *et al.* 1998; Stoppa-Lyonnet *et al.* 2000; Johannsson *et al.* 1998). In addition, because *BRCA1* and *BRCA2* are involved in DNA repair, especially double-strand DNA breaks, the effect of adjuvant therapies (both radiation therapy and chemotherapy) may differ in hereditary breast cancer compared with sporadic cases (Khanna & Jackson 2001; Turner *et al.* 1999; Kerr & Ashworth 2001). This uncertainty needs to be resolved because clinicians are already beginning to offer more radical surgical treatment to women at high genetic risk on the basis of hypothesis and of imperfect and methodologically flawed studies. There is a need for good unbiased data to provide clear answers to the question of risk of death from the primary diagnosis versus risk of a second primary for each type of hereditary breast cancer, so that questions of treatment and prophylaxis can be given appropriate weight in the management decisions of patient and treating clinicians.

There is little useful information in the literature about any of these issues (Phillips *et al.* 1999; Phillips & McKay 2001). In the UK at present, most young women diagnosed with breast cancer have not had a genetic test. Technical challenges and cost limit the ability to perform rapid molecular genetic testing. Current data suggest that 5–10% of women diagnosed with breast cancer aged 40 years or younger will have a *BRCA1* gene mutation: the published frequencies of mutation detection, in similar age groups, range from 2.6–15% (Loman *et al.* 2001; Papelard *et al.* 2000; Malone *et al.* 2000; Turchetti *et al.* 2000; Eccles *et al.* 1998; Peto *et al.* 1999; Newman *et al.* 1998). Variations in prevalence of mutation carriers will depend on the sensitivity of the analysis technique used and on the method of ascertainment of the population being studied. For example, if *BRCA1 per se* confers a poor prognosis, studies where potential recruits have been omitted because of their early death will underestimate the prevalence of mutation carriers. In the UK there is no identified prominent founder mutation to simplify mutation analysis. Thus most newly diagnosed breast cancer cases will be treated in a conventional manner without knowledge of the patient's genetic status except for knowledge of the family history. As technology moves on and genetic testing becomes more readily available, treatment decisions may be increasingly influenced by knowledge of the patient's genetic make-up.

Recent studies have examined the use of gene expression profiling to determine prognosis for breast and other cancers. In future, such methods may help to direct and individualise adjuvant therapies for maximum therapeutic benefit (Van 't Veer *et al.* 2002; Iwao *et al.* 2002; Bertucci *et al.* 2002).

## Summary

Progress in knowledge of breast cancer genetics has been rapid as technology advances. However, clinical studies, which will allow these advances in knowledge to be used to improve and advance clinical management, are lagging behind. High-risk genes that predispose to breast cancer are relatively uncommon, making collaboration within and between countries important if we are to further our understanding of risk assessment and risk management. More frequent but lower-penetrance genes are still being discovered and may interact with each other and with environmental risk factors in complex ways. Advances in technology may allow these lower-penetrance genes to be used clinically but at present they have no such use. Assessment of risk is complex and no single method provides a clear-cut estimate. The measures that are frequently advocated for risk reduction are often of uncertain efficacy, although current research focused on assessing screening and preventive strategies may clarify some of these issues. Conveying risk to individuals is also beset with complexities because of the psychology of risk perception and decision making. This is also an area where much more research is needed so that a comprehensive clinical service can be offered.


## *References*

Antoniou, A. C., Pharoah, P. D., McMullan, G., Day, N. E., Ponder, B. A. & Easton, D. (2001). Evidence for further breast cancer susceptibility genes in addition to BRCA1 and BRCA2 in a population-based study. *Genetic Epidemiology* **21**, 1–18.

Armstrong, K. & Weber, B. (2001). Breast cancer screening for high-risk women: too little, too late? *Journal of Clinical Oncology* **19**, 919–920.

Armstrong, K., Schwartz, J. S., Randall, T., Rubin, S. C. & Weber, B. L. (2004). Hormone replacement therapy and life expectancy after prophylactic oophorectomy in women with *BRCA1/2* mutations: a decision analysis. *Journal of Clinical Oncology* **22**, 1045–1054.

Begg, C. B. (2002). On the use of familial aggregation in population-based case probands for calculating penetrance. *Journal of the National Cancer Institute* **94**, 1221–1226.

Bertucci, F., Nasser, V., Granjeaud, S., Eisinger, F., Adelaide, J., Tagett, R., Loriod, B., Giaconia, A., Benziane, A., Devilard, E. *et al.* (2002). Gene expression profiles of poor-prognosis primary breast cancer correlate with survival. *Human Molecular Genetics* **11**, 863–872.

Black, W. C., Haggstrom, D. A., Gilbert, W. H. (2002). All-cause mortality in randomized trials of cancer screening. *Journal of the National Cancer Institute* **94**, 167–173.

Boddy, A. V. & Ratain, M. J. (1997). Pharmacogenetics in cancer etiology and chemotherapy. *Clinical Cancer Research* **3**, 1025–1030.

Brekelmans, C. T., Seynaeve, C., Bartels, C. C., Tilanus-Linthorst, M. M., Meijers-Heijboer, E. J., Crepin, C. M., van Geel, A. A., Menke, M., Verhoog, L. C., van den Oeweland, O. A. *et al.* (2001). Effectiveness of breast cancer surveillance in BRCA1/2 gene mutation carriers and women with high familial risk. *Journal of Clinical Oncology* **19**, 924–930.

Chang-Claude, J., Becher, H., Caligo, M., Eccles, D., Evans, G., Haites, N., Hodgson, S., Moller, P., Weber, B. H. & Stoppa-Lyonnet, D. (1999). Risk estimation as a decision-making tool for genetic analysis of the breast cancer susceptibility genes. EC Demonstration Project on Familial Breast Cancer. *Disease Markers* **15**, 53–65.

Claus, E. B., Risch, N. & Thompson, W. D. (1994). Autosomal dominant inheritance of early onset breast cancer. *Cancer* **73**, 643–651.

Davies, D. R., Armstrong, J. G., Thakker, N., Horner, K., Guy, S. P., Clancy, T., Sloan, P., Blair V, Dodd, C., Warnes T. W. *et al.* (1995). Severe Gardner syndrome in families with mutations restricted to a specific region of the APC gene. *American Journal of Human Genetics* **57**, 1151–1158.

de Jong, M. M., Nolte, I. M., te Meerman, G. J., van der Graaf, W. T., Oosterwijk, J. C., Kleibeuker, J. H., Schaapveld, M. & de Vries, E. G. (2002). Genes other than BRCA1 and BRCA2 involved in breast cancer susceptibility. *Journal of Medical Genetics* **39**, 225–242.

Eccles, D., Marlow, A., Royle, G., Collins, A. & Morton, N. E. (1994). Genetic epidemiology of early onset breast cancer. *Journal of Medical Genetics* **31**, 944–949.

Eccles, D. M., Englefield, P., Soulby, M. A. & Campbell, I. G. (1998). BRCA1 mutations in southern England. *British Journal of Cancer* **77**, 2199–2203.

Eccles, D. M., Evans, D. G. & Mackay, J. (2000). Guidelines for a genetic risk based approach to advising women with a family history of breast cancer. UK Cancer Family Study Group (UKCFSG). *Journal of Medical Genetics* **37**, 203–209.

Eccles, D., Simmonds, P., Goddard, J., Coultas, M., Hodgson, S., Lalloo, F., Evans, G. & Haites, N. (2001). Familial breast cancer: an investigation into the outcome of treatment for early stage disease. *Family Cancer* **1**, 65–72.

Eccles, D. M., Dowsett, M., Howell, A. *et al.* (2002). The Raloxifene plus Zoladex (RAZOR) trial for breast cancer risk reduction. *Cancer Epidemiology Biomarkers* **11**, C108 (part 2).

Emery, J. *et al.* (1999). Screening for ovarian cancer. *The Lancet* **354**, 509.

Evans, D. G. R., Burnell, L. D., Hopwood, P. & Howell, A. (1993). Perception of risk in women with a family history of breast cancer. *British Journal of Cancer* **67**, 612–614.

Evans, D., Lalloo, F., Shenton, A., Boggis, C. & Howell, A. (2001). Uptake of screening and prevention in women at very high risk of breast cancer. *The Lancet* **358**, 889–890.

Fisher, B., Costantino, J. P., Wickerham, D. L., Redmond, C. K., Kavanah, M., Cronin, W. M., Vogel, V., Robidoux, A., Dimitrov, N., Atkins, J. *et al.* (1998). Tamoxifen for prevention of breast cancer: report of the National Surgical Adjuvant Breast and Bowel Project P-1 Study. *Journal of the National Cancer Institute* **90**, 1371–1388.

Grann, V. R., Jacobson, J. S., Thomason, D., Hershman, D., Heitjan, D. F., Neugut, A. I. (2002). Effect of prevention strategies on survival and quality-adjusted survival of women with BRCA1/2 mutations: an updated decision analysis. *Journal of Clinical Oncology* **20**, 2520–2529.

Harper, P. (1993). General aspects of genetic counselling. In *Practical Genetic Counselling*, 4th edition, chapter 1, p. 3. Oxford: Butterworth-Heinemann.

Harper, P. (1998). Working party on cancer genetics services in the UK. DHSS discussion document.

Hartmann, L. C., Schaid, D. J., Woods, J. E., Crotty, T. P., Myers, J. L., Arnold, P. G., Petty, P. M., Sellers, T. A., Johnson, J. L. & McDonnell, S. K. *et al.* (1999). Efficacy of bilateral prophylactic mastectomy in women with a family history of breast cancer. *New England Journal of Medicine* **340**, 77–84.

Hodgson, S., Milner, B., Brown, I., Bevilacqua, G., Chang-Claude, J., Eccles, D., Evans, G., Gregory, H., Moller, P., Morrison, P. *et al.* (1999). Cancer genetics services in Europe. *Disease Markers* **15**, 3–13.

Hogg, R. & Friedlander, M. (2004). Biology of epithelial ovarian cancer: implications for screening women at high genetic risk. *Journal of Clinical Oncology* **22**, 1315–1327.

Hopwood, P. (2000). Breast cancer risk perception: what do we know and understand? *Breast Cancer Research* **2**, 387–391.

IBIS investigators (2002). First results from the International Breast Cancer Intervention Study (IBIS-1): a randomised prevention trial. *The Lancet* **360**, 817–824.

Iwao, K., Matoba, R., Ueno, N., Ando, A., Miyoshi, Y., Matsubara, K., Noguchi, S. & Kato, K. (2002). Molecular classification of primary breast tumors possessing distinct prognostic properties. *Human Molecular Genetics* **11**, 199–206.

Jacobs, I. J., Skates, S. J., MacDonald, N., Menon, U., Rosenthal, A. N., Prys-Davies, A., Woolas, R., Jeyarajah, A. R., Sibley, K., Lowe, D. G. & Oram, D. H. (1999). Screening for ovarian cancer: a pilot randomised controlled trial. *The Lancet* **353**, 1207–1210.

Janezic, S. A., Ziogas, A., Krumroy, L. M., Krasner, M., Plummer, S. J., Cohen, P., Gildea, M., Barker, D., Haile, R. *et al.* (1999). Germline BRCA1 alterations in a population based series of ovarian cancer cases. *Human Molecular Genetics* **8**, 889–897.

Johannsson, O. T., Ranstam, J., Borg, A. & Olsson, H. (1998). Survival of BRCA1 breast and ovarian cancer patients: a population-based study from southern Sweden. *Journal of Clinical Oncology* **16**, 397–404.

Julian-Reynier, C. M., Bouchard, L. J., Evans, D. G., Eisinger, F. A., Foulkes, W. D., Kerr, B., Blancquaert, I. R., Moatti, J. P. & Sobol, H. H. (2001). Women's attitudes toward preventive strategies for hereditary breast or ovarian carcinoma differ from one country to another: differences among English, French, and Canadian women. *Cancer* **92**, 959–968.

Kauff ND, Satagopan JM, Robson ME, Scheuer L, Hensley M, Hudis CA, Ellis NA, Boyd J, Borgen PI, Barakat RR, Norton L, Castiel M, Nafa K, Offit K 2002 Risk-reducing salpingo-oophorectomy in women with a BRCA1 or BRCA2 mutation. *New England Journal of Medicine* **346**, 1609–1615.

Kerlikowske, K., Carney, P. A., Geller, B., Mandelson, M. T., Taplin, S. H., Malvin, K., Ernster, V., Urban, N., Cutter, G., Rosenberg, R. & Ballard-Barbash R (2000). Performance of screening mammography among women with and without a first-degree relative with breast cancer. *Annals of Internal Medicine* **133**, 855–863.

Kerr, P. & Ashworth, A. (2001). New complexities for BRCA1 and BRCA2. *Current Biology* **11**, R668–R676.

Khanna, K. K. & Jackson, S. P. (2001). DNA double-strand breaks: signaling, repair and the cancer connection. *Nature Genetics* **27**, 247–254.

Kollias, J., Sibbering, D. M., Blamey, R. W., Holland, P. A. M., Obuszko, Z., Wilson, A. R. M., Evans, A. J., Ellis, I. O. & Elston, C. W. (1998). Screening women aged less than 50 years with a family history of breast cancer. *European Journal of Cancer* **34**, 878–883.

Langston, A. A., Malone, K. E., Thompson, J. D., Daling, J., Ostrander, E. A. (1996). BRCA1 mutations in a population-based sample of young women with breast cancer. *New England Journal of Medicine* **334**, 137–142.

Lloyd, S., Watson, M., Waites, B., Meyer, L., Eeles, R., Ebbs, S. & Tylee, A. (1996). Familial breast cancer: a controlled study of risk perception, psychological morbidity and health beliefs in women attending for genetic counselling. *British Journal of Cancer* **74**, 482–487.

Loman, N., Johannsson, O., Kristoffersson, U., Olsson, H. & Borg, A. (2001). Family history of breast and ovarian cancers and BRCA1 and BRCA2 mutations in a population-based series of early-onset breast cancer. *Journal of the National Cancer Institute* **93**, 1215–1223.

Lucassen, A., Watson, E., Eccles, D. (2001). Advice about mammography for a young woman with a family history of breast cancer. *British Medical Journal* **322**, 1040–1042.

MacKarem, G., Roche, C. A. & Hughes, K. S. (2001). The effectiveness of the gail model in estimating risk for development of breast cancer in women under 40 years of age. *Breast Journal* **7**, 34–39.

Malone, K. E., Daling, J. R., Neal, C., Suter, N. M., O'Brien, C., Cushing-Haugen, K., Jonasdottir, T. J., Thompson, J. D. & Ostrander, E. A. (2000). Frequency of BRCA1/BRCA2 mutations in a population-based sample of young breast carcinoma cases. *Cancer* **88**, 1393–1402.

McDonnell, S. K., Schaid, D. J., Myers, J. L., Grant, C. S., Donohue, J. H., Woods, J. E., Frost, M. H., Johnson, J. L., Sitta, D. L., Slezak, J. M. *et al.* (2001). Efficacy of contralateral prophylactic mastectomy in women with a personal and family history of breast cancer. *Journal of the National Cancer Institute* **19**, 3938–3943.

Meijers-Heijboer, H., van den Oeweland, O. A., Klijn, J., Wasielewski, M., de Snoo, A., Oldenburg, R., Hollestelle, A., Houben, M., Crepin, E., Veghel-Plandsoen, M., Elstrodt, F. *et al.* (2002a). Low-penetrance susceptibility to breast cancer due to CHEK2(*)1100delC in noncarriers of BRCA1 or BRCA2 mutations. *Nature Genetics* **31**, 55–59.

Meijers-Heijboer, E. J., Verhoog, L. C., Brekelmans, C. T., Seynaeve, C., Tilanus-Linthorst, M. M., Wagner, A., Dukel, L., Devilee, P., van den Ouweland, A. M., van Geel, A. N. & Klijn, J. G. (2000b). Presymptomatic DNA testing and prophylactic surgery in families with a BRCA1 or BRCA2 mutation. *The Lancet* **355**, 2015–2020.

Newman, B., Mu, H., Butler, L.M., Millikan, R.C., Moorman, P.G. & King, M.C. (1998). Frequency of breast cancer attributable to BRCA1 in a population-based series of American women. *Journal of the American Medical Association* **279**, 915–921.

Papelard, H., de Bock, G. H., van Eijk, R., Vliet Vlieland, T. P., Cornelisse, C. J., Devilee, P. & Tollenaar, R. A. (2000). Prevalence of BRCA1 in a hospital-based population of Dutch breast cancer patients. *British Journal of Cancer* **83**, 719–724.

Peto, J., Collins, N., Barfoot, R. *et al.* (1999). Prevalence of BRCA1 and BRCA2 gene mutations in patients with early-onset breast cancer. *Journal of the National Cancer Institute* **91**, 943–949.

Phillips, K. A., Andrulis, I. L. & Goodwin, P. J. (1999). Breast carcinomas arising in carriers of mutations in BRCA1 or BRCA2: are they prognostically different?. *Journal of Clinical Oncology* **17**, 3653–3663.

Phillips, K. A. & McKay, M. J. (2001). Breast conservation in BRCA1 or BRCA2 mutation carriers with early stage breast cancer. *Australasian Radiology* **45**, 200–204.

Porter, D. E., Cohen, B. B., Wallace, M. R., Smyth, E., Chetty, U., Dixon, J. M., Steel, C. M. & Carter, D. C. (1994). Breast cancer incidence, penetrance and survival in probable carriers of BRCA1 gene mutations in families linked to BRCA1 on chromosome 17q12–21. *British Journal of Surgery* **81**, 1512–1515.

Powles, T. J., Tillyer, C. R., Jones, A. L. *et al.* (1990). Prevention of breast cancer with tamoxifen: an update on the Royal Marsden pilot programme. *European Journal of Cancer* **26**, 680–684.

Rebbeck, T. R., Friebel, T., Lynch, H. T., Neuhausen, S. L., van't Veer, L., Garber, J. E., Evans, G. R., Narod, S. A., Isaacs, C., Matloff, E., Daly, M. B., Olopade, O. I., Weber, B. L. (2004). Bilateral prophylactic mastectomy reduces breast cancer risk in *BRCA1* and *BRCA2* mutation carriers: the PROSE Study Group. *Journal of Clinical Oncology* **22**, 1055–1062.

Rebbeck, T. R., Lynch, H. T., Neuhausen, S. L., Narod, S. A., Van't Veer, L., Garber, J. E., Evans G, Isaacs, C., Daly, M. B., Matloff, E. *et al.* (2002). Prophylactic oophorectomy in carriers of BRCA1 or BRCA2 mutations. *New England Journal of Medicine* **346**, 1616–1622.

Rockhill, B., Spiegelman, D., Byrne, C., Hunter, D. J. & Colditz, G. A. (2001). Validation of the Gail *et al.* model of breast cancer risk prediction and implications for chemoprevention. *Journal of the National Cancer Institute* **93**, 358–366.

Spiegelman, D., Colditz, G. A., Hunter, D. & Hertzmark, E. (1994). Validation of the Gail *et al.* model for predicting individual breast cancer risk. *Journal of the National Cancer Institute* **86**, 600–608.

Stoppa-Lyonnet, D., Ansquer, Y., Dreyfus, H., Gautier, C., Gauthier-Villars, M., Bourstyn, E., Clough, K., Magdelenat, H., Pouillart, P., Vincent-Salomon, A., Fourquet, A. & Asselain, B. Institute Curie Breast Cancer Group (2000). Familial invasive breast cancers: worse outcome related to BRCA1 mutations. *Journal of Clinical Oncology* **18**, 4053–4059.

Turchetti, D., Cortesi, L., Federico, M., Bertoni, C., Mangone, L., Ferrari, S. & Silingardi, V. (2000). BRCA1 mutations and clinicopathological features in a sample of Italian women with early-onset breast cancer. *European Journal of Cancer* **36**, 2083–2089.

Turner, B. C., Harrold, E., Matloff, E., Smith, T., Gumbs, A. A., Beinfield, M., Ward, B., Skolnick, M., Glazer, P. M., Thomas, A. & Haffy, B. (1999). BRCA1/BRCA2 germline mutations in locally recurrent breast cancer patients after lumpectomy and radiation therapy: implications for breast-conserving management in patients with BRCA1/BRCA2 mutations. *Journal of Clinical Oncology* **17**, 3017–3024.

Van't Veer, L. J., Dai, H., van de Vijver, M. J., He, Y. D., Hart, A. A., Mao, M., Peterse, H. L., van der Kooy, K., Marton M. J., Witteveen, A. T. *et al.* (2002). Gene expression profiling predicts clinical outcome of breast cancer. *Nature* **415**, 530–536.

Verhoog, L. C., Brekelmans, C. T. M., Seynaeve, C., van den Bosch, L. M. C., Dahmen, G., van Geel, A. N., Tilanus-Linthorst, M. M. A., Bartels, C. C. M., Wagner, A., van den Ouweland, A. M. W. *et al.* (1998). Survival and tumour characteristics of breast-cancer patients with germ-line mutations of BRCA1. *The Lancet* **351**, 316–321.

Webb, M. J. (1993). Screening for ovarian cancer. Still a long way to go. *British Medical Journal* **306**, 1015–1016.

Wonderling, D., Hopwood, P., Cull, A., Douglas, F., Watson, M., Burn, J. & McPherson, K. (2001). A descriptive study of UK cancer genetics services: an emerging clinical response to the new genetics. *British Journal of Cancer* **85**, 166–170.

# PART 2

# Imaging, biopsy and endoscopy

# Chapter 4

# Current status of magnetic resonance imaging in the detection of malignancy and in the assessment of treatment response

*Lindsay W. Turnbull*

## Introduction

Using gadolinium-based intravenous contrast agents, fast imaging techniques and dedicated receiver coils, dynamic contrast-enhanced magnetic resonance imaging (DCE-MRI) is becoming an invaluable tool in the diagnosis and treatment of breast disease. This technique is termed 'dynamic' as it relies on rapid data acquisition before, during and after the bolus administration of an MR-specific contrast agent. Using this method of data acquisition, sensitivities for symptomatic cases are now in excess of 95% and specificities greater than 90% for invasive breast cancer (Fischer 1999; Tan 1999).

The high sensitivity and specificity of DCE-MRI relies on the use of intravenous gadolinium, which passes into the extravascular space and accumulates in tissues with high vascularity. The justification for using gadolinium is that most cancers induce neovascularisation. A carcinoma larger than 3 mm in diameter secretes pro-angiogenic molecules, which increase the vascularity of the region by recruiting new vessels. Other factors that encourage tissue enhancement are expansion of the extracellular space, increased interstitial pressure and increased capillary permeability due to an abnormal basement membrane or cytokinin mediated effects. These result in more rapid accumulation of gadolinium in cancers than in benign lesions.

## Techniques

The methods of analysis of the DCE-MRI data generated are numerous and are based on the pattern of contrast uptake and the morphology of the lesion obtained from post-contrast, fat-suppressed or subtracted images. Kuhl *et al.* (1999) reported on the classification accuracy of experienced radiologists subjectively assessing signal-intensity time curves, grade from I to III, and obtained a diagnostic efficacy of 86%, with a sensitivity of 91% and a specificity of 83%, respectively. This is similar to an earlier report by Knowles *et al.* (1998) who quoted an accuracy rate of 76%, but the specificity value rose to 91% with the addition of morphological information, emphasising the importance of using both data sources.

Many techniques have been used to maximise diagnostic efficacy, and empirical techniques are the simplest, least labour intensive, and the most widely applied. They are used either alone or in combination, to examine contrast uptake relative to background, at pre-determined time points, which have been shown previously to provide best lesion discrimination (Buckley *et al.* 1994; Gribbestad *et al.* 1994; Greenstein Orel *et al.* 1995; Hulka *et al.* 1995; Liney *et al.* 1999). However, these are subject to some inaccuracies resulting from timing and speed of bolus injection and seldom allow for spurious data points secondary to artefacts.

There is now increasing interest in the use of additional techniques to optimise and automate DCE-MRI analysis to speed up analysis and aid the radiologist. These including: textural analysis (Gibbs *et al.* 2003); independent component analysis which uses a statistical algorithm to separate mixed signal sources of unknown nature to enable extraction of spatial and temporal features (Yoo *et al.* 2002); use of geometric indices, particularly spherical shape index (Shahar *et al.* 2002); and most commonly, the use of neural networks. Neural networks have been used in several different ways. Abdolmaleki *et al.* (2001) used a jack-knife method to extract and analyse quantitative data from signal intensity time profiles to predict pathological outcome, and achieved a better diagnostic accuracy rate (89%) than the radiologist (79%). Using a classic feed-forward back-propagation neural network with three layers, Vergnaghi *et al* (2001) analysed three-dimensional MR data and correctly identified the curves with a sensitivity of 76% and a specificity of 90%. They used a neural network clustering approach to prevent discarding of information from the complete dynamic time series and concluded that it contributed to the diagnosis of indeterminate breast lesions.

## Locoregional staging

There is now substantial evidence of a good correlation between the findings at MRI and histology of resected specimens, with results exceeding those obtained by X-ray mammography or ultrasound (Davies 1996; Esserman 1999; Balen 1997). Davies *et al.* used a 3D fast spoilt gradient echo, contrast-enhanced, fat-suppressed sequence and demonstrated an excellent correlation between the largest cancer diameter measured by MR and histopathology, compared with poorer correlation coefficients and larger standard errors for X-ray mammography and ultrasound. Ando *et al.* (1997) presented similar data demonstrating a good correlation between histopathology and direct invasion of mammary tissue, satellite nodule formation and intraductal tumour extension. Current evidence suggests that chest wall invasion can be diagnosed with confidence (Deutch 1993; Fischer 1994; Whitney 1993).

## Multi-focal/multi-centric disease

Previous studies of surgical treatment for primary breast cancer without subsequent radiotherapy, have demonstrated an increased risk of local tumour recurrence of

25–40% (Leopold *et al.* 1989; Kurtz *et al.* 1990) when the initial disease is multi-focal or multi-centric, compared with an 11% recurrence rate when the initial tumour is uni-focal. A higher rate of inadequate/indeterminate resection margins in specimens with multiple malignant foci may account for these findings. From detailed sectioning of mastectomy specimens it is known that additional tumour foci are present in 30–63% of women mammographically suspected of having uni-focal disease and that 10–50% of multi-centric foci lie out with the index quadrant of the breast (Holland *et al.* 1985; Vaidya *et al.* 1996). Although controversy exists over the clinical importance of multi-centric foci and the clinical impact of MR-detected multi-centric foci is not known, their detection is at present still considered important (Kramer 1998; Davidson 1997; Drew 1999).

It is essential that care be exercised in the diagnosis of multi-focal disease. A preliminary report by Balen *et al.* (1997) commented on inappropriate mastectomy in up to 28% of patients. In a further report Krämer *et al.* (1998) used multiple 3D MR acquisitions obtained at 90 second intervals and demonstrated good sensitivity at 89%, but 17% of women had an incorrect diagnosis of multi-centric disease. Of note, both studies used 3D imaging at 60–90 second intervals after contrast injection, and the reduced temporal resolution may have contributed to the false-positive results.

## Clinical management

Limited reports of the role of DCE-MRI in the clinical management of patients scheduled for breast conservation surgery are available. Tan *et al.* (1999) examined 83 patients scheduled for breast conserving surgery and found management to be definitively altered in 18%, with 13% of women undergoing additional surgery. However, no factors were demonstrated, which could predict alteration in outcome from either patient or tumour characteristics, mammographic results or the timing of MRI. In a further larger study in 1999 by Fischer *et al.* (463 women with 548 cancers) management was changed in 14.3% of women owing to detection of more extensive or multi-centric disease. Of the 54 patients with multi-focal/multi-centric disease, 48% had BI-RADS overall breast composition pattern 4 and 52% pattern 3, but again no criterion for defining special subgroups of women with multi-focal or multi-centric disease seen by MR alone were detected.

The cost-effectiveness of MRI in the clinical management of primary breast cancer is still unknown and can only be answered by a randomised controlled clinical trial. The ongoing NHS R&D Health Technology Assessment funded COMICE trial will address the issues of relative accuracy rates for depicting tumour margins, by comparing the re-operation and mastectomy rates following primary excision, between those planned by conventional triple assessment and those planned by a combination of triple assessment and DCE-MRI. It also aims to examine the uncertainty surrounding identification of multi-centric disease preoperatively, determination of the risk factors for referral for MRI, the impact of MRI on clinical management and quality of life and patient satisfaction, and the medium-term ipsilateral breast tumour recurrence rate. This trial will report in 2007 and will inform those responsible for provision of future healthcare requirements.

## Lobular carcinoma

Infiltrating lobular carcinoma accounts for 5–10% of all breast cancers (Sariego 1993). As a result of the natural history of lobular breast cancer, the diagnosis and staging can be difficult. Clinical examination is characterised by ill-defined thickening or induration in the breast, and the mammographic and ultrasound appearance is frequently subtle and the extent of disease difficult to determine (Bochmann 1996; Francis 2001). Failure to stage accurately may lead to inappropriate surgery, especially when the disease is multi-focal.

The sensitivity of DCE-MRI for the detection of invasive lobular carcinoma is consistently high averaging at approximately 95% (Kneeshaw 2003; Francis 2001) and performs better than X-ray mammography, ultrasound or clinical assessment. Several recent publications have indicated improved detection of multi-focal lobular carcinoma by DCE-MRI relative to other imaging modalities. Davidson *et al.* (1997) reported improved accuracy of DCE-MRI over mammography in delineating multi-focal/multi-centric disease (86% versus 50%). In a study by Kneeshaw *et al.* (2003) DCE-MRI detected multi-focality in 100% of patients with histologically confirmed multi-focal disease. Of the eight patients in whom X-ray mammography and ultrasound failed to identify multi-focal disease, the MRI findings changed clinical management in 40%.

## Occult tumours

Recent reports also suggest that MRI may be helpful in detecting clinically and mammographically occult breast tumours. Olsen *et al.* (2000) reported on the ability of DCE-MRI to detect occult malignancy and thereby facilitate breast conserving surgery. Of the 40 women examined, MRI identified a primary tumour in 70%, of whom 95% had tumour present within the subsequent surgical specimen. Overall the results of MRI allowed preservation of the breast in 46% of women.

## Microcalcifications

Most microcalcifications within the breast are secondary to benign conditions, but approximately 20–30% of cases are due to malignant processes even when no palpable mass is detected (Kopans 1998). Clustered microcalcifications on X-ray mammography are a highly sensitive sign of ductal carcinoma *in situ* (DCIS), but the specificity ranges from 10% to only 35% (Basset 1992). Some patterns of microcalcification classified by size, shape and distribution fall into the indeterminate group, when a confident diagnosis of benign or malignant disease cannot be made. Routine management of these cases includes stereotactic biopsy, although there is a recognised failure rate of approximately 5% primarily because of lesion location relative to the patient's size and many of these cases will progress to open surgical radio-localised biopsy.

Early studies suggested that DCE-MRI could not be used to assess microcalcifications (Westerhof 1998; Gilles 1996). However, in a similar manner to invasive disease, DCIS can induce angiogenesis, and increased contrast uptake in either a focal or branching pattern has been reported. Previous MR studies have reported variable accuracy for classification of microcalcification. Westerhof *et al.* (1998), investigating mammographically suspicious microcalcifications, reported a sensitivity of 45%, specificity of 72%, a positive predictive value of 71%, negative predictive value 46% and accuracy of 56%. In a further study, Gilles *et al.* (1995) reported a sensitivity of 95%, but a specificity of only 51%. The basic method of assessing contrast uptake as either present or absent could potentially account for the low reported specificity. By contrast, Kneeshaw *et al.* (2003), in a study of 88 patients, used objectively derived empirical and pharmacokinetic parameters to compare benign and malignant microcalcifications. Using these techniques, DCE-MRI had an overall accuracy at 77.5%. When combined with morphological input as part of a radiological report, DCE-MRI was equal to X-ray mammography in terms of sensitivity (85.7%) but had a superior specificity, positive predictive value (PPV) and negative predictive value (NPV), and an overall accuracy rate of 81.7%. Moreover, when combined with the results of triple assessment using logistic regression analysis, an accuracy rate of 91% was achieved with the radiological DCE-MRI report, the empirically derived enhancement index and the results of ultrasound being important distinguishing parameters. These results would indicate a role for MRI in the management of patients in whom the results of conventional triple assessment are equivocal.

## Magnetic resonance screening

Despite the promise of MRI for detecting mammographically occult lesions, no large-scale studies are available that would validate the application in asymptomatic patients. The false negative rate of screening mammography in patients with dense breasts is not known, but cancer is less likely to be detected in these women (Bird 1992). In older women with palpable cancer, 87% are seen at mammography. In women less than 50 years of age, only 56% of malignancies are visible at mammography. Indeed, the sensitivity of screening mammography in younger women has been reported between 60 to 84% compared with 86 to 95% in older women (Tabar, 1992; Peeters, 1989).

A meta-analysis (Shapiro, 1994) of eight prospective, randomised clinical trials of mammography has shown that screened women older than 50 years have a 25–30% reduction in mortality, whereas women younger than 50 have a non-significant reduction of 10–15%. Suggested explanations for this difference in mortality have included the greater difficulty in early detection of cancer in pre-menopausal women with radio-dense breasts. The use of MRI in pre-menopausal asymptomatic women is as yet unproven. Parenchymal enhancement was most frequently seen during weeks 1 and 4 but resolved either during different phases of the same or in subsequent menstrual cycles. None of the patients underwent biopsy, the evanescent changes being ascribed to fluctuating hormone levels. Menstrual cycle-dependent changes in contrast uptake were simultaneously reported by Müller-Schimphle *et al.* (1997). Patients showed significantly less parenchymal enhancement in days 7–20 of the menstrual cycle compared with days 21–26, whereas patients in the age range 35–50 years demonstrated significantly greater enhancement than either older or younger age groups. These studies have been largely responsible for the timing of MR breast examinations in this patient group, with most centers scanning patients between days 6–16 of the menstrual cycle wherever possible.

Only by a prospective comparative study of pre-menopausal women known from either genetic testing or family history to be at genetic risk of breast cancer, will the usefulness of MR breast imaging in this age group be evaluated. A national multi-centre MRC study comparing the relative sensitivity and specificity of MRI and mammography is in progress in the UK (MARIBS) (Leach, 1997). This study comprises an initial high sensitivity screening measurement, followed by a high specificity measurement in equivocal cases, allowing a multi-parametric analysis encompassing morphometric assessment, the kinetics of contrast agent uptake and determination of quantitative pharmacokinetic parameters. It is hoped that this multi-feature analysis will provide an alternative management option for high risk women for whom prophylactic bilateral mastectomy is not desired.

## Response to treatment

Neoadjuvant systemic chemotherapy has been shown to decrease primary breast tumour size in up to 90% of patients (Kling 1997), potentially facilitating breast-conserving surgery, as well as reducing the risk of tumour dissemination during surgery (Jacquillat 1989). Its use, followed by breast conserving surgery, is the preferred means of treatment for patients with locally advanced disease at presentation. Disadvantages of this treatment, however, include cost and toxic side effects to patients, potential delays in starting effective therapy and obscuring pathological tumour staging.

In a study by Weatherall *et al.* (2001), 20 patients with breast cancer were evaluated after chemotherapy by using MRI to assess the size of cancer residua and the results compared with histological measurements of the viable tumour. The study also compared the preoperative tumour size, as determined by clinical examination and X-ray-mammography with subsequent histology. They reported an excellent correlation coefficient between tumour size as measured by MRI and histopathology at 0.93, whereas the values for clinical examination and X-ray mammography were considerably lower at 0.72 and 0.63, respectively.

Another study by Balu-Maestro *et al* (2002) also included ultrasonography in the evaluation. They found that MRI was the most reliable modality for the evaluation of tumour size post chemotherapy; MRI correctly estimated 63% of cases versus, respectively, 52, 38 and 43% for clinical examination, mammography and ultrasound. MRI also correctly identified all five cases of complete response to chemotherapy, 43/55 partial responders, 12 non-responders, and among the 32 patients who underwent mastectomy, MRI also correctly revealed multi-focal disease in 12/15 cases, whereas mammography and ultrasound were accurate in only 6/15 cases.

However, many of the newer therapies are cytostatic and measurement of tumour size or volume is an inappropriate indicator of response, and as a consequence there is a need to develop other surrogate markers of response. Hayes *et al.* (2002) examined changes in the temporal pattern of signal enhancement, the rate ($K_{trans}$) and amplitude of enhancement and the volume transfer constant of the contrast agent between the blood plasma and the extravascular extracellular space, in 15 breast cancer patients before and after the first cycle of neoadjuvant chemotherapy. Of particular note in this study was the negative correlation between pre-treatment $K_{trans}$ value and the reduction in value observed post chemotherapy.

MR spectroscopy provides a non-invasive biochemical measure of metabolism and has also been shown to assist in lesion characterisation (Cecil 2001). Malignant lesions demonstrate elevation of composite choline levels arising from increased cellular proliferation. Cecil *et al.* (2001) reported elevated choline levels in 19 of 23 confirmed cancers, and in a larger study of 100 malignant and 53 benign tumours by Katz-Brull *et al.* (2002) the detection of composite choline signal in H-1 MR spectra resulted in sensitivity and specificity values of 83 and 85%, respectively. However, in a sub-group of 20 younger patients the sensitivity and specificity values approached 100%. So far, no studies have been reported examining the role of MR spectroscopy in the assessment of treatment response, but information on cellular lipid and energy metabolism obtained from H-1 and P-31 metabolites has been examined in other solid tumours and shows promise in predicting response.

At the present time complete imaging response after neoadjuvant chemotherapy does not rule out the need for resection of the tumour bed. Microscopic tumour foci may remain and the surgical specimen gives histological information important for prognosis and management decisions, as well as reducing the risk of local recurrence.

## Conclusions

In summary, MRI shows considerable promise for improved management of patients with primary breast malignancy. The comparative and cost-effectiveness of this technique with respect to other imaging modalities is currently under evaluation, but interest will centre around alteration in surgical management, in particular reduction in the requirement for re-operation for positive resection margins; the role of MRI in assessment of microcalcification; and assessment of the efficacy of neoadjuvant chemotherapy.

## References

Abdolmaleki, P., Buadu, L.D. & Naderimansh, H. (2001). Feature extraction and classification of breast cancer on dynamic magnetic resonance imaging using artificial neural network. *Cancer Letters* **171**, 183–191.

Ando, Y., Fukatsu, H., Ishigaki, T., Endo, T. & Mikazaki, M. (1997). Evaluation of breast cancer vascularity using MR mammography. In *Proceedings of the 5th International Society of Magnetic Resonance in Medicine*, Vancouver, 12–18 April 1997, Abstract No. 1045.

Balen, F.G., Hall-Craggs, M.A., Mumtaz, H., Wilkinson, I. & Scheidau, A. (1997). MRI of invasive lobular carcinoma of the breast. In: *Proceedings of the UK Radiological Congress*, Birmingham, May 1997, p. 51.

Balu-Maestro, C., Chapellier, C., Bleuse, A., Chanalet, I., Chauvel, C. & Largiller, R. (2002). Imaging in evaluation of response to neoadjuvant breast cancer treatment benefits of MRI. *Breast Cancer Research and Treatment* **72**, 145–152.

Basset, L. W. (1992). Mammographic analysis of microcalcifications. *Radiology Clinics of North America* **30**, 93–105.

Bird, R. E., Wallace, T. W. & Yankaskas, B. C. (1992). Analysis of cancers missed at screening mammography. *Radiology* **184**, 613–617.

Bochmann, D., Bahnsen, J., Loning, T. & Bocker, W. (1996). Lobular cancer transformation of the human breast. Mammography diagnosis and clinical relevance. *Gerburtshilfe und Frauenheikunde* **56**, 204–80.

Buckley, D. L, Kerslake, R. W, Blackband, S. J. & Horsman, A. (1994). Quantitative analysis of multi-slice Gd-DTPA enhanced dynamic MR images using an automated simplex minimisation procedure. *Magnetic Resonance in Medicine* **32**, 646–651.

Cecil, K. M., Schnall, M. D., Siegelman, E. S. & Lenkinski, R. E. (2001). The evaluation of human breast lesions with magnetic resonance imaging and proton magnetic resonance spectroscopy. *Breast Cancer Research and Treatment* **68**, 45–54.

Davidson, T., Mumtaz, H., Hall-Craggs, M. A., Kissin, M. W., Thurell, W. & Taylor, I. (1997). Impact of magnetic resonance imaging in determining surgical management in breast cancer. *Breast* **6**, 177–182.

Davies, P. L., Staiger, M. J., Harris, K. B., Ganott, M. A., Klementaviciene, J., McCarthy, K. S. & Tobon, H. (1996). Breast cancer measurements with magnetic resonance imaging, ultrasonography and mammography. *Breast Cancer Research and Treatment* **37**, 1–9.

Deutch, B. M., Merchant, T. E., Schwartz, L. H., Powell, C. M., Liberman, I., Dershaw, D. D. (1993). Local staging of breast cancer by using MR imaging. [Abstract.] *Radiology* **189**(P), 301.

Drew, P. J., Chatterjee, S., Turnbull, L. W., Read, J., Carleton, P. J., Fox, J. N., Monson, J. R. T. & Kerin, M. J. (1999). Dynamic contrast enhanced magnetic resonance imaging of the breast is superior to triple assessment for the preoperative detection of multi-focal disease. *Annals of Surgical Oncology* **6**, 599–603.

Esserman, L., Hylton, N., Yassa, L. *et al.* (1999). Utility of magnetic resonance imaging in the management of breast cancer: evidence for improved preoperative staging. *Journal of Clinical Oncology* **17**, 110–119.

Fischer, U., Vosshenrich, R., Kopka, M., von Heyden, D., Oestmann, J. W. & Grabbe, E. H. (1994) Preoperative MR mammography in patients with breast cancer: impact on therapy. [Abstract.] *Radiology* **193**(P), 121.

Fischer, U., Kopka, L. & Grabbe, E. (1999). Breast carcinoma: effect of preoperative contrast-enhanced MR imaging on the therapeutic approach. *Radiology* **213**, 881–888.

Francis, A., England, D. W., Rowlands, D. C., Wadley, M., Walker, C. & Bradley, S. A. (2001). The diagnosis of invasive lobular breast cancer. Does MRI have a role? *The Breast* **10**, 38–40.

Gilles, R., Zafrani, B., Guinebretiere, J. M. *et al.* (1995). Ductal carcinoma in situ: MR imaging-histopathological correlation. *Radiology* **1996**, 415–419.

Gilles, R., Meunier, N. & Lucudarme, O. (1996). Clustered breast microcalcifications: evaluation by dynamic contrast-enhanced subtraction MRI. *Journal of Computer Assisted Tomography* **20**, 14.

Greenstein Orel, S., Schnall, M. D., Powell, C. M. *et al.* (1995). Staging of suspected breast cancer: Effect of MR imaging and MR-guided biopsy. *Radiology* **1996**, 115–122.

Gribbestad, I. S., Nilsen, G., Fjosne, H. E. *et al.* (1994). Comparative signal intensity measurements in dynamic gadolinium-enhanced MR mammography. *Journal of Magnetic Resonance Imaging* **4**, 477–480.

Hayes, C., Padhani, A. R. & Leach, M. O. (2002). Assessing changes in tumour vascular function using dynamic contrast-enhanced magnetic resonance imaging. *NMR in Biomedicine* **15**, 154–163.

Holland, R., Veling, S. H. J., Mravunav, M., Hendricks, J. H. C. L. (1985). Histological multifocality of Tis, T1-1 breast carcinomas: implications for clinical trials of breast conserving surgery. *Cancer* **56**, 979–990.

Hulka, C. A., Smith, B. L., Sgroi, D. C. *et al.* (1995). Benign and malignant breast lesions: differentiation with echo-planar MR imaging. *Radiology* **197**, 33–38.

Jacquillat, C., Weil, M., Auclerc, G. *et al.* (1989). Neoadjuvant chemotherapy in conservative breast cancer treatment: a study of 205 patients. *Bulletin du Cancer* **74**, 694.

Katz-Brull, R., Lavin, P. T. & Lenkinski, R. E. (2002). Clinical utility of proton magnetic resonance spectroscopy in characterising breast lesions. *Journal of the National Cancer Institute* **94**, 1197–1203.

Kling, K. M., Ostrzega, N., Schmitt, P. (1997). Breast conservation after induction chemotherapy for locally advanced breast cancer. *American Surgeon* **63**, 861–864.

Kneeshaw, P. J., Turnbull, L.W., Smith, A. & Drew, P. J. (2003). Dynamic contrast-enhanced magnetic resonance imaging aids the surgical management of invasive lobular breast cancer. *European Journal of Surgical Oncology* **29**, 32–37.

Kneeshaw, P. J., Lowry, M., Hubbard, A., Turnbull, L. W. & Drew, P. J. (2003). DCE-MRI is able to differentiate benign from malignant breast disease associated with screening detected microcalcifications. *Annals of Surgical Oncology* **10**, S52.

Knowles, A. J., Issa, B., Burton, S., Liney, G. P., Gibbs, P., Turnbull, L. W. (1998). Classification of benign and malignant disease by neural network analysis of dynamic imaging. *Proceedings of Radiology* **1400**, 83.

Kopans, D. B. (1998). The mammographic appearance of breast cancer. In *Breast imaging*, 2nd edn (ed. J. Ryan), pp. 375–408. 388 pages. Philadelphia and New York: Lippincott-Raven.

Krämer, S., Döinghaus, K., Schulz-Wendtland, R., Lang, N. & Bautz, W. (1997). The role of MR-mammography in the diagnosis of multicentricity in breast cancer. In *Proceedings of the UK Radiological Congress*, Birmingham, May 1997, p. 51.

Krämer, S., Schulz-Wendtland, R., Hagedorn, K., Bautz, W. & Lang, N. (1998). Magnetic resonance imaging and its role in the diagnosis of multicentric breast cancer. *Anticancer Research* **18**, 2163–2164.

Kuhl, C. K., Mielcareck, P., Klaschik, S., Leutner, C., Wardelmann, E., Gieseke, J., Schild, H. H. (1999). Dynamic breast MR imaging: are signal intensity time course data useful for differential diagnosis of enhancing lesions? *Radiology* **211**, 101–110.

Kurtz, J. M, Jacquemier, J., Amalric, R. *et al.* (1990). Breast-conserving therapy for macroscopic multiple cancers. *Annals of Surgery* **212**, 38–44.

Leach, M. (1997). National study magnetic resonance imaging to screen women at genetic risk of breast cancer. *The Lancet* **350**, 6.

Leopold, K. A., Recht, A., Schnitt, S. J. *et al.* (1989). Results of conservative surgery and radiation therapy for multiple synchronous cancers of one breast. *International Journal of Radiation Oncology, Biology, Physics* **16**, 11–16.

Liney, G. & Turnbull, L. W. (1999) Assessment of several quantitative measurements of dynamic contrast enhanced MRI in the differentiation of primary breast tumours. *Journal Diagnostic Radiography and Imaging* **2**, 81–87.

Muller-Schimpfle, M., Ohmenhauser, K., Stoll, P., Dietz, K., Clausenn, C. D. (1997). Menstrual cycle and age: Influence of parenchymal contrast medium enhancement in MR imaging of the breast. *Radiology* **203**, 145–149.

Munot, K., Dall, B., Achuthan, R., Parkin, G., Lane, S. & Horgan, K. (2002). Role of magnetic resonance imaging in the diagnosis and single-stage surgical resection of invasive lobular carcinoma of the breast. *British Journal of Surgery* **89**, 1296–1301.

Olsen, J. A., Morris, E. A., Van Zee, K. J., Lineham, D. C., Borgen, P. I. (2000). Magnetic resonance imaging facilitates breast conservation for occult breast cancer. *Annals of Surgical Oncology* **7**, 411–415.

Peeters, P. H. M., Verbeek, A. L. M., Straatman, H., Holland, R., Hendricks, J. H. C. L., Mravunac, M., Rothengatter, C., Vandijkmilatz, A. & Were, J. M. (1989). Evaluation of overdiagnosis of breast cancer in screening with mammography – results of the Nijmegen program. *International Journal of Epidemiology* **18**, 295–299.

Sariego, J., Byrd, M., Kerstein, M. & Matsumoto, T. (1993). Factors influencing survival in infiltrating lobular carcinoma of the breast. *American Surgeon* **59**,405–409.

Shahar, K. H., Solaiyappan, M. & Bluemke, D. A. (2002). Quantitative differentiation of breast lesions based on three-dimensional morphology from magnetic resonance imaging. *Journal of Computer Assisted Tomography* **25**, 1047–1053.

Shapiro, S. (1994). Screening – assessment of current studies. *Cancer* **74**, 231–238.

Tabar, L., Fagerberg, G., Duffy, S. W., Day, N. E., Gad, A. & Grontoft, O. (1992). Update of the Swedish Two-County Program of Mammographic Screening for Breast Cancer. *Radiology Clinics of North America* **30**, 187–210.

Tan, J. E., Orel, S. G., Schnall, M. D., Schultz, D. J. & Solin, L. J. (1999). Role of magnetic resonance imaging and magnetic resonance imaging-guided surgery in the evaluation of patients with early-stage breast cancer for breast conserving treatment. *American Journal of Clinical Oncology* **22**, 414–418.

Vaidya, J. S., Vyass, J. J., Chinoy, R. F., Merchant, N. H., Sharma, O. P. & Mittra, I. (1996). Multi-centricity of breast cancer: whole organ analysis and clinical implications. *British Journal of Cancer* **74**, 820–824.

Vergnaghi, D., Monti, A., Setti, E. & Musumeci, R. (2001). A use of neural network to evaluate contrast enhancement curves in breast magnetic resonance images. *Journal of Digital Imaging* **14**, 58–59.

Weatherall, P. T., Evans, G. F., Metzger, G. J., Saborrian, M. H., Leitch, A. M. (2001). MRI vs histological measurement of breast cancer following chemotherapy: Comparison with X-ray mammography and palpation. *Journal of Magnetic Resonance Imaging* **13**, 868–875.

Westerhof, J. P., Fischer, U., Moritz, J. D. & Oestmann, J. W. (1998). MR imaging of mammographically detected clustered microcalcifications: is there any value? *Radiology* **207**, 75–81.

Whitney, W. S., Herfkens, R. J., Silverman, J., Ikeda, D., Brumbaugh, J. & Jeffreys, S. (1993). Gadolinium-enhanced spectral-spatial MR imaging for evaluation of breast carcinoma. (Abstract.) *Radiology* **189**(P), 136.

Yoo, S. S., Choi, B. G., Han, J. Y. & Kim, H. H. (2002). Independent component analysis for the examination of dynamic contrast-enhanced breast magnetic resonance imaging data – preliminary study. *Investigative Radiology* **37**, 647–654.

# Chapter 5

# Early progress in breast duct micro-endoscopy

*Nicolas Beechey-Newman and Ashutosh Kothari*

## Introduction

With more than one million cases of breast cancer being diagnosed worldwide annually, breast cancer no longer remains the problem of the developed countries, but has assumed truly pandemic proportions. Although adjuvant treatment modalities such as systemic therapy yield considerable improvements in survival from breast cancer, additional measures are clearly required if the number of deaths are to be reduced substantially. Research into prevention and cure may provide the answers eventually. For the present, however, the early detection and treatment offers the best chance of significantly reducing mortality from breast cancer.

Despite the early work of Sartorius *et al.* (1977), demonstrating that the breast consists of 15–20 radially arranged lobules each opening at the nipple through a major duct, right up until the turn of the 20th century, the breast has always been considered as a solid organ. Breast duct micro-endoscopy promises a revolutionary method of breast imaging for the 21st century, which for the first time will allow the assessment of the part of the breast that is of most importance to us – the duct epithelium.

The mammary gland is an unusual organ in that most of its development takes place at puberty and subsequently through pregnancy and lactation. Almost 90% of all breast cancers are described histopathologically as invasive ductal or lobular carcinomas. It is now established that these histologically distinct breast epithelial tumour types originate from the epithelial lining of the intralobular ducts and terminal ducto-lobular units (TDLU). Almost without exception breast carcinomas express protein characteristics of ductal luminal epithelial cells. Studies into the natural history of breast cancer have revealed that the journey from the first signs of epithelial cell atypia to frank invasive malignancy may take several years. In this process of transformation, up to and including the stage of ductal carcinoma *in situ* (DCIS), the problem is confined entirely within the breast duct and is amenable to simple local surgical treatment. Once the invasive stage of cellular neoplasia is reached then the paradigm that it should be regarded as a systemic disease rather than a loco-regional entity has some truth. The histological recognition and classification of these pre-invasive states has been advanced greatly over the past two decades. However, the most significant benefits from the application of these advances may still be to come.

None of the imaging modalities available for the diagnosis of early breast cancer today give us direct access to the ductal epithelium, which is the point of origin of all breast carcinomas. Holland *et al.* (1990) demonstrated that only 50% of micro-papillary or cribriform DCIS is associated with micro-calcification, and it fails to show *in situ* malignancy in the region of the nipple in 70% of the cases. Other pre-malignant conditions such as atypical ductal hyperplasia (ADH) are rarely if ever detected by any of the existing imaging modalities. It follows therefore that an imaging technique that offers direct visualisation of the mammary ductal epithelia has the potential to provide greater accuracy in the diagnosis of benign and malignant pathology.

## Development of breast endoscopy

Endoscopic visualisation of the human mammary ductal system has been sporadically reported over the past decade. Rapid and groundbreaking developments in the field of optics have now made the previously unseen labyrinth of mammary ducts accessible to direct examination.

The technique of examining mammary ducts by endoscopes introduced through the nipple has been developing since 1991 when Okazaki *et al.* (1991) reported using a 0.45 mm fibre-optic scope to visualise the internal features of the ectatic ducts of 52 patients with a nipple discharge. Adequate visualisation was achieved in 90% of their cases. Although their scope had no working channel for biopsy or brushings, the authors removed the scope and lavaged the ductal system to obtain cytology samples. Because of the absence of an operating channel they could not perform simultaneous insufflation during the procedure. Love & Barsky (1996) have described the use of 0.4 mm endoscopes on human subjects, but encountered difficulties due to the lack of an operating channel to insufflate the duct and keep it distended during the procedure. In the same year Makita *et al.* (1991) described successful visualisation of the breast ducts in 22 patients with nipple discharge, and obtained a biopsy in 15 of these by removing the scope and sampling through the outer channel. The procedure was accomplished by using an endoscope that was very large in comparison to those that are available today. The instrument consisted of an outer cannula of 1.7 mm (16G) in diameter and a 1.25 mm non-fibre-optic scope that fitted through the centre. This design overcame the problem of not having an operating channel at the expense of a comparatively large external diameter. Berna *et al.* (1991) performed mammary duct endoscopy using a 1.9 mm neonatal cysto-urethroscope with a working channel. The scope was introduced over a guide wire through the working channel and insufflation with saline was useful in obtaining clear vision. However, they reported that because of the cumbersome size of their scope they could not visualise ducts of less than 2 mm.

Large scopes, limited optics and the inability to biopsy and insufflate have been the technical obstacles to successful mammary duct endoscopy. Technology has progressed a great deal since these early attempts, leading to the development of a new generation of micro-endoscopes with excellent optics along with the ability to visualize and insufflate/irrigate packaged into extremely small external diameters. The Depth of Field Micro-Minimally Invasive (DOFI® MMI, Acueity Inc., California, USA) consists of a 0.89 mm external diameter solid rod rigid endoscope with a 0.35 mm working channel that provides depth of perception during visualisation. Dietz *et al.* (2000) used similar older generation endoscopes of 1.2 mm diameter to successfully conduct feasibility studies on sowbelly mammary ductal systems, before proceeding to human subjects.

## Instrumentation: a new technology

### A typical micro-endoscopy system

Invariably almost all the micro-endoscopy systems available commercially today are composed of three basic components: the endoscope, the camera unit and a monitor to view the images in real-time. Although a video unit is not usually included in the package it is an essential component for maintaining individual patient records. In our experience, we have noted that the use of digital video imaging greatly enhances the quality and clarity of recorded images.

### Types of micro-endoscope

For any mammary endoscope to qualify as a 'micro-endoscope' the external diameter of the scope has to be less than 1 mm. There are various technical issues critical to the design and function of these very small endoscopes. Owing to the extremely small external diameters of the micro-endoscopes, specialized optics are necessary to carry the images from the tip of the micro-endoscope to the camera. Most systems use novel arrangements of fibre-optics. However, as the endoscopes get ever smaller the problem of pixelation becomes more troublesome, with compromise of the ultimate picture quality. More recently, solid rod technology has been incorporated into some micro-endoscopes. The advantage of these solid rod lenses is that they do not require that the image is broken up for transmission through the most narrow part of the scope and the images are therefore of higher quality with no pixelation.

Extremely small diameter scopes of down to 0.3 mm (Karlheinz Hinze Optoengineering GmbH & Co., Hamburg, Germany) external diameter are now available, but because of their very small calibre these instruments usually do not have a working channel or lavage/isufflation option. Slightly larger endocopes of 0.89 mm maximum external diameter (Acueity Inc.) have a working channel incorporated within the body of the micro-endoscope and hence allow for not only insufflation but also the possibility of obtaining ductal lavage specimens for cytology. Tissue biopsy with the help of specifically designed purpose-built micro-instrumentation negotiated through these operating channels is currently under development. The ability to take tissue samples is critical to the further development of breast duct micro-endoscopy as it enables histopathological correlation of the epithelial abnormalities that are seen.

Although the procedure is minimally invasive and does not breach any epithelial barriers it is of course still necessary to use sterile instrumentation. Not surprisingly the delicate optics of certain micro-endoscopes will not lend themselves easily to gas/chemical/heat sterilisation. Some manufacturers have therefore designed completely disposable micro-endoscopes in such a way that the sheath has its own built in fibre-optics which couple to the external camera. A separate sterilisable optical system that can be threaded through a reusable/resterilisable external sheath system is another available option.

Medical endoscopes generally are either rigid or flexible. Flexible scopes are designed to enhance manoeuvrability and in the breast to negotiate the complicated ductal system. However, considering the external size constraints required for breast endoscopy, suitable flexible scopes are extremely fragile and easily damaged. The costs of these systems are also a prohibitive factor. Rigid or semi-rigid endoscopes, on the other hand, are much cheaper to manufacture, especially if a single use design is employed. For the breast, one must remember that the tissue is soft and the breast an easily deformable organ; hence the rigidity of the scopes is not necessarily a limiting factor in negotiating the ductal tree and in practical terms seems to be a distinct advantage. The endoscope can in fact be very easily manoeuvred through the ducts and the straightening that results tends to aid visibility.

## Procedure

The patient is placed on the examination table in the supine position. The nipple is dekeratinised with alcohol and/or dekeratinising cream. Some duct orifices can be identified by the manual expression, and/or aspiration of pathological discharge. Some ducts will have copious amounts of fluid discharge, some may only have a small drop, and many ducts (often the majority) may have none at all. The ducts with no discharge are obviously the most difficult to identify and the use of magnifying loops ($\times$ 3.5) can be of limited help. The position of the orifice; for example, at the 10 o'clock position, either centrally, or peripherally, should be accurately recorded.

### Anaesthesia

For procedures done in the office or outpatient department, local anaesthesia will be the only type of anaesthetic required. For intra-operative cases, often, the patient will be heavily sedated, or even under a general anaesthetic. The description below applies to outpatients who are wide awake, with no sedation.

A nipple block with placement of 1% lidocaine without epinephrine is performed. The local anaesthetic is injected in a peri-areolar fashion in a relatively superficial plane. The amount of local anaesthetic required is usually about 10 ml.

There may be an indication for using topical anaesthesia. The Japanese and Chinese have a long experience of using topical anaesthesia as their only anaesthetic. It is possible to apply Eutectic Mixture of Local Anesthetics (EMLA) cream approximately half an hour before the procedure. The patient can be given a small amount of EMLA cream to place under an adhesive dressing before she comes to the clinic. Additional anaesthesia can be given as the procedure progresses. Occasionally, a patient will describe some discomfort as the scope is advanced. Placing 1% lidocaine through the sheath, or endoscope, will immediately provide anaesthesia to the ductal tree.

## Dilation of the nipple orifice

Once the appropriate fluid-producing orifice is identified, the diameter of the orifice needs to be increased to accommodate the scope. There are several different techniques for achieving this result.

A. The ViaDuct system has a tapered dilator as part of the apparatus. The dilator is placed through the endoscopic sheath. The dilator and sheath are then slowly advanced into the appropriate orifice. Care must be taken to not disrupt the duct as the dilator is advanced. In many cases, the dilator is sufficient to enter the duct. There is a sphincter approximately 1 cm from the skin surface. This sphincter can be quite tight and can actually go into spasm. Care should be taken to dilate this sphincter with slow advance of the dilator. Once the sheath has passed through this sphincter, further advancement of the scope will be quite easy.

B. A specially designed atraumatic mammary duct dilator has been developed. Employing this instrument it is almost impossible to perforate the duct.

C. If the dilator within the sheath is not sufficient for duct entry, graduated lacrimal duct probes can be used. Starting with the small 4-0 dilator, the size of the probes is slowly increased to the 3-0, 2-0, 0, 1 and the #2 dilator. The #2 dilator is approximately the same size as a scope. Again, care should be taken to advance the dilators quite slowly to avoid perforation of the ductal wall.

D. An alternative method to ductal access is placement of a Prolene suture; usually a 2-0 or 0 size is used. The Prolene is placed into the orifice and a #25 Angiocath is then advanced over the Prolene. The Angiocath can dilate the orifice in a gentle fashion. The size of the Angiocath is then increased to a #22 gauge and then #20 gauge size in succession. Use of the #20 gauge Angiocath will provide adequate access for placement of the scope. The type of access used will vary from patient to patient.

E. If the above methods are unsuccessful, graduated orthopedic wires can be used. They do come in graduated sizes and can be used in the same way the lacrimal duct probes are used.

## Scope preparation

After the nipple orifice has been accessed, the scope is prepared. The light cord and camera coupler are attached. The scope is then focused and white balanced. The scope should then be oriented so the operating physician knows which movement of the scope corresponds to the view on the monitor. The scope is then flushed with saline or lignocaine.

## Accessories

The surgeon should have available syringes of various sizes, lidocaine 1% without epinephrine, specimen containers for lavage and biopsy samples.

## Endoscopy

Continuous infusion of irrigant should be provided to dilate the ductal system. The usual amount of fluid is between 1 and 3 ml per minute. Saline can be used for irrigation. Alternatively, lidocaine diluted in saline can also be used.

The ductal system is evaluated visually and the scope is advanced carefully under direct vision. Many times the ductal anatomy is normal with glistening white epithelium seen. Typically, ducts that contain some type of pathology may be more dilated than normal ducts. Discharge, usually white in colour, or a particulate matter can be seen within normal ducts and may not be pathological. As the scope is advanced, bifurcations will be encountered. Keeping track of the path will enable the operator to return to the same site if pathology is seen. Additional still photos can be taken of areas of abnormal ductal lining.

## Sampling

Lavage specimens can be taken at any point during the endoscopic evaluation using the irrigation/working channel or by removing the optics from the outer sheath. A gentle suction should remove adequate fluid though this rarely more than 0.5 ml. If aspirate is not forthcoming, some irrigating solution can be placed through the side port of the scope and immediately re-aspirated. Intraluminal biopsy can be performed, though current availability of such fine forceps is restricted to research and development programmes.

## Typical findings during breast micro-endoscopy

The external openings of mammary ducts on the nipple are not as well demarcated as one would like to believe. In practice they are occasionally quite difficult to locate, as they not placed in any sort of symmetrical pattern on the nipple. Previous anatomical studies do not agree on the number of such openings that one would encounter on the nipple, but figures range from 8 to 20. The rugosity of the nipple skin makes visualisation more difficult as do the keratin plugs that usually occlude the ostia. We found that the use of magnifying surgical loops ($\times$ 3.5 magnification) did not add significantly to our pick up rate of the number of ducts orifices identified per specimen.

The first part of each duct is the lactiferous sinus, which is comparatively wide and about 1 cm in length. At its distal end (away from the nipple skin) the lactiferous sinus narrows significantly as it becomes the main duct proper and at this point there is a noticeable narrowing or sphincter which may prove difficult to negotiate particularly with larger scopes. Normal ductal epithelium was usually visualised as a pearlescent white shiny, smooth surface. In some cases flimsy adhesions partially occluded the ducts, these, however, could be broken in most instances and the scope navigated further down the duct. However, those ducts that were narrowed concentrically were very difficult to negotiate. They did not distend despite forceful insufflation and attempts to force the scope through often led to false passages. Exiting the confines of a duct or false passages were fairly easy to identify as the images changed suddenly, from the shiny smooth ductal epithelium to a cavernous honeycomb like appearance of the breast adipose tissue.

As the scope is navigated through the ductal tree bifurcations are encountered. There is no symmetry or uniformity with regards to the depth when the ducts begin to arborise. Occasionally a bifurcation is encountered as close as 2 cm from the surface and on other occasions it is possible to traverse up to 4 cm within a major duct without encountering any sub-divisions. We also regularly noted duct trifurcations but with less frequency than we encountered duct bifurcations. We have been unable to detect any sort of spatial pattern to the duct divisions or branching.

## Complications

The micro-endoscope is useful for office diagnosis, preoperative evaluation, and intra-operative surgical assistance. The most crucial point in the entire endoscopic process is the dilation of the appropriate nipple orifice without disturbing the integrity of the ductal system. If the ductal wall is traversed by the dilator or lacrimal duct probe placing the scope will result in extra-ductal placement. This is usually determined by seeing the scope within the fat tissue. The clean white glistening walls of the duct are not seen, and are instead replaced by a yellowish honeycomb or cobweb like architecture representing the loose fibro-adipose connective tissue of the breast. Another clue is that the pressure required to irrigate is noticeably less when the scope is outside the ducts. Free-flowing irrigation fluid usually means that the scope is outside the ducts and the irrigant is filling the extra-ductal breast tissue. There have been no major scope-related complications in patients throughout the past decade, even when investigators have used endoscopes of diameter up to 2 mm. Once the ductal system is entered, visual inspection, cell and tissue sampling and surgical guidance are easily accomplished.

## Results: evaluation of the technique

Although there are as yet no clinical results relating to micro-endoscopy in breast disease data relating to the efficacy of the technique per se is becoming available. In our unit preliminary pre-clinical studies to explore the efficacy of breast duct micro-endoscopy were carried out on *ex vivo* mastectomy specimens. In one sample a total of 35 mastectomy specimens were assessed. The micro-endoscopic examination was conducted by the same two trained investigators on each occasion. The median age of the cohort was 55.5 years (range 32–83 years). None of the patients had overt pathological nipple discharge indicating that mostly normal calibre ducts were evaluated. Twenty-nine mastectomies were performed for primary carcinoma, two for a locally advanced breast cancer, two for DCIS and two were prophylactic mastectomies.

Cannulation of the ductal system with the endoscope was achieved in all the 35 specimens. A total of 115 ducts were cannulated in all, the median number of ducts per specimen being three (range one to eight). For this investigation we have defined the first 2 cm of the mammary ducts as the 'proximal ducts'. Visualisation of the proximal duct only was achieved in 12/35 (34%), whereas distal navigation beyond 2 cm was achieved in 23/35 (66%) of specimens. Imaging of the duct system deeper than 5 cm was possible in 18/115 ducts (16%). False passages were created in 16% of duct examinations and in all these cases further attempts at negotiating that duct were abandoned.

Abnormalities of the mammary ducts were seen in 40% of breast specimens examined. Detailed morphological/pathological correlation of these abnormalities is technically difficult if it is to be done accurately, but is vital if duct micro-endoscopy is to be useful for the diagnosis of malignant disease. Accurate marker studies have been developed to address this problem and are currently underway. In the meantime a morphological classification of duct abnormalities has been established. This divides visible abnormalities into three categories: papillomatous lesions, obstructing lesions and epithelial surface abnormalities. Papillomatous lesions may be defined as single or multiple discreet, rounded lesions adherent to the duct wall at only one point of its circumference and allowing the passage of the micro-endoscope passed the lesion. Obstructing lesions fill the duct lumen sufficient to prevent further passage of the scope and appear adherent to the duct wall at more than one point or circumferentially. Epithelial surface changes are defined as an irregular alteration of the duct wall in either colour or surface texture and allowing free passage of the micro-endoscope.

## Indications

In these very early days of breast duct micro-endoscopy there are few definite and no proven indications for the technique. Duct endoscopy was first devised to investigate nipple discharge. Preliminary studies have shown that duct micro-endoscopy is an effective way to identify duct papillomas and the technique is used clinically for this in a few centres around the world. Duct micro-endoscopy is particularly effective in patients with single-duct discharge. The discharging duct is always pathologically ectatic, making cannulation and visualisation of the duct rewarding. Most duct papillomas that cause nipple discharge are located within 3–4 cm of the nipple and are readily seen shortly after entering the duct and usually before any duct divisions have occurred. Although it is not yet possible to remove a papilloma from within the duct by using the micro-endoscope, the exact location of the lesion is indicated by transillumination through the skin from the tip of the micro-endoscope. This facilitates an open papillectomy through a small well-placed incision with minimal damage to adjacent ducts.

All other indications for duct micro-endoscopy are at present either the subject of current experimentation or are wholly speculative. The technique has been included as part of a large American trial investigating the efficacy of nipple discharge cytology. Patients with abnormal discharge cytology undergo duct micro-endoscopy in addition, but because this is an observational trial only with no further surgical intervention, the vital correlation with the underlying histology is unlikely to be known for most of the patients taking part in the study. Further reports from the USA have described the use of micro-endoscopy to ensure adequate surgical margins during tumourectomy for invasive malignancy. The micro-endoscope is advanced along the principal duct that drains from the area of the cancer. This is facilitated by the observation that careful expression can usually produce at least a little discharge from a duct system that is affected by tumour. Examination of this duct gives a clear visual indication of unsuspected disease away from the main palpable tumour and can help the surgeon to carry out the tumourectomy with adequate margins of excision.

Work at Guy's Hospital, London, is looking at the application of micro-endoscopy to assess the extent of DCIS before definitive surgery. The aim of the procedure is to measure the extent of the disease, multifocality/multicentricity, and the presence of associated epithelial change such as atypical ductal hyperplasia (ADH). The meticulous histopathological surveys of Holland *et al.* (1990) have shown how frequently DCIS is underestimated by mammography, and in particular how often the changes extend to the nipple. Results from this work indicated that 70% of changes close to the nipple are mammographically occult. It is hoped that breast micro-endoscopy will provide additional pre-operative information about the extent of DCIS and may also indicate in which patients the nipple can be safely preserved. The information will enable the most appropriate surgical technique (mastectomy or wide local excision) to be recommended for each patient.

One of the greatest hopes for the future is that duct micro-endoscopy will provide a means of screening patients at high risk of developing breast cancer. This may include women with proven gene mutations, women with a strong family history of breast cancer, and patients who have already had breast cancer on one side and are at a 4–5 times relative risk of developing contra-lateral malignancy. The aim of breast micro-endoscopy in all these instances should be to recognise pre-invasive breast duct epithelial change, allow for its accurate characterisation and facilitate therapy at this stage so that invasive breast cancer is avoided. In some cases immediate therapy may not be necessary and a repeat examination after six months or a year may be all that is required. Although several trials have been set-up to address this indication, proof of efficacy will take a long time to establish.

Other indications for micro-endoscopy include the investigation of suspicious lesions found by using conventional imaging but for which standard biopsy techniques have have been inconclusive. Currently it is not possible to guide an endoscope to a predetermined area of the breast but preliminary research in our unit has suggested ways in which this may be achieved.

## Future technical developments

With the realisation that breast duct micro-endoscopy may have a useful role, increasing technological effort has been applied to making the procedure easier and more effective. Current work could be described as employing first-generation instruments, but there seems little doubt that the technology, which seems new to us now, can be greatly improved in years to come if the technique continues to look promising.

The micro-endoscopes that are currently being evaluated for breast use are a little under 1 mm in external diameter. At this size the investigation of pathologically ectatic duct is simple, but ducts of normal calibre present more of a problem. There is little doubt that smaller micro-endoscopes would greatly facilitate the visualisation of normal calibre ducts and would enable the endoscopist to effectively assess the important minor duct tributaries, which are currently unseen. Work is already advanced on producing micro-endoscopes of 0.5 mm or less. These instruments have comparatively larger working channels than first generation instruments, though the optical resolution has yet to be assessed. Nonetheless, to achieve these smaller scopes the optics have continued to improve, with the result that image resolution is likely to be further enhanced.

Intra-luminal tissue biopsy is vital if breast micro-endoscopy is to be used to assess malignant disease. Prototype accessories capable of passing down the working channel without first removing the optics are soon to be commercially available. Cytology brushes are also required to improve the currently poor cell yield associated with duct lavage.

## Conclusion

Although breast endoscopy has been possible for more than a decade it is only over the past three years that the technique has started to attract serious interest. The advent of significant advances in optics and endoscope design has for the first time made possible medical grade micro-endoscopes with an external diameter of less than 1 mm. These instruments have an operating channel for insufflation and biopsy, and an optical resolution that makes the detailed examination of the morphology of the epithelial surface of the mammary ducts a reality. It has been clearly demonstrated that not only ectatic ducts but ducts of normal calibre can be examined. The procedure is minimally invasive and can be performed under local anaesthetic. Perforation of the duct occurs in around 15% of ducts examined but there are no adverse sequelae associated with this and the procedure has proven to be free of any significant complications.

Breast duct micro-endoscopy is at its earliest stage of evaluation and as such its place in the clinical diagnosis and treatment of both benign and malignant breast disease can only be guessed at. Small series have already demonstrated how micro-endoscopy can be used to identify and guide the surgery for duct papillomas. Epithelial abnormalities of various types have been noted in patients with malignancy but further work is required to characterise these epithelial changes and relate them to accepted histopathological criteria.

## *References*

Berna, J. D., Garcia-Medina, V. & Kunni, C. C. (1991). Ductoscopy: a new technique for ductal exploration. *European Journal of Radiology* **12**, 127–129.

Dietz, J. R., Kim, J. A., Malycky, J. L., Levy, L. & Crowe, J. (2000). Feasibility and technical considerations of mammary ductoscopy in human mastectomy specimens. *The Breast Journal* **6**, 161–165.

Holland, R, Hendriks, J., Verbeek, A., Mravunac, M. & Schuurmanns Stekhoven, J. (1990). Extent, distribution, and mammographic/histological correlations of breast ductal carcinoma in situ. *The Lancet* **335**, 519–522.

Love, S. M. & Barsky, S. H. (1996). Breast-duct endoscopy to study stages of cancerous breast disease. *The Lancet* **348**, 997–999.

Makita, M., Sakatomo, G., Akiyama, F. *et al.* (1991). Duct endoscopy and endoscopic biopsy in the evaluation of nipple discharge. *Japanese Journal of Breast Cancer Research and Treatment* **18**, 179–188.

Okazaki, A., Okazaki, M., Asaishi, K. *et al.* (1991). Fibreoptic ductoscopy of the breast: a new diagnostic procedure for nipple discharge. *Japanese Journal of Clinical Oncology* **21**, 188–196.

Sartorius, O., Morris, P., Benedict, D. *et al.* (1977). Contrast ductography for recognition and localisation of benign and malignant breast lesions: an improved technique. In *Breast carcinoma: the radiologist's expanded role* (ed. W. Logan), pp. 281–300. New York: Wiley.

# Chapter 6

# Should needle core biopsy replace fine-needle aspiration cytology of the breast?

*Andrew H. S. Lee, Sarah E. Pinder, Ian O. Ellis and Christopher W. Elston*

The ability to obtain a preoperative diagnosis has had a major impact on the management of breast disease. Traditionally, a clinical abnormality was managed by a diagnostic surgical biopsy. Either a frozen section was performed, followed by definitive surgery if the result was malignant, or the biopsy was reported routinely with definitive surgery at a later date if necessary. From the late 1980s, soon after the introduction of the UK National Health Service Breast Screening Programme, fine-needle aspiration cytology (FNAC) was the favoured method of non-operative diagnosis. More recently, after the introduction of improved automated core biopsy devices, core biopsy has become the sampling method of choice in many units including our own. In this chapter the reasons for this change, and the benefits and disadvantages associated with it are discussed.

The aims of non-operative diagnosis are: (1) for patients with breast cancer to undergo only one surgical procedure; (2) to facilitate counselling of patients; (3) to reduce the number of diagnostic surgical biopsies for benign breast disease; and (4) to allow improved planning of operating lists and bed occupancy. To achieve this the pathologist needs to be able to: (1) diagnose malignancy reliably, (2) distinguish invasive and *in situ* carcinoma, (3) make definite benign diagnoses, and (4) explain clinical and radiological abnormalities including calcification.

## Technique of performing FNAC and core biopsy

FNAC is quick to perform and cheap. The only equipment required is a venepuncture needle (gauge 22 or finer), a syringe and slides. Skill is required to sample the lesion, and to spread the aspirate on to the slide well. The slides are stained with Giemsa, Papanicolaou or, less commonly, with haematoxylin and eosin. Experienced aspirators performing a sufficiently large number of procedures have higher success rates with fewer inadequate specimens (Dixon *et al.* 1984; Brown and Coghill 1991; Snead *et al.* 1997). Regular audit and feedback are important in maintaining low inadequate rates (Snead *et al.* 1997). Skill and experience are also important in achieving high standards of reporting for FNAC specimens. Immediate reporting is possible, with a result available in about 20 minutes if the pathologist is present in the clinic. Other factors that influence the success of FNAC include the size and the cellularity of the lesion (Barrows *et al.* 1986; Brown and Coghill 1991), and the number of passes of the needle (Pennes *et al.* 1990). The most frequent complications are haematomas, which can largely be prevented by firm pressure after withdrawing the needle, and fainting. Pneumothorax is very rare. Seeding of carcinoma cells along the needle track is described, but of uncertain significance.

Needle core biopsy can be readily performed by clinicians and can easily be reported in most pathology laboratories. A core of tissue 1–2 cm long and 1–3 mm in width is produced. Specimens are fixed and processed, and paraffin sections cut and stained with haematoxylin and eosin. Spring-loaded needle biopsy devices are easier to use, associated with less patient discomfort, achieve a higher sampling success rate and produce better quality specimens than manual devices (McMahon *et al.* 1992). Compared with FNAC, core biopsy is more expensive and takes longer to perform, and the report is usually not available until the next day. Both methods, however, are cheaper, quicker and easier for the patient than open surgical biopsy. As with FNAC, the accuracy of core biopsy increases with larger numbers of samples (Liberman *et al.* 1994b; Rich *et al.* 1999). Both FNAC and core biopsy can be used freehand or with ultrasonographic or stereotactic guidance. Haematoma is more frequent after core biopsy than FNAC, but is usually not clinically significant. As with FNAC, fainting, pneumothorax and seeding of tumour cells can occur. It is possible to remove all of a lesion, particularly calcification, with core biopsy. This problem can be overcome by insertion of a clip (currently possible only with the mammotome), which can guide any further procedures.

The major difference between FNAC and core biopsy is the extra architectural information provided by core biopsy. FNAC yields individual cells and small groups of cells, so that only the cytological features can be examined. In core biopsy a sample of tissue is obtained, so that the interrelationship of the epithelium, myoepithelial cells, basement membrane and stroma can be assessed, in addition to the cytological features. Thus more diagnostic information can be obtained from core biopsy.

Five diagnostic categories are recommended for reporting FNAC and core biopsy specimens (Non-operative diagnosis subgroup, 2001) (Table 6.1). Categories 3–5 are similar for the two methods. Categories 1 and 2 are not equivalent for the two methods. FNAC cannot distinguish normal from benign epithelium, so both are grouped together as C2. With core biopsy, however, it is possible to separate normal (B1) and benign changes (B2). Some fine needle aspirations (FNAs) are inadequate (C1), most commonly because there are too few epithelial cell groups for assessment.

## Diagnosis of malignancy

### Symptomatic patients

With skilled aspirators and pathologists, FNAC of palpable lesions can achieve excellent results. In one large series the absolute sensitivity rate was 88%, complete sensitivity rate 91%, specificity 89%, false-negative rate 3.6% and false-positive rate

**Table 6.1** Diagnostic categories for fine-needle aspiration cytology and needle core biopsy of the breast

| *Fine-needle aspiration cytology* | *Needle core biopsy* |
| --- | --- |
| C1 Inadequate | B1 Normal |
| C2 Benign | B2 Benign |
| C3 Atypia probably benign | B3 Lesion of uncertain malignant potential |
| C4 Suspicious of malignancy | B4 Suspicious of malignancy |
| C5 Malignant | B5 Malignant |

0.2%, with a positive predictive value of a malignant diagnosis of 99.8% (Zajdela *et al.* 1975) – see Table 6.2 for definitions. In most studies the complete sensitivity rate is over 80%, but it can be as low as 65% or as high as 98% (Giard and Hermans 1992). The reported range of specificity for benign lesions is also wide. For palpable lesions, the absolute and complete sensitivities for detecting carcinoma are similar for FNAC and core biopsy. Ballo and Sneige (1996) found similar absolute sensitivity rates for FNAC (92%) and core (90%), but higher complete sensitivity rate for FNAC (97% vs 90%). Poole *et al.* (1996) found that the sensitivity for FNAC (absolute sensitivity rate 80%, complete sensitivity rate 85%) was lower than for core biopsy (absolute and complete sensitivity rates of 88%). Combining the two methods gave even better results (absolute sensitivity rate 97%, complete sensitivity rate 100%). Cheung *et al.* (1987) had very similar results for FNAC and core biopsy.

The positive predictive value of a malignant diagnosis is high for both techniques. False-positive results are uncommon with FNAC (< 1%), and even less common with core biopsy. FNAC has lower sensitivity for certain types of carcinoma such as invasive lobular and tubular carcinoma and ductal carcinoma *in situ* (DCIS) (Lamb and Anderson 1989; Brown and Coghill 1991; Ciatto *et al.* 1993), which can be explained by low cellularity or the low degree of pleomorphism making definite diagnosis difficult. There is a higher chance of a 'suspicious' diagnosis in these tumour types (Bondeson and Lindholm 1990; Deb *et al.* 2001). The diagnosis of invasive lobular carcinoma is easier on core biopsy (Sadler *et al.* 1994). One study found that, in patients with an initial inadequate FNAC, subsequent core biopsy provided useful information in 90%, but only 45% of repeat FNACs did so (Carty *et al.* 1994). The sensitivity for a definite diagnosis of carcinoma was also much higher with core biopsy than repeat FNAC (89% vs 10%).

A literature review of ultrasonically guided FNAC and core biopsy found that absolute sensitivity was less with FNAC (83%) compared with core (97%), although the complete sensitivities were similar (95% and 98%) (Britton 1999). The specificity was lower for FNAC (84% vs 99%). The inadequate rate in cancer was a little higher with FNAC (2% vs 0%).

**Table 6.2** Definitions of quality assurance standards

| | |
|---|---|
| Absolute sensitivity | The number of carcinomas diagnosed as C5 or B5, expressed as a proportion of the total number of carcinomas sampled. It is assumed that all lesions called C5/B5, but which are not excised, are carcinomas |
| Complete sensitivity | The number of carcinomas diagnosed as C5/B5, C4/B4 or C3/B3 expressed as a proportion of the total number of carcinomas sampled |
| Specificity (full) | The number of correctly identified benign lesions (the number of C2/B2 results minus the number of false negatives) expressed as a proportion of the total number of benign lesions sampled. It is assumed that lesions that are diagnosed as C3/B3, but which are not excised, are benign |
| Positive predictive value of a C5/B5 diagnosis | The number of correctly identified cancers (number of C5 or B5 results minus the number of false-positive results) expressed as a percentage of the total number of positive results (C5 or B5) |
| False-negative case | A case that subsequently turns out (over the next 3 years) to be carcinoma having had a negative cytology or core result. (This will by necessity include some patients where a different area from the lesion was sampled but who turn up with an interval cancer) |
| False-positive case | A case that was given a C5 or B5 result which turns out at open surgery to be a benign lesion (including atypical hyperplasia) |
| False-negative rate | The number of false-negative results expressed as a percentage of the total number of carcinomas sampled |
| False-positive rate | The number of false-positive results expressed as a percentage of the total number of carcinomas sampled |
| Miss rate in cancer | The total of B1 or B2 cores (or C1 or C2 FNACs) in patients who are later shown to have cancer as a percentage of the total number of carcinomas sampled |

Core biopsy clearly outperforms FNAC for stereotactic procedures (Britton 1999). The absolute sensitivity (90% vs 62%), complete sensitivity (95% vs 83%) and specificity (98% vs 87%) were all better for core biopsy. The inadequate rate in cancer was higher with FNAC (5% vs 1.5%).

## Screening patients

A survey of the results of FNAC and core biopsy in the NHS Breast Screening Programme (NHSBSP) was performed for the year 1996–1997 (Britton and McCann 1999). At this time, most of the procedures were FNAC (77%) rather than core. The median results of this survey are shown in Tables 6.3 and 6.4. The absolute sensitivity was much higher for core biopsy, although the complete sensitivities were similar for the two methods. The specificity of core biopsy was also much higher. The positive predictive value of a malignant diagnosis and the false-positive rate were similar for both methods. The false-negative rate was higher for core biopsy. The inadequate rate from cancers was a little higher for FNA. A definite benign or malignant result was more likely with core (85%) than with FNAC (62%). An earlier survey of FNAC in the NHSBSP found that many units were not achieving the guidelines. A common problem was low sensitivity combined with a high false-negative rate and a high inadequate rate from lesions that were subsequently found to be cancer (Wells *et al.* 1999). The authors suggested that this was the result of problems with accurate localisation of lesions for aspiration. In our early experience with core biopsy, combining FNA and core biopsy in screening assessment improved the rate of diagnosis of carcinoma (87%) compared with FNA alone (61%) or core biopsy alone (74%) (Litherland *et al.* 1996). The increase in sensitivity was particularly marked for DCIS. Preliminary results from a NHSBSP survey for 1995–1999 (Non-operative diagnosis subgroup, 2001) show similar results to the 1996–1997 survey (Tables 6.3 and 6.4). More recent results from Nottingham are also included in Tables 6.3 and 6.4; for core biopsy the sensitivity and specificity are higher, and the inadequate rate from cancers is lower compared with FNAC. Others have described similar results (Shannon *et al.* 2000). It is possible to achieve a preoperative diagnosis rate for cancer in screening patients well above the guideline of 70% with almost exclusive use of core biopsy. The overall figure in Nottingham for 1999–2000 was 89%, with rates of 95% for invasive carcinoma and 74% for DCIS.

## Distinction of invasive and *in situ* carcinoma

The distinction between *in situ* and invasive carcinoma is important because staging of the axilla is appropriate for invasive carcinoma, but not for pure DCIS. FNAC cannot distinguish *in situ* from invasive carcinoma. Some features, such as stromal fragments and tubular structures, are seen more in invasive carcinoma than in *in situ* carcinoma (Sneige 1998), but a definitive distinction using features of the aspirate is not possible. With core biopsy, the positive predictive value of a diagnosis of invasion is virtually 100%, but about 20% of patients with a diagnosis of DCIS on core will have invasion in the subsequent surgical resection specimen (Jackman *et al.* 1994; Liberman *et al.* 1995; Meyer *et al.* 1999).

The majority of lesions are diagnosed as inadequate (C1), benign (C2) or malignant (C5) with FNAC, or as normal (B1), benign (B2) or malignant (B5) with core biopsy.

**Table 6.3** Fine-needle aspiration cytology in assessment of screening patients

| | NHSBSP minimum standards 1993[a] | NHSBSP minimum standards 2001[b] | NHSBSP preferred standards 2001[b] | NHSBSP survey 1996–1997[c] | NHSBSP survey 1995–1999[b] | NCH 1996–1999 |
|---|---|---|---|---|---|---|
| Absolute sensitivity (%) | > 60 | > 60 | > 70 | 54 | 57 | 68 |
| Complete sensitivity (%) | > 80 | > 80 | > 90 | 82 | 81 | 81 |
| Specificity (full) (%) | > 60 | > 55 | > 65 | 58 | 58 | 50 |
| Positive predictive value of C5 (%) | > 95 | > 98 | > 99 | 100 | 99.6 | 100 |
| False negative (%) | < 5 | < 6 | < 4 | 6 | 6 | 7 |
| False positive (%) | < 1 | < 1 | < 0.5 | 0 | 0.2 | 0 |
| Inadequate rate from cancers (%) | – | < 10 | < 5 | 11 | 10 | 12 |
| Miss rate (C1 + C2) from cancers (%) | – | – | – | – | – | 19 |
| Suspicious rate (%) | < 20 | < 20 | < 15 | Approx. 15 | 16 | 8 |

NHSBSP, National Health Service breast screening programme; NCH, Nottingham City Hospital.
[a]Cytology sub-group of the National Coordinating Committee for Breast Cancer Screening pathology (1993).
[b]Non-operative diagnosis subgroup of the National Coordinating Committee for Breast Cancer Screening pathology (2001).
[c]Britton and McCann (1999). Median values are given for the two surveys.

**Table 6.4** Core biopsy in screening patients

| | NHSBSP minimum standard 2001[a] | NHSBSP preferred standard 2001[a] | NHSBSP survey 1996–1997[b] | NHSBSP survey 1995–1999[a] | NCH 1999–2000 |
|---|---|---|---|---|---|
| Absolute sensitivity (%) | > 70 | > 80 | 75 | 76 | 90 |
| Complete sensitivity (%) | > 80 | > 90 | 77 | 84 | 97 |
| Specificity (full) (%) | > 75 | > 85 | 84 | 81 | 93 |
| Positive predictive value of B5 (%) | > 99 | > 99.5 | 100 | 100 | 100 |
| False positive (%) | < 0.5 | < 0.1 | 0 | 0 | 0 |
| Miss rate (B1 + B2 ) from cancer (%) | < 15 | < 10 | | 15 | 7 |
| Suspicious rate (%) | < 10 | < 5 | Approx. 4 | 5 | 7 |

NHSBSP, National Health Service breast screening programme; NCH, Nottingham City Hospital.
[a]Non-operative diagnosis subgroup of the National Coordinating Committee for Breast Cancer Screening pathology (2001).
[b]Britton and McCann (1999). Median values are given for the two surveys.

However, for a small proportion of lesions, borderline categories need to be used. C3 is used for aspirates that have predominantly benign features, but also show nuclear pleomorphism or discohesion, so that malignancy cannot be excluded. C4 (suspicious of malignancy) is used when there are cells with malignant features, but the specimen is scanty, poorly prepared or poorly preserved, or the atypical cells are mixed with numerous benign cells, or the atypia is insufficient for a definite diagnosis of malignancy. The B3 category consists of lesions that appear benign, but can show heterogeneity, or lesions associated with an increased risk of malignancy. Radial scars, some atypical intra-acinar epithelial proliferations and papillary lesions are included in this group. B4 is used for biopsies with atypical cells suggestive of carcinoma, but poor preservation or insufficient sampling of the abnormality prevents a definite diagnosis of malignancy. In Nottingham we use these borderline categories in about 8% of FNAs (C3: 3.6%; C4: 3.9%), with subsequent biopsy showing malignancy in 32% of C3 lesions and 81% of C4 lesions undergoing surgical biopsy (Deb *et al.* 2001). The frequency of B3 and B4 reports with core biopsy is a little lower (B3: 3.1%, B4: 1.1%) (Lee *et al.* 2003). The positive predictive values are 26% for a B3 diagnosis and 86% for a B4 diagnosis. Patients with a 'borderline' diagnosis need multidisciplinary discussion. Most will need further investigation; either a repeat core biopsy or a diagnostic surgical biopsy. Definitive therapeutic surgery should not be performed on the basis of a C3 or C4 FNAC result or B3 or B4 core biopsy diagnosis.

## Assessment of calcification

FNAC and core biopsy have an important role in the assessment of mammographically detected calcification, with the aim of explaining the calcification. The assessment of calcification in a core biopsy is quite sophisticated. The core specimen radiograph shows whether the calcification has been sampled (Liberman *et al.* 1994a). This should be compared with the mammogram to ensure that it is representative of the lesion of interest. Histological calcification is then sought, and any associated pathology identified. Comparison of the size and appearance of the radiological and histological calcification is then undertaken. Thus, there is a clear sequence of evidence from the calcification on the mammogram to the histological changes associated with the calcification. The sensitivity for diagnosing malignancy associated with calcification is less than for malignancy that presents as a mass lesion on mammography (Liberman *et al.* 1994b; Rich *et al.* 1999). The sensitivity increases with increasing numbers of flecks of calcification in the core samples (Bagnall *et al.* 2000). In contrast with core biopsy, calcification is rarely seen in FNAC, so there is less certainty that the correct area has been sampled. If the cytology is malignant, and this is in keeping with the other components of the triple assessment, a confident diagnosis can be made. However, there is less certainty with a benign cytological diagnosis of an area of calcification.

## Definite benign diagnosis

FNA cannot reliably distinguish normal breast tissue from most benign lesions, so definite benign diagnoses are generally difficult, and there is an element of uncertainty whether a lesion has been sampled. With core biopsy, the extra architectural information seen in the histological section often enables definite diagnosis of benign lesions such as fibroadenomas. This greater certainty of diagnosis gives more confidence when a lesion is not excised.

## Immunohistochemistry

Immunohistochemistry is much easier to perform on core biopsies than FNAC. It is possible to carry out immunohistochemistry on FNAC specimens, but extra slides need to be made at the time of aspiration and immediately fixed. With core biopsy, it is easy to cut more sections for further stains. Immunohistochemical staining for oestrogen receptor is possible with both FNAs (Weintraub *et al.* 1987) and core biopsies (Jacobs *et al.* 1998). There is good agreement between oestrogen receptor status on either FNAC or core biopsy and surgical excision specimens (Weintraub *et al.* 1987; Jacobs *et al.* 1998). Most diagnoses are based on routinely stained aspirates or sections, but immunohistochemistry is useful in certain diagnostic situations. Cytokeratins can confirm the suspicion of paucicellular invasive lobular carcinoma or show epithelial differentiation in a spindle cell carcinoma. Stains for myoepithelial cells and basement membrane can be useful for distinguishing invasive and *in situ* carcinoma, and tubular carcinomas from sclerosing lesions. Lymphocyte markers are useful in the diagnosis of lymphomas.

## Prognostic factors

Histological grading and typing of carcinomas are easier on core biopsy, because of the extra architectural information seen in the histological section. Histological grade is based on three features (Elston and Ellis 1991). Nuclear pleomorphism can be assessed on both FNAC and core biopsy, but tubule formation and mitoses can be assessed more accurately on core biopsy (Wallgren *et al.* 1976; Howell *et al.* 1994). Core biopsy grade agrees with that of the resection specimen in about 70–80% of tumours (Di Loreto *et al.* 1996; Harris *et al.* 2003; Sharifi *et al.* 1999), with a tendency to undergrade on core as a result of underestimation of the mitotic count. Grading is possible on FNAC but largely relies on nuclear features (size, pleomorphism and presence of nucleoli), with some methods including cellular cohesion. The accuracy of cytological grading (about 50–60%) is less than that on core biopsy (Hunt *et al.* 1990; Howell *et al.* 1994; Robinson *et al.* 1994). Although histological typing is possible with FNAC, e.g. mucinous carcinoma can be recognised by the combination of malignant cells and extracellular mucin, more types can be recognised with core biopsy, because of the additional architectural information. Vascular invasion cannot be recognised on FNAC, and is rarely seen on core biopsy compared with the resection specimen.

The advantages of core biopsy (Table 6.5) have led many breast units, including ours, to assess most lesions using this method. One difficulty with this is that in a small number of patients core biopsy is either contraindicated or may be difficult: (1) lesion near chest wall; (2) patient on anticoagulation; (3) very small lesion (< 3 mm); (4) lesion near vessel; (5) lesion near implant; (6) very dense breasts; or (7) urgent result required. If core biopsy is not possible, either FNA or surgical biopsy has to be performed. One approach is to abandon FNAC (Britton *et al.* 1997) and perform more diagnostic surgical biopsies.

**Table 6.5** Comparison of FNAC and core biopsy in the assessment of breast lesions

| | |
|---|---|
| Diagnosis of malignancy | |
|     Symptomatic patients | Both methods good |
|     Screening | Core better |
| Distinction of invasive and *in situ* carcinoma | Possible with core, but not with FNAC |
| Making definite benign diagnosis | Easier with core |
| Assessment of calcification | Core better |
| Immunohistochemistry | Easier with core |
| Procedure | FNAC quicker |
| Speed of result | FNAC quicker |
| Reporting specimen | FNAC requires specialist training |
| Carcinoma grading and typing | More accurate with core |
| Cost | FNAC cheaper |
| Complications | Low for both |

An alternative approach is to continue to use FNAC in a smaller number of patients. Since the introduction of automated core biopsy in our unit, there has been a dramatic decrease in the number of FNAC specimens from 2400 in 1995 to 400 in the year 2000. The proportion of inadequate FNACs has increased from 31% in 1995 to 54% in the year 2000. This results partly from the different lesions now being aspirated; in 1995 24% of lesions aspirated were clinically or radiologically malignant compared with 13% in 2000. It is also recognised that inadequate rates are higher in aspirators who perform a smaller number of FNAs (Snead *et al.* 1997). Another problem with low numbers of FNAs is maintaining the competence of the pathologist. Since 1995 the number of FNAs reported as malignant in Nottingham has dropped from about 400 to 40 per year. By comparison the number of core biopsies is now about 2000 per year with about 600 malignant diagnoses. For the UK National Health Service cervical screening programme, there are minimum numbers of slides that need to be seen in a laboratory and by individual screeners and individual pathologists

(Quality assurance guidelines for the cervical screening programme. 1996). We have found that our confidence is reduced as we are reporting smaller numbers of breast FNAs. Our strategy is to have a low threshold for obtaining a second opinion from a colleague. Double reporting would be an alternative approach. The reduction in the number of FNAs has particular implications for trainee histopathologists, who may have difficulty reaching the level of experience and expertise that those working in the early years of the NHSBSP achieved.

## Triple approach

It is important to remember that both FNAC and core biopsy have limitations, and that both provide less information than excision biopsy. A major factor is the skill with which the lesion of interest is localised and sampled; just over half our core biopsies are taken using ultrasonographic (45%) or stereotactic (10%) guidance. Even with the 'gold standard' of open surgical biopsy, it is possible to miss the lesion (Jackman and Marzoni 1997). The results of FNAC and core biopsy must be considered in combination with the clinical and radiological findings, ideally in the context of multidisciplinary meetings. Using FNAC, this triple approach improves the overall sensitivity and specificity of assessment of both palpable (Thomas *et al.* 1978; Dixon *et al.* 1984; Di Pietro *et al.* 1987) and impalpable lesions (Lamb *et al.* 1987; Azavedo *et al.* 1989). It is important that, as with FNAC, needle core biopsy is performed as part of triple assessment, rather than with the intention of achieving a definitive diagnosis, even though this is possible in most cases. In Nottingham every patient undergoing FNAC or core biopsy is given a clinical category (Table 6.6), based on the clinical and radiological features (Ellis *et al.* 1993), which is written on the specifically designed non-operative specimen request card.

## Conclusions

Both FNAC and needle core biopsy have good sensitivity for the diagnosis of malignancy in symptomatic patients. In screening patients the absolute sensitivity for carcinoma and specificity are higher for core. The distinction between *in situ* and invasive carcinoma cannot be made with FNAC, but is possible in most core specimens. FNAC cannot reliably distinguish normal breast tissue from benign lesions, whereas the architectural information provided by core biopsy often enables definite diagnosis of benign lesions. The assessment of calcification is more sophisticated using core biopsy. Immunohistochemistry and assessment of prognostic factors are more easily performed on core biopsy.

The advantages of core biopsy have led many breast units, including ours, to assess most lesions using this method. In a small number of patients core biopsy is either contraindicated or may be difficult, so that either FNAC or surgical biopsy has to be performed. A problem with infrequent use of FNAC is maintenance of competence of both the aspirator and the pathologist. Neither FNAC nor core biopsy

**Table 6.6** Clinical and radiological diagnostic patient categories

| | |
|---|---|
| Category A | A lesion that is clinically or radiologically malignant or suspicious of malignancy. Surgical excision of the lesion is required, with the core biopsy or FNA directing whether the surgery is therapeutic or diagnostic |
| Category B | A lesion that is clinically or radiologically likely to be benign. To avoid surgery, the core biopsy must provide a benign diagnosis that explains the clinical and radiological features, or the FNA show an adequate population of benign epithelial cells |
| Category C | Clinical examination and imaging show an abnormality that is almost certainly benign. Multidisciplinary discussion is required for patients with B3, B4, B5, C3, C4 or C5 result. An inadequate FNAC is acceptable for lesions in this group |
| Category D | Follow-up of patient with malignant disease |

If there is a discrepancy between the clinical and radiological category the worse category is used, so that a lesion that is category B clinically and category A on imaging would be called category A.

is perfect. It is essential that the results of both techniques are assessed in the light of the clinical and imaging findings, ideally in the context of multidisciplinary meetings.

## *References*

Azavedo, E., Svane, G., Auer, G. (1989). Stereotactic fine-needle biopsy in 2594 mammographically detected non-palpable lesions. *The Lancet* **i**, 1033–1036.

Bagnall, M. J. C., Evans, A. J., Wilson, A. R. M., Burrell, H., Pinder, S. E., Ellis, I. O. (2000). When have mammographic calcifications been adequately sampled at needle core biopsy? *Clinical Radiology* **55**, 548–553.

Ballo, M. S., Sneige, N. (1996). Can core needle biopsy replace fine-needle aspiration cytology in the diagnosis of palpable breast carcinoma. *Cancer* **78**, 773–777.

Barrows, G. H., Anderson, T. J., Lamb, J. L., Dixon, J. M. (1986). Fine-needle aspiration of breast cancer. Relationship of clinical factors to cytology results in 689 primary malignancies. *Cancer* **58**, 1493–1498.

Bondeson, L., Lindholm, K. (1990). Aspiration cytology of tubular breast carcinoma. *Acta Cytologica* **34**, 15–20.

Britton, P. D. (1999). Fine needle aspiration or core biopsy. *The Breast* **8**, 1–4.

Britton, P. D., McCann, J. (1999). Needle biopsy in the NHS Breast Screening Programme 1996/97: how much and how accurate? *The Breast* **8**, 5–11.

Britton, P. D., Flower, C. D. R., Freeman, A. H. *et al.* (1997). Changing to core biopsy in an NHS breast screening unit. *Clinical Radiology* **52**, 764–767.

Brown, L. A., Coghill, S. B. (1991). Fine needle aspiration cytology of the breast: factors affecting sensitivity. *Cytopathology* **2**, 67–74.

Carty, N. J., Ravichandran, D., Carter, C., Mudan, S., Royle, G. T., Taylor, I. (1994). Randomized comparison of fine-needle aspiration cytology and Biopty-Cut needle biopsy after unsatisfactory initial cytology of discrete breast lesions. *British Journal of Surgery* **81**, 1313–1314.

Cheung, P. S., Yan, K. W., Alagaratnam, T. T. (1987). The complimentary role of fine needle aspiration cytology and Tru-cut biopsy in the management of breast masses. *Australian and New Zealand Journal of Surgery* **57**, 615–620.

Ciatto, S., Cariaggi, P., Bulgaresi, P., Confortini, M., Bonardi, R. (1993). Fine needle aspiration cytology of the breast: review of 9533 consecutive cases. *The Breast* **2**, 87–90.

Cytology Sub-Group of the National Co-ordinating Committee for Breast Screening Pathology (1992). *Guidelines for Cytology Procedures and Reporting in Breast Cancer Screening.* Sheffield: NHSBSP Screening Publications.

Deb, R. A., Matthews, P., Elston, C. W., Ellis, I. O., Pinder, S. E. (2001). An audit of 'equivocal' (C3) and 'suspicious' (C4) categories in fine needle aspiration cytology of the breast. *Cytopathology* **12**, 219–226.

Di Loreto, C., Puglisi, F., Rimondi, G. *et al.* (1996). Large core biopsy for diagnostic and prognostic evaluation of invasive breast carcinomas. *European Journal of Cancer* **32A**, 1693–1700.

Di Pietro, S., Fariselli, G., Bandieramonte, G. *et al.* (1987). Diagnostic efficacy of the clinical–radiological–cytological triad in solid breast lumps: results of a second prospective study on 631 patients. *European Journal of Surgical Oncology* **13**, 335–340.

Dixon, J. M., Anderson, T. J., Lamb, J., Nixon, S. J., Forrest, A. P. M. (1984). Fine needle aspiration cytology, in relationships to clinical examination and mammography in the diagnosis of a solid breast mass. *British Journal of Surgery* **71**, 593–596.

Ellis, I. O., Galea, M. H., Locker, A. *et al.* (1993). Early experience in breast cancer screening: emphasis on development of protocols for triple assessment. *The Breast* **2**, 148–153.

Elston, C. W., Ellis, I. O. (1991). Pathological prognostic factors in breast cancer. I. The value of histological grade in breast cancer: experience from a large study with long-term follow-up. *Histopathology* **19**, 403–410.

Giard, R. W. M., Hermans, J. (1992). The value of aspiration cytologic examination of the breast. *Cancer* **69**, 2104–2110.

Harris, G. C., Denley, H. E., Pinder, S. E. *et al.* (2003). Correlation of histologic prognostic factors in core biopsies and therapeutic excisions of invasive breast carcinoma. *American Journal of Surgical Pathology* **27**, 11–15.

Howell, L. P., Gandour-Edwards, R., O'Sullivan, D. (1994). Application of the Scarff–Bloom–Richardson tumor grading system to fine-needle aspirates of the breast. *American Journal of Clinical Pathology* **101**, 262–265.

Hunt, C. M., Ellis, I. O., Elston, C. W., Locker, A., Pearson, D., Blamey, R. W. (1990). Cytological grading of breast carcinoma – a feasible proposition? *Cytopathology* **1**, 287–295.

Jackman, R. J., Marzoni, F. A. (1997). Needle-localized breast biopsy: why do we fail? *Radiology* **204**, 677–684.

Jackman, R. J., Nowels, K. W., Shepard, M. J., Finkelstein, S. I., Marzoni, F. A. (1994). Stereotaxic large-core needle biopsy of 450 nonpalpable breast lesions with surgical correlation in lesions with cancer or atypical hyperplasia. *Radiology* **193**, 91–95.

Jacobs, T. W., Siziopikou, K. P., Prioleau, J. E. *et al.* (1998). Do prognostic marker studies on core needle biopsy specimens of breast carcinoma accurately reflect the marker status of the tumour? *Modern Pathology* **11**, 259–264.

Lamb, J., Anderson, T. J. (1989). Influence of cancer histology on the success of fine needle aspiration of the breast. *Journal of Clinical Pathology* **42**, 733–735.

Lamb, J., Anderson, T. J., Dixon, M. J., Levack, P. A. (1987). Role of fine needle aspiration cytology in breast cancer screening. *Journal of Clinical Pathology* **40**, 705–709.

Lee, A. H. S., Denley, H. E., Pinder, S. E. *et al.* (2003). Excision biopsy findings in patients with breast core biopsies reported as suspicious of malignancy (B4) or lesion of uncertain malignant potential (B3). *Histopathology* in press.

Liberman, L., Evans, W. P., Dershaw, D. D. *et al.* (1994a). Radiography of microcalcifications in stereotaxic mammary core biopsy specimens. *Radiology* **190**, 223–225.

Liberman, L., Dershaw, D. D., Rosen, P. P., Abramson, A. F., Deutch, B. M., Hann, L. E. (1994b). Stereotaxic 14-gauge breast biopsy: how many core biopsy specimens are needed? *Radiology* **192**, 793–5.

Liberman, L., Dershaw, D. D., Rosen, P. P. *et al.* (1995). Stereotactic core biopsy of breast carcinoma: accuracy at predicting invasion. *Radiology* **194**, 379–381.

Litherland, J. C., Evans, A. J., Wilson, A. R. M. *et al.* (1996). The impact of core-biopsy on pre-operative diagnosis rate of screen detected breast cancer. *Clinical Radiology* **51**, 562–565.

McMahon, A. J., Lutfy A. M., Matthew, A. *et al.* (1992). Needle core biopsy of the breast with a spring-loaded device. *British Journal of Surgery* **79**, 1042–5.

Meyer, J. E., Smith, D. N., Lester, S. C. *et al.* (1999). Large-core needle biopsy of nonpalpable breast lesions. *Journal of the American Medical Association* **281**, 1638–1641.

Non-operative diagnosis subgroup of the National Coordinating Committee for Breast Cancer Screening Pathology (2001). *Guidelines for Non-operative Diagnostic Procedures and Reporting in Breast Cancer Screening.* Sheffield: NHSBSP.

Pennes, D. R, Naylor, B., Rebner, M. (1990). Fine needle aspiration biopsy of the breast. Influence of the number of passes and the sample size on the diagnostic yield. *Acta Cytologica* **34**, 673–676.

Poole, G. H., Willsher, P. C., Pinder, S. E., Robertson, J. F. R., Elston, C. W., Blamey, R. W. (1996). Diagnosis of breast cancer with core-biopsy and fine needle aspiration cytology. *Australian and New Zealand Journal of Surgery* **66**, 592–594.

Quality assurance guidelines for the cervical screening programme (1996). Report of a working party convened by the NHS Cervical Screening Programme and chaired by Dr John Pritchard. Sheffield: NHSCSP Publications.

Rich, P. M., Michell, M. J., Humphreys, S., Howes, G. P., Nunnerley, H. B. (1999). Stereotactic 14G core biopsy on non-palpable breast cancer: what is the relationship between number of core samples taken and the sensitivity for detection of malignancy? *Clinical Radiology* **54**, 384–389.

Robinson, I. A., McKee, G., Nicholson, A. *et al.* (1994). Prognostic value of cytological grading of fine needle aspirates from breast carcinomas. *The Lancet* **343**, 947–949.

Sadler, G. P., McGee, S., Dallimore, N. S. *et al.* (1994). Role of fine-needle aspiration cytology and needle-core biopsy in the diagnosis of lobular carcinoma of the breast. *British Journal of Surgery* **81**, 1315–1317.

Shannon, J., Douglas-Jones, A. G., Dallimore, N. S. (2001). Conversion to core biopsy in preoperative diagnosis of breast lesions: is it justified by results? *Journal of Clinical Pathology* **54**, 762–765.

Sharifi, S., Peterson, M. K., Baum, J. K., Raza, S., Schnitt, S. J. (1999). Assessment of pathologic prognostic factors in breast core needle biopsies. *Modern Pathology* **12**, 941–945.

Snead, D. R. J., Vryenhoef, P., Pinder, S. E. *et al.* (1997). Routine audit of breast fine needle aspiration (FNA) cytology specimens and aspirator inadequate rates. *Cytopathology* **8**, 236–247.

Sneige, N. (1998). Is a diagnosis of infiltrating versus in situ ductal carcinoma of breast possible on fine-needle aspiration specimens? *Cancer* **84**, 186–191.

Thomas, J. M., Fitzharris, B. M., Redding, W. H. *et al.* (1978). Clinical examination, xeromammography, and fine-needle aspiration cytology in diagnosis of breast tumours. *British Medical Journal* **ii**, 1139–1141.

Wallgren, A., Silfversward, C., Zajicek, J. (1976). Evaluation of needle aspirates and tissue sections as prognostic factors in mammary carcinoma. *Acta Cytologica* **20**, 313–318.

Wells, C. A., Perera, R., White, F. E., Domizio, P. (1999). Fine needle aspiration cytology in the UK breast screening programme: a national audit of results. *The Breast* **8**, 261–266.

Weintraub, J., Weintraub, D., Redard, M., Vassilakos, P. (1987). Evaluation of estrogen receptors by immunocytochemistry on fine-needle aspiration biopsy specimens from breast tumours. *Cancer* **60**, 1163–1172.

Zajdela, A., Ghossein, N. A., Pilleron, J. P., Ennuyer, A. (1975). The value of aspiration cytology in the diagnosis of breast cancer: experience at the Fondation Curie. *Cancer* **35**, 499–506.

# Chapter 7

# Biopsy of the breast: technical approaches and the advent of HER2 and EGFR immunohistochemistry and a look into the near future

*Andrew M. Hanby and Valerie Speirs*

## Introduction

As we move further into the 21st century the place of the histopathologist in the diagnosis, determination of treatment and as a pivotal player in the development of new therapies for breast cancer is surprisingly secure. With the cracking of the human genome the optimists may have felt that knowledge of the genome alone may be enough to tackle disease and arguably render histopathological analysis redundant. Happily, such predictions seem premature. As a result now, there are as many, if not more, histopathological challenges in the analysis of breast cancer. These manifest as changes in the spectrum and quality of material received, in the form of novel imaging techniques and approaches to obtaining a biopsy. They also include the reliable assessment of molecular markers of predictive value, such as HER2, the anticipation of new targets and the problems we may face in measuring these. Finally there is the grail of a better breast cancer taxonomy and the ability to predict outcome and direct therapy with more precision.

## The impact of new imaging technologies on breast carcinoma pathology: what is here now and what might be coming

The mainstay of breast imaging remains ultrasonography and mammography. The most prevalent theme of change is in the nature of the diagnostic material removed, with a gradual move away from fine-needle aspiration cytology (FNAC) to core biopsies (Denley *et al.* 2001). The core biopsy not only allows for the confident delineation of *in situ* from invasive in malignant samples, but also the ability to return to the material to examine for the expression of predictive markers; immunohistochemistry can be used upon cytological preparations, but material is inevitably limited (Denley *et al.* 2001). The ability to reach a successful diagnosis has been considerably augmented by the introduction of several new biopsy techniques able to take larger samples.

## The mammotome

The most widely available of these new biopsy systems is the mammotome, which is able to retrieve large samples, even remove whole fibroadenomas, without breast mutilation (Fine *et al.* 2002). This equipment is of significant benefit in certain defined circumstances where a definitive result may avoid expensive surgery. Unfortunately, clear sight of the global financial benefits can be lost where the cost of the expensive needles is borne by radiology and the savings made in the surgery departments. For the pathologist, the larger samples can be of considerable benefit in analysing certain lesions, but the removal of larger lesions imposes a significant increase in workload and the attempted removal of malignant lesions is highly risky because analysis of resection margins and tumour size is rendered impossible.

## Magnetic resonance imaging

Advances in other imaging strategies may also help defined lesions that are poorly seen using conventional strategies. Notable among these is magnetic resonance imaging (MRI), whose utility in the imaging of covert lesions is increasingly documented (Drew *et al.* 1999). Pre-eminent among covert malignant lesions are lobular carcinomas, which can often be poorly defined in extent, or even invisible to mammography and ultrasonography but more obvious by MRI (Munot *et al.* 2002). The ability of MRI to detect and define the extent of breast carcinomas and evaluate its cost-effectiveness is being tested formally in the COMICE trial. This study includes the evaluation of the pathology of lesions imaged during the trial and it seems reasonable to speculate that there might be enhanced delineation of invasive lobular carcinoma as previous studies have already shown (Munot *et al.* 2002). MRI-guided biopsies (Kinkel & Vlastos 2001) are increasingly available in the UK. However, their use may be hampered by a general lack of overall MRI capacity.

## Breast duct endoscopy

The ability to look directly into the breast ducts through the nipple is interesting and is being pioneered in several centres, particularly for the investigation of nipple symptoms (Yamamoto *et al.* 2001; Dooley 2002). It remains to be seen whether this technique will gain wide acceptance in the clinic. However, not only might it impact on the spectrum of biopsied lesions, but it could also help us identify what the truly 'early' lesions in breast cancer really are. It is, however, very early days for this technique.

All of these technologies have the ability to impact on the spectrum of disease seen in the breast pathology laboratory and to increase the quality and quantity of material available to be examined further for the expression of predictive markers.

# Predictive markers

## Oestrogen receptor

Whereas prognosis is focused on relating knowledge of clinicopathological criteria to likely survival outcome, prediction is all about determining the likelihood of tumour response to certain specific therapies based on the assessment of expressed molecular markers.

Although the concept of targeted therapies appears 'trendy', the specific targeting of the oestrogen receptor (ER), the paradigm of this approach, has been in existence for a long time. In the early years of tamoxifen use ER levels were determined by ligand-binding assays, but often treatment was given regardless of the result. This assay was limited because it relied on fresh tissue the composition of which was not always known; furthermore, the receptor was prone to degradation if the tissue was not handled carefully. With the introduction of robust antibodies able to localise the receptor in fixed tissues, the evaluation of ER status moved from the biochemistry to the histopathology laboratory (Barnes & Millis 1995).

The history of the introduction of widespread ER testing includes important lessons that are necessary to be learnt so as to develop accurate processes for the analysis of new predictive markers. The most significant was revealed in a paper detailing an analysis of the results of the UK NEQAS-ICC scheme, which audits the quality of immunohistochemistry in laboratories around in the UK and 25 other countries. The authors found a significant level of understaining in weak positive tumours, with only 37% of laboratories detecting this appropriately and approximately one-third of laboratories failing to register any staining at all (Rhodes *et al.* 2000). Because it is recognised that tamoxifen has had a major impact on survival in breast cancers, it is reasonable to propose that these false-negative results would have had real impact on patient prospects.

Any predictive marker needs to be assessed by a laboratory with rigourous practice and the results assessed by a pathologist who is not only able to identify the tumour but who also can see the warning signs of a poor technical result. Appropriate controls should be included, both positive which should be positive and negative which should be negative. Because of the idiosyncrasies of individual sections, effort should also be made to find positive internal controls; usually some benign breast epithelium is included in the sample and this should include some positive nuclei. Many laboratories also stain for progesterone receptor, a molecule whose gene expression is upregulated by ER, and thus whose expression can act as a surrogate marker of ER function (Ravdin *et al.* 1992). Less frequently, other molecules whose genes contain an oestrogen response element (ERE) are used in a similar fashion, for example TFF1, previously known as pS2 (Prest *et al.* 2002).

## HER2/c-erbB2

This molecule is a member of the EGFR/type 2 tyrosine kinase growth factor receptor family. Unlike the other members of its family, it has no known specific ligand and is believed to act through the formation of heterodimers with other members of the group.

Its functions in normal are disparate and in mice have been shown to include induction of differentiation and regulation of lactation (Jones & Stern 1999). In some breast cancers over-expression of the molecule occurs almost always as a result of amplification of the gene on chromosome arm 17q (Berger *et al.* 1988). This amplification is seen in tumours that typically are high grade and is observed in between 80% and 90% of Paget's disease of the nipple (Lammie *et al.* 1989; Kothari *et al.* 2002), an observation that may relate to this gene's ability to induce motility and epidermotropism (Schelfhout *et al.* 2000). Although over-expression of HER2 has correlated with poor survival, multivariate analysis shows that its assessment gives no additional information over and above established indicators of breast cancer prognosis, tumour size, grade and nodal status. The last observation possibly results from the existence of an aggressive population of HER2-negative high-grade invasive carcinomas (Barnes *et al.* 1992). However, this generalisation may not extend to very selected populations and for certain comparisons; for example, in a recent Finnish study HER2 amplification was superior to ER as a prognostic factor in small (less than 5 mm) well-differentiated, node-negative primary breast cancers (Joensuu *et al.* 2003).

The importance of the assessment of the expression of this molecule has changed dramatically with the introduction of trastuzumab (Herceptin), a humanised version of a monoclonal antibody to HER2. This agent has been able to induce significant tumour responses in cohorts of patients who have failed first- and second-line chemotherapy (Cobleigh *et al.* 1999), usually in combination with other agents such as taxols (Norton *et al.* 1999). Most responses have occurred in patients who show high levels of surface expression of the molecule (3+) and/or demonstrable gene amplification by fluorescent *in situ* hybridisation (FISH), some of which may only be 2+ by immunohistochemistry. Targeting to the right patients is important; set against the proven benefits for the right patients is cardiotoxicity for some, particularly when combined with doxorubicin (Slamon *et al.* 2001), and the high cost of the agent. Thus demonstration of HER2 over-expression is essential before treatment.

As appropriate targeting is essential and given the lessons from the ER experience, a cautious approach is advised in instigating laboratory testing. The range of antibodies that bind to HER2 is wide (Press *et al.* 1994), as is the diversity of methodology (Allred & Swanson 2000) and these vary in efficacy, with only a subset having the appropriate mix of sensitivity and specificity to be useful reagents/approaches (Press *et al.* 1994). Pathologists can opt to use a validated 'off the shelf' antibody which needs to be appropriately titrated or, alternatively, use a kit such as the Herceptest whose reagent quality and concentrations are tightly controlled to give a potentially greater level of reliability, but at a financial cost. Interestingly, although this test has a high degree of specificity, its sensitivity has been questioned (Allred & Swanson 2000). The assessment of HER2 is a further level of difficulty above ER. For the latter, the principal question is: is the tumour positive or not? For HER2 it is more complex: is the tumour positive at the 3+ levels or 2+ with proven gene amplification? HER2 is normally expressed on the surface of epithelial cells and inadequate titration will reveal this; thus a non-amplified tumour may be scored 3+; however, 3+ staining of co-existent benign epithelium will act as a clue to inappropriate positivity. Illustrations of the scoring patterns and their definitions can be found on the Dako website at http://wwwdakousa.com.herinfo/hctsumm.htm. Occasionally, cytoplasmic or even nuclear staining will be detected, but should be ignored for scoring purposes (Press *et al.* 1994). There are also some interesting quirks to be aware of. For example, some benign apocrine lesions over-express HER2 without associated amplification of the gene (Selim *et al.* 2002). Other histology clues may alert the pathologist to an inappropriate result. For example, a 3+ immunohistochemical test as evidence of amplification would be unusual in a tubular carcinoma; equally, a negatively stained slide displaying Paget's disease of the nipple should also alert the pathologist to a potential false-negative result.

Our practice is to use two antibodies. New batches are used to stain cases with known HER2 copy numbers by FISH and titrated such that known 0, 1, 2 and 3+ cases stain appropriately. Cell lines with known copy number and staining levels can also be used for this (Koeppen *et al.* 2001), and these are used by the UK NEQAS-ICC scheme to assess laboratory performance in this regard. All batches of routine work contain a positive (3+) control and both test and control slides are dated so they can be matched. Close attention is paid to the histological context and if this appears odd, the two antibodies give disparate results or the level of staining is 2+, the sample is subjected to FISH testing.

As can be seen from this overview, the testing for HER2 as a predictive marker is not completely straightforward and given the implications of the results, not to be performed lightly. Until now, most laboratories have been able to avail themselves of central facility testing at one of the UK reference centres; with the instigation of charges it is clear that several additional laboratories in the UK will take on this testing, some offering a centrally funded regional service. It is recommended that such work needs to be done under tight standard operating procedures (SOPs), in laboratories performing at least 250 tests a year (Roche *et al.* 2002) and according to national guidelines. All laboratories performing these tests should participate in a recognised quality assurance scheme, which in the UK is represented by UK NEQAS-ICC. Important guidelines for testing for HER2 in the UK have been published (Ellis *et al.* 2002).

## EGFR

At least two drugs able to target EGFR-1, the prototypic member of its family are in the early stages of trialling (Baselga & Hammond 2002). Early work on these drugs, gefitinib (Iressa) and erlotinib (Tarceva), has focused on non-small-cell lung cancer. Some breast cancer is known to over-express, without gene amplification, EGFR-1 and treatment of these tumours using these new agents is currently the subject of several new trials. Clearly, consideration needs to be given to whether and how this molecule is assessed. EGFR-1, like the other members of the family, is expressed on the cell surface and can be localised by immunohistochemical techniques. So far, it seems the levels of expression do not correlate with likelihood of response, not surprising given the complexities of interactions of these agents with other members of the family (Normanno *et al.* 2003). Thus, at the moment, there is no evidence to support regular testing for the expression of EGFR-1 as a predictive marker of response to these new drugs. This does not mean that this will remain the case and in the meantime the search goes on for good antibodies able to work in formalin-fixed, paraffin-embedded tissues, the commonest and most available manifestation of archived pathological material.

## Other potential predictive markers

The determination of a predictive marker depends on its expression levels being indicative of probable or possible response to a specific agent. Any molecule that is differentially over-expressed in a tumour compared with benign tissues has the potential to be used as a target which novel agents can be developed against; therefore the list of potential predictive markers is enormous. Targeted therapies hold the key to cancer cure, and pathology has an important role to play in identifying molecules that are important in this context. For example, c-kit has recently been observed to be over-expressed in malignant phyllodes tumours (Sawyer *et al.* 2002). Over-expression of c-kit associated with activating mutations is seen in gastrointestinal stromal tumours, which as a consequence respond to the c-kit targeting drug imatinib (Glivec) (Miettinen *et al.* 2002). Whether malignant phyllodes tumours respond remains speculative, particularly because mutations cannot be demonstrated; nevertheless this is one of many examples of potential novel target molecules that ultimately pathologists may have to test for.

## The future of breast cancer taxonomy: how will we recognise different treatment groups?

Research into the biology and pathology of breast cancer is enormously confounded by the diversity of the group of diseases it represents. The taxonomy we currently use has been arrived at in a 'hit-and-miss' fashion, over a prolonged period of time and is almost wholly based on the correlation of morphology and clinical outcomes data. The wide range of morphologies observed is matched by both diverse clinical behaviour and by similarly diverse cytogenetic/molecular changes. We do know that certain specific types of breast carcinoma, for example lobular (Berx *et al.* 1996) and mucinous carcinomas (O'Connell *et al.* 1998), are underpinned by specific molecular abnormalities, which can conceivably explain their biology. By extrapolation it may be inferred that some of the less molecularly defined but distinct morphologies seen in the broad mass of breast carcinomas may also be telling us something: 'if they look different, then perhaps they *are* different'. Because there may be wide biological differences in different breast cancer types, it is important to delineate these. The molecular signature of these groups may include determinants of response to different treatment strategies, and therefore it is important to recognise the 'response taxonomy'. The current taxonomy of breast cancer, although good, is not perfect. Notably, approximately 75% of breast carcinomas are ductal carcinomas of no special type (NST), and yet closer examination reveals clear differences within this group. For example, the results of cytogenetic studies indicate that grade I tumours are more similar to lobular carcinomas than the rest than to higher-grade ductal carcinomas (Nishizaki *et al.* 1997; Roylance *et al.* 1999) and that progression of grade I to grade III tumours is likely to be rare (Roylance *et al.* 1999). Thus, grade is as much a determinant of tumour type as an indicator of a clone of malignancy. It follows that cohorts investigating the expression of molecular markers should have enough samples of each tumour grade to be able to study the expression of the marker and its relationship to outcome within the grade groups as well as between them. Within-grade studies can reveal useful, otherwise hidden data. For example, E-cadherin expression was found to be positively correlated with poor outcome, contrary to the results from smaller pan-grade studies (Gillett *et al.* 2001; Lynch *et al.* 2002).

## The future

The quest for new markers and their analysis in large patient cohorts has been considerably accelerated by cDNA arrays which can, and have, analysed large numbers of gene expression levels (Sorlie *et al.* 2001), some potential targets that then can be localised immunohistochemically or by *in situ* hybridisation on tissue microarrays. These methods will be further augmented by the increasing introduction of proteomic array technology. Whether these approaches will make conventional morphological analysis redundant remains to be seen (Yeatman 2003). However, these array methods have already demonstrated considerable prognostic power (Vijver *et al.* 2002). The vast amount of data is subject to bioinformatics/AI analysis, which conceivably could include morphological data. In this way distinct clusters with distinct morphologies and different drug-response profiles might be defined, so allowing histopathological triage of tumours into different groups which then may be subject to more focused costly analysis. This is, of course, purely speculative and the results of further studies which will specifically test such possibilities are awaited with great interest.

## References

Allred, D. C. & Swanson, P. E. (2000). Testing for erbB-2 by immunohistochemistry in breast cancer. *American Journal of Clinical Pathology* **113**, 171–175.

Barnes, D. M., Bartkova, J., Camplejohn, R. S., Gullick, W. J., Smith, P. J. & Millis, R. R. (1992). Overexpression of the c-erbB-2 oncoprotein: why does this occur more frequently in ductal carcinoma in situ than ininvasive mammary carcinoma and is this of prognostic significance? *European Journal of Cancer* **28**, 644–648.

Barnes, D. M. & Millis, R. R. (1995). In *Progress in pathology*, vol. 2 (ed. N. Kirkham, & N. R. Lemoine), pp. 89–114. Churchill Livingstone.

Baselga, J. & Hammond, L. A. (2002). HER-targeted tyrosine-kinase inhibitors. *Oncology* **63**(Suppl.) **1**, 6–16.

Berger, M. S., Locher, W., Saurer, S., Gullick, W. J., Waterfield, M. D., Groner, B. & Hynes, N. E. (1988). Correlation of c-erbB-2 gene amplification and protein expression in human breast carcinoma with nodal status and nuclear grading. *Cancer Research* **48**, 1238–1243.

Berx, G., Cleton-Jansen, A. M., Strumane, K., Leeuw, W. J. F. d., Nollet, F., Roy, F. v. & Cornelisse, C. (1996). E-cadherin is inactivated in a majority of invasive human lobular breast cancers by truncation mutations throughout its extracellular domain. *Oncogene* **13**, 1919–1925.

Cobleigh, M. A., Vogel, C. L., Tripathy, D., Robert, N. J., Scholl, S., Fehrenbacher, L., Wolter, J. M., Paton, V., Shak, S., Lieberman, G. & Slamon, D. J. (1999). Multinational study of the efficacy and safety of humanized anti-HER2 monoclonal antibody in women who haveHER2-overexpressing metastatic breast cancer that has progressed after chemotherapy for metastatic disease. *Journal of Clinical Oncology* **17**, 2639–2648.

Denley, H., Pinder, S. E., Elston, C., Lee, A. & Ellis, I. (2001). Preoperative assessment of prognostic factors in breast cancer. *Journal of Clinical Pathology* **54**, 20–24.

Dooley, W. C. (2002). Routine operative breast endoscopy during lumpectomy. *Annals of Surgical Oncology* **9**, 920–923.

Drew, P. J., Chatterjee, S., Turnbull, L. W., Read, J., Carleton, P., Fox, J. N., Monson, J. R. & Kerin, M. J. (1999). Dynamic contrast enhanced magnetic resonance imaging of the breast is superior to triple assessment for the pre-operative detection of multifocal breast cancer. *Annals of Surgical Oncology* **6**, 599–603.

Ellis, I. O., Bartlett, J., Dowsett, M., Humphries, S., Jasani, B., Miller, K., Pinder, S. E., Rhodes, A. & Walker, R. (2004). Best Practice No 176: Updated recommendations for HER2 testing in the UK. *Journal of Clinical Pathology* **57**(3), 233–237.

Fine, R., Boyd, B., Whitworth, P., Kim, J., Harness, J. & Burak, W. E. (2002). Percutaneous removal of benign breast masses using a vacuum-assisted hand-held device with ultrasound guidance. *American Journal of Surgery* **184**, 332–336.

Gillett, C. E., Miles, D. W., Ryder, K., Skilton, D., Liebman, R. D., Springall, R. J., Barnes, D. M. & Hanby, A. M. (2001). Retention of the expression of E-cadherin and catenins is associated with shorter survival in grade III ductal carcinoma of the breast. *Journal of Pathology*, **193**, 433–441.

Joensuu, H., Isola, J., Lundin, M., Salminen, T., Holli, K., Kataja, V., Pylkkanen, L., Turpeenniemi-Hujanen, T., Smitten, K. V. & Lundin, J. (2003). Amplification of erbB2 and erbB2 expression are superior to estrogen receptor status as risk factors for distant recurrence in pT1N0M0 breast cancer: a nationwide population-based study. *Clinical Cancer Research* **9**, 923–930.

Jones, F. E. & Stern, D. F. (1999). Expression of dominant-negative ErbB2 in the mammary gland of transgenic mice reveals a role in lobuloalveolar development and lactation. *Oncogene* **18**, 3481–3490.

Kinkel, K. & Vlastos, G. (2001). MR imaging: breast cancer staging and screening. *Seminars in Surgical Oncology* **20**, 187–196.

Koeppen, H. K. W., Wright, B. D., Burt, A. D., Quirke, P., Mcnicol, A. M., Dybdal, N. O., Sliwkowski, M. X. & Hillan, K. J. (2001). Overexpression of HER2/neu in solid tumours: an immunohistochemical survey. *Histopathology* **38**, 96–104.

Kothari, A. S., Beechey-Newman, N., Hamed, H., Fentiman, I. S., D'Arrigo, C., Hanby, A. M. & Ryder, K. (2002). Paget disease of the nipple: a multifocal manifestation of higher-risk disease. *Cancer* **95**, 1–7.

Lammie, G. A., Barnes, D. M., Millis, R. R. & Gullick, W. H. (1989). An immunohistochemical study of the presence of c-erbB-2 protein in Paget's disease of the nipple. *Histopathology* **15**, 505–514.

Lynch, J., Pattekar, R., Barnes, D. M., Hanby, A. M., Camplejohn, R. S., Ryder, K. & Gillett, C. E. (2002). Mitotic counts provide additional prognostic information in grade II mammary carcinoma. *Journal of Pathology* **196**, 275–279.

Miettinen, M., Majidi, M. & Lasota, J. (2002). Pathology and diagnostic criteria of gastrointestinal stromal tumors (GISTs): a review. *European Journal of Cancer* **38**, S39–S51.

Munot, K., Dall, B., Achuthan, R., Parkin, G., Lane, S. & Horgan, K. (2002). Role of magnetic resonance imaging in the diagnosis and single-stage surgical resection of invasive lobular carcinoma of the breast. *British Journal of Surgery* **89**, 1296–1301.

Nishizaki, T., DeVries, S., Chew, K. 3rd, Ljung, B. M., Thor, A. & Waldman, F. M. (1997). Genetic alterations in primary breast cancers and their metastases: direct comparison using modified comparative genomic hybridization. *Genes, Chromosomes and Cancer* **19**, 267–272.

Normanno, N., Maiello, M. R. & Luca, A. D. (2003). Epidermal growth factor receptor tyrosine kinase inhibitors (EGFR-TKIs): simple drugs with a complex mechanism of action? *Journal of Cellular Physiology* **194**, 13–19.

Norton, L., Slamon, D., Leyland-Jones, B. Wolter, J., Fleming, T., Eirmann, W., Baselga, J., Mendelsohn, J., Bajamonde, A., Ash, M. & Shak, S. (1999). Overall survival (OS) advantage to simultaneous chemotherapy (CRx) plus the humanized anti-HER2 monoclonal antibody herceptin (H) in HER2-overexpressing (HER2+) metastatic breast cancer. *Proceedings of the American Society of Clinical Oncology* **18**, abstract 483.

O'Connell, J. T., Shao, Z., Drori, E., Basbaum, C. B. & Barsky, S. H. (1998). Altered mucin expression is a field change that accompanies mucinous (colloid) breast carcinoma histogenesis. *Human Pathology* **29**, 1517–1523.

Press, M. F., Hung, G., Godolphin, W. & Slamon, D. J. (1994). Sensitivity of HER-2/neu antibodies in archival tissue samples: potential source of error in immunohistochemical studies of oncogene expression. *Cancer Research* **54**, 2771–2777.

Prest, S. J., May, F. E. & Westley, B. R. (2002). The estrogen-regulated protein, TFF1, stimulates migration of human breast cancer cells. *FASEB Journal* **16**, 592–594.

Ravdin, P. M., Green, S., Dorr, T. M., McGuire, W. L., Fabian, C., Pugh, R. P., Carter, R. D., Rivkin, S., Borst, J. R. & Belt, R. J. (1992). Prognostic significance of progesterone receptor levels in estrogen receptor-positive patients with metastatic breast cancer treated with tamoxifen: results of a prospective Southwest Oncology Group study. *Journal of Clinical Oncology* **10**, 1284–1291.

Rhodes, A., Jasani, B., Barnes, D. M., Bobrow, L. G. & Miller, K. D. (2000). Reliability of immunohistochemical demonstration of oestrogen receptors in routine practice: interlaboratory variance in the sensitivity of detection and evaluation of scoring systems. *Journal of Clinical Pathology* **53**, 125–130.

Roche, P. C., Suman, V. J., Jenkins, R. B., Davidson, N. E., Martino, S., Kaufman, P. A., Addo, F. K., Murphy, B., Ingle, J. N. & Perez, E. A. (2002). Concordance between local and central laboratory HER2 testing in the breast intergroup trial N9831. *Journal of the National Cancer Institute* **94**, 855–857.

Roylance, R., Gorman, P., Harris, W., Liebmann, R., Barnes, D., Hanby, A. & Sheer, D. (1999). Comparative genomic hybridization of breast tumors stratified by histological grade reveals new insights into the biological progression of breast cancer. *Cancer Research* **59**, 1433–1436.

Sawyer, E. J., Hanby, A. M., Rowan, A. J., Gillett, C. E., Thomas, R. E., Poulsom, R., Lakhani, S. R., Ellis, I. O, Ellis, P. & Tomlinson, I. P. (2002). The Wnt pathway, epithelial-stromal interactions, and malignant progression in phyllodes tumours. *Journal of Pathology* **196**, 437–444.

Schelfhout, V. R. J., Coene, E. D., Delaey, B., Thys, S., Page, D. L. & Potter, C. R. D. (2000). Pathogenesis of Paget's disease: epidermal heregulin-alpha, motility factor, and the HER receptor family. *Journal of the National Cancer Institute* **92**, 622–628.

Selim, A. G., El-Ayat, G. & Wells, C. A. (2002). Expression of c-erbB2, p53, Bcl-2, Bax, c-myc and Ki-67 in apocrine metaplasia and apocrine change within sclerosing adenosis of the breast. *Virchows Archiv* **441**, 449–455.

Slamon, D. J., Leyland-Jones, B., Shak, S., Fuchs, H., Paton, V., Bajamonde, A., Fleming, T., Eiermann, W., Wolter, J., Pegram, M., Baselga, J. & Norton, L. (2001). Use of chemotherapy plus a monoclonal antibody against HER2 for metastatic breast cancer that overexpresses HER2. *New England Journal of Medicine* **344**(11),783–792.

Sorlie, T., Perou, C. M., Tibshirani, R., Aas, T., Geisler, S., Johnsen, H., Hastie, T., Eisen, M. B., Rijn, M. v. d., Jeffrey, S. S. *et al.* (2001). Gene expression patterns of breast carcinomas distinguish tumor subclasses with clinical implications. *Proceedings of the National Academy of Sciences of the United States of America* **98**, 10,869–10,874.

van de Vijver, M. J., He, Y. D., van't Veer, L. J., Dai, H., Hart, A. A., Voskuil, D. W., Schreiber, G. J., Peterse, J. L., Roberts, C., Marton, M. J., Parrish, M., Atsma, D., Witteveen, A., Glas, A., Delahaye, L., van der Velde, T., Bartelink, H., Rodenhuis, S., Rutgers, E. T., Friend, S. H. & Bernards, R. (2002). A gene-expression signature as a predictor of survival in breast cancer. *New England Journal of Medicine* **347**, 1999–2009.

Yamamoto, D., Ueda, S., Senzaki, H., Shoji, T., Haijima, H., Gondo, H. & Tanaka, K. (2001). New diagnostic approach to intracystic lesions of the breast by fibreoptic ductoscopy. *Anticancer Research* **21**, 4113–4116.

Yeatman, T. J. (2003). The future of clinical cancer management: one tumor, one chip. *American Surgeon* **69**, 41–44.

# PART 3

# Surgical intervention

# Chapter 8

# Management of the axilla including sentinel node biopsy

*Robert Mansel*

Surgical management of the axilla has been and remains a controversial area (Fentiman and Mansel 1991). The introduction of breast screening programmes and the consequent reduction in tumour size has called into question the need to remove all the axillary nodes in order to treat the axilla when only 25% of screen detected patients have involved axillary nodes. The development of sampling techniques and sentinel node biopsy has added fuel to the fire of debate.

## Axillary node clearance

Removal of the axillary nodes has been a standard part of mastectomy and this practice seemed logical when large tumour sizes meant that more than 50% of axillae contained axillary metastases. Large series of complete axillary clearance taking all three levels of the axilla have shown that a mean of 20 nodes are recovered during the pathological examination (Veronesi *et al.* 1993). The exact number of nodes retrieved depends on both the technique employed and the diligence of the pathologist. However, it has been shown by the Danish Co-operative group that recovery of more than ten nodes (i.e. equivalent to full axillary clearance) gives the maximal survival if all those 10 nodes are negative (Axelsson *et al.* 1992). If fewer than 10 negative nodes were removed the survival was less than in the >10 negative node groups. The worst survival occurs when no nodes are recovered from the axilla. This is an unusual event in node clearance operations but much more common in sampling operations. In addition to the excellent prognostic information given by nodal histology, there is a therapeutic benefit as the local recurrence rate is low in classic axillary node clearance. Large series of axillary clearance operations have given local recurrence rates of 0–5% (Cabanes *et al.* 1992; Shukla *et al.* 1999).

The question remains as to the significance of nodal deposits: are these simply markers of an aggressive cancer or do they represent an orderly progression of the cancer? These two concepts outline the two recent paradigms of cancer metastasis, i.e. that of the centripetal spread espoused by Halsted and the early systemic spread promulgated by Fisher. Of course these two ideas come from different time frames and disease conditions, as Halsted was dealing with advanced cancers while Fisher was studying smaller tumours at an 'earlier' stage in their life history. Fisher maintains that positive nodes are merely a marker for existing systemic disease and do not in themselves contribute to that systemic disease, whereas the Halstedian concept implies spread first to the lymph nodes followed by more distant spread. Fisher has described high local recurrence in the axilla when no surgery or radiotherapy was given but no difference in survival in the face of high levels of recurrent disease (Fisher *et al.* 1985). He has used this argument to support the concept that breast cancer does not metastasise from nodes but from the primary tumour in the first instance. However, the survival differences between recurrence free and recurrent disease patients would be quite small because we know that approximately 40% of patients with breast cancer will die whatever treatment is given and that their demise is caused by distant metastases at the time of primary surgery. This would mean that very large numbers are needed to show these small differences and the National Surgical Adjuvant Breast and Bowel Project (NSABP) trials are under-powered to show a small survival difference.

In a publication in the late 1990s, the Cardiff Breast Unit examined this problem in a study of patients operated on in the same unit by one surgeon with Halstedian philosophy compared with another surgeon who believed the Fisherian concept. The trial (although not randomised formally) showed a 12% difference in survival in favour of the Halstedian surgeon. These results were obtained before the days of routine chemotherapy (Shukla *et al.* 1999). It is likely that routine postoperative chemotherapy would narrow these differences. Indeed, in the Oxford overview reported in 2000 there was a small but significant survival advantage in those patients who did not suffer local recurrence compared with the high local recurrence groups (Oxford Overview 2000, unpublished data). One interpretation may be that, in a small number of patients, distant metastases can occur from sites of local recurrence. The implication of this is that reducing the local recurrence rate should also increase survival by a small amount.

## The morbidity of axillary clearance

Although axillary clearance is an effective operation from the point of view of local control, there is a major issue in relation to morbidity. In the past, less attention was paid to this morbidity in the face of a life-threatening disease. However, with the advent of better prognosis tumours as a result of screening, the issue of morbidity has become more prominent. The increasing emphasis on good cosmesis from breast conservation and quality of life issues has also raised awareness of axillary morbidity. The principal problems are sensory changes caused by surgical damage to the intercostobrachial nerve and the threat of arm swelling as a result of lymphatic stasis after removal of the axillary nodes. Table 8.1 shows the subjective and objective rates of these complications, which are very common. Other common symptoms post-clearance are arm weakness and shoulder stiffness. In most patients these complications are mild or transient but in a small number of patients severe paraesthesia or swelling can seriously affect the quality of the patient's life. If this occurs there is no effective curative treatment and the conditions are likely to persist for the remainder of the patient's life. It is for these reasons that alternatives to axillary clearance such as axillary sampling have been sought, especially for the good prognosis, node-negative tumours.

**Table 8.1** The morbidity of axillary clearance

| Symptom | Subjective (%) | Objective (%) |
| --- | --- | --- |
| Arm swelling | 40 | 20 |
| Sensory change | 90 | 70 |
| Shoulder stiffness | 30 | 20 |
| Arm weakness | 40 | 25 |

From Ivens *et al.* (1992) and Kissen *et al.* (1986)

## Axillary sampling

In an effort to reduce axillary morbidity, the Edinburgh Breast Unit devised a partial removal of axillary nodes (axillary sampling). This operation requires removal of at least four nodes in order to give a reasonable qualitative assessment of the status of the axilla. These nodes are located by palpation, usually at level I in the axilla. The Edinburgh Breast Unit has conducted randomised trials of axillary sampling against axillary clearance and has shown that, if at least four nodes are removed, there is a good qualitative match with the results of axillary positivity as determined by axillary clearance (Forrest *et al.* 1995). If any of the sampled nodes proves to be malignant, the axilla is treated by postoperative radiotherapy. Long-term follow-up of these trials has shown that the morbidity of axillary sampling is less than clearance if the patient does not receive radiotherapy. However, if the sampled nodes are positive and the axilla is then irradiated, the long-term morbidity is similar to that of axillary clearance in terms of arm swelling and shoulder function. Thus, sampling does offer a lower rate of morbidity for patients with negative nodes. However, axillary sampling has not been adopted by the majority of surgeons and axillary clearance remains the operation of choice. Some of the reticence around sampling may involve the idea that removing some of the nodes may result in missing other cancer-containing nodes nearby, which were too small to be detected by palpation. Indeed, this potential problem has been shown to be a fact in reality as the Edinburgh trials of sampling versus clearance have shown higher rates of local recurrence in the sampling group, although the absolute rates are still modest at around 7–9%. The Danish Co-operative group has also shown that survival is lower if fewer than 10 negative nodes are removed (Axelsson *et al.* 1992).

The philosophy behind axillary sampling is the fact that a majority of patients and, in breast screening, a large majority of patients, will turn out to be node negative after axillary clearance, meaning that the node-negative patients in retrospect undergo a high-morbidity operation (Table 8.2). These facts have led to a search for a less morbid method of determining axillary status.

**Table 8.2** Rates of positive axillae in different diseases

| Cancer | Percentage axillary positivity |
| --- | --- |
| Ductal carcinoma *in situ* (DCIS) | 2 |
| Screen-detected carcinoma | 20 |
| Early symptomatic carcinomas | 35 |
| Advanced breast cancer | 40–60 |

## Sentinel node biopsy

Sentinel node biopsy is a targeted form of node sampling. In this technique a combination of isotope-tagged colloid and blue dye is injected around the tumour and both flow with the lymph fluid to the first draining node (first echelon) in the axilla. The first node is usually found at level I (lateral to the pectoralis major muscle) but may occasionally be at a higher level. Although the technique was first described and developed for melanoma, there was little interest until 1992 when Morton *et al.* from UCLA published their comprehensive studies in melanoma. This paper described a high success rate in identification of the sentinel lymph node with a low false-negative rate (negative histological sentinel node in an axilla/groin with other positive nodes present). This seminal paper also described the surgical learning curve. Subsequent progress in sentinel node biopsy was very rapid with increasing numbers of papers being described year on year describing the technique in melanoma, breast cancer and latterly in parathyroid/gastrointestinal cancers.

Since this was a new technique all these early papers describe simple audit studies and incorporate the learning curves of many surgeons (Mansel *et al.* 2000). Widely varying rates of success in finding a sentinel node are described, from 66% for blue dye alone to 97–100% for the combined isotopic/blue dye technique. The false-negative rates have varied from 0% to 30%. Krag *et al.* (1998) carried out a multicentre audit of sentinel node biopsy in breast cancer and showed individual surgeon false-negative rates of up to 29%.

However, the technique has shown great reliability in negative predictive value because the chance of finding a positive node in an axilla containing a negative sentinel node is less than 1 in 1000 nodes (Turner *et al.* 1997). These are very encouraging results but to date no randomised trials of sentinel node biopsy have been published, although there are ongoing trials in the USA and Europe. Many of the issues around the technique relate to the reproducibility in individual surgeons' hands. The Krag study suggested that some surgeons would have difficulty in learning the technique, but in the USA sentinel node biopsy is spreading widely without formal accreditation of the procedure. A consensus meeting in 1999 in the USA suggested that at least 30 cases should be done after a training course in order to achieve reproducible results.

In the UK the MRC funded an audit trial (the ALMANAC trial – Principal Investigator: Professor RE Mansel) which mandates that each surgeon must perform 40 cases with full data recording and comparison with a standard axillary procedure, either clearance or sampling of the four nodes. This study is running in approximately 14 centres with 24 surgeons involved and had recruited over 1000 patients by September 2003. This study has now completed a randomised trial comparing sentinel node biopsy alone against standard axillary surgery, but only those surgeons who achieved 90% success rate and a 5% or less false-negative rate of $\leq 5\%$ in their 40 audit cases were allowed to enter patients into the randomised trial. This trial has randomised over 250 cases with a target of 1200 patients. Patients who had a positive sentinel node in the test arm of the trial could have either radiotherapy or a second operation to clear the axilla. Currently, two-thirds of these patients are having further surgery and one-third are having axillary radiotherapy.

The end-points of the study are morbidity, psychological morbidity, quality of life and the health economics of the procedure. The study should define the utility of this operation in the staging of the axilla in breast cancer and the results will be reported on availability.

## *References*


Axelsson, C. K., Mourisden, H. T., Zedeler, K. (1992). Axillary dissection of level I and II lymph nodes is important in breast cancer classification. *European Journal of Cancer* **28**, 1415–1418.

Cabanes, P., Salmon, R., Vilcoq, J. *et al.* (1992). Value of axillary dissection in addition to lumpectomy and radiotherapy in early breast cancer. *The Lancet* **339**, 1245.

Fentiman, I., Mansel, R. E. (1991). The axilla – not a no-go zone. *The Lancet* **337**, 221–223.

Fisher, B., Redmond, C., Fisher *et al.* (1985). Ten year results of a randomised clinical trial of comparing radical mastectomy and total mastectomy with or without radiation. *New England Journal of Medicine* **312**, 674–681.

Forrest, A. P. M., Everington, D., McDonald, C. C., Steele, R. J. C., Chetty, U., Stewart, H. J. (1995). The Edinburgh randomised trial of axillary sampling or clearance after mastectomy. *British Journal of Surgery* **82**, 1504–1508.

Ivens, D., Hoe, A. I., Podd, T. J. *et al.* (1992). Assessment of morbidity from complete axillary dissection. *British Journal of Cancer* **66**, 136–138.

Kissin, M. W., Querci della Rovere, G., Easton, D., Westbury, G. (1986). Risk of lymphoedema following the treatment of breast cancer. *British Journal of Surgery* **73**, 580–584.

Krag, D., Weaver, D., Asikaga, T. *et al.* (1998). The sentinel node in breast cancer – A multi centre validation study. *New England Journal of Medicine* **339**, 941–946.

Mansel, R. E., Khonji, N., Clarke, D. (2000). History, present status and future of sentinel node biopsy in breast cancer. The Mary Beves Lecture. *Acta Oncologica* **127**, 265–268.

Morton, D. L., Wen, D. R., Wong, J. H. *et al.* (1992). Technical details of intraoperative lymphatic mapping for early stage melanoma. *Archives of Surgery* **127**, 392–399.

Shukla, H. S., Melhuish, J., Mansel, R. E., Hughes, L. E. (1999). Does local therapy affect survival rates in breast cancer. *Annals of Surgical Oncology* **6**, 455–460.

Turner, R., Ollila, D. W., Krasne, D. L., Guiliano, A. E. (1997). Histopathological validation of the Sentinel Lymph Node Hypothesis for breast carcinoma. *Annals of Surgery* **226**, 271–27.

Veronesi, U., Galimberti, V., Zurrida, M., Greco, M., Luini, A. (1993). Prognostic significance of number and level of axillary node metastases in breast cancer. *The Breast* **2**, 224–8.

Chapter 9

# Perspectives in the training and skills of the oncoplastic breast surgeon

*Richard M. Rainsbury*

## A new inter-specialty training initiative

Breast surgery is now an established subspecialty of general surgery in the UK, but the traditional model of the general surgeon with a subspecialty interest in breast surgery is changing. On the one hand, shorter training programmes, the European Working Time Directive, better outcomes, and mounting patient, provider and professional expectations are leading to greater specialisation. On the other hand, today's trainees with a subspecialty interest in breast surgery are acquiring a new range of skills and competencies, with more than 80% prioritising training in breast reconstruction (Rainsbury & Browne 2001). Heightened trainee expectations are generating innovative new initiatives that cross traditional boundaries between breast and plastic surgery, encouraging the acquisition of hybrid skills. Growing collaboration between the British Association of Surgical Oncology and the British Association of Plastic Surgeons has resulted in a new cross-specialty training programme in oncoplastic breast surgery. Oncoplastic breast surgery combines the best principles of tumour resection to achieve wide, tumour-free margins, with the best principles of breast reconstruction to optimise cosmetic outcomes while minimising complications.

This initiative represents a radical departure from current practice, where the breast surgeon performs the resection of the tumour, and the plastic surgeon performs the reconstruction, often at a later date. The oncoplastic breast surgeon is trained in all aspects of diagnosis, resection, reconstruction and clinical management, a new model which has several potential advantages. First, the patient is saved the need for two admissions and two operations, with the associated physical discomfort, psychological morbidity and the financial penalties of prolonged convalescence and time off work. Second, planning of the treatment episode is more straightforward as everything is managed by one multidisciplinary team rather than by two often physically separated units. Lastly, the costs to the provider are reduced considerably by the reduction in the number of treatment episodes and subsequent follow-up visits.

The cross-specialty training initiative has three fundamental aims: to improve the service to patients, to facilitate interspecialty training at all levels and to increase recruitment into breast surgery. The first tranche of senior breast and plastic trainees was appointed to nine large multidisciplinary oncoplastic breast units in 2002. These posts have been selected to provide comprehensive oncological and reconstructive training experience, with structured educational supervision, assessment and feedback to inform future developments in this new field. As the boundaries between breast and plastic surgery begin to break down, both specialties are learning new operative skills which enable the surgeon to combine resection with immediate reconstruction. Skin-sparing mastectomy combined with immediate breast reconstruction and breast-sparing reconstruction represent two important developments in this field.

## Skin-sparing mastectomy

Skin-sparing mastectomy allows the surgeon to preserve as much of the skin envelope of the breast as possible, thereby reducing the size of the mastectomy scar to a point where it can be concealed by a subsequent nipple/areola reconstruction (the 'scarless mastectomy'). The breast can be removed and reconstructed through a variety of different incisions, including a small central peri-areolar aperture which allows the removal and reconstruction of the entire breast within the undisturbed skin envelope (Peyser *et al.* 2000). This enables the surgeon to reproduce a symmetrical breast with a life-like shape and ptosis, avoiding the sometimes unsightly scars resulting from skin-sacrificing procedures. The larger, more ptotic breast can be removed through a standard breast reduction incision, which reduces the area of the skin envelope and enables the reconstruction of a smaller breast mound. This is combined with simultaneous or subsequent contralateral breast reduction to achieve symmetry.

The cosmetic results from this type of approach can be outstanding, with some patients enjoying a reconstruction that is almost indistinguishable from the native breast. These procedures can be performed without compromising the surgical or oncological safety of mastectomy (Carlson *et al.* 1997; Kroll *et al.* 1997), but two risks of this approach include ischaemia of the skin envelope and local recurrence. Skin envelope necrosis has been reported in 5–10% of patients and the risk is increased significantly in smokers (Carlson *et al.* 1997; Peyser *et al.* 2000). The reported rate of local recurrence after skin-sparing mastectomy is very low, although the procedure has been used most frequently for prophylaxis, pre-invasive and small invasive tumours (Slavin *et al.* 1998; Kroll *et al.* 1999). The incidence of local recurrence after skin-sparing mastectomy increases with time, and when used for the treatment of more advanced tumours (Figure 9.1) (Rivadeneira *et al.* 2000). Recent studies have highlighted the cosmetic advantages of skin-sparing mastectomy and immediate reconstruction (Slavin *et al.* 1998), but a prospective comparison of the surgical and cosmetic outcomes of skin-sparing mastectomy versus non-skin-sparing mastectomy has yet to be performed.

In the absence of such data, the proportion of patients requiring contralateral procedures to achieve symmetry provides a useful surrogate measure of cosmetic result (Peyser *et al.* 2000). With increasing experience and the use of tissue expanders

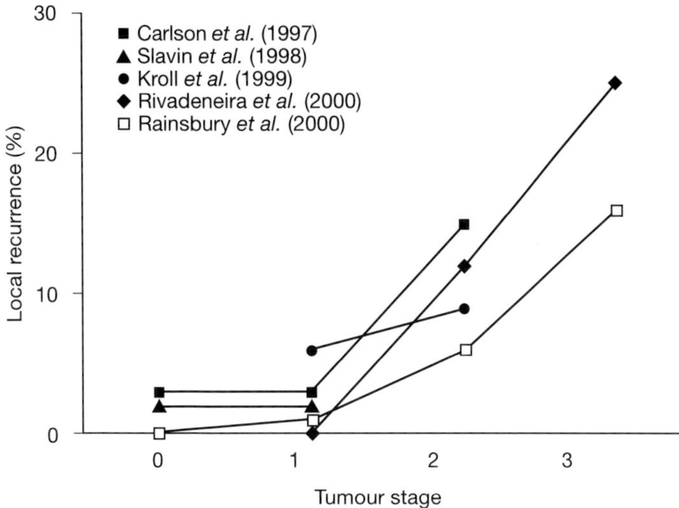



**Figure 9.1** Local recurrence after skin-sparing mastectomy: effect of stage

to enable postoperative volume adjustment, skin-sparing mastectomy will help to avoid contralateral surgery altogether. The technique lends itself to reconstruction using a variety of different methods, including subpectoral, latissimus dorsi and TRAM-flap procedures. Careful patient selection, meticulous technique and high-quality lighting and equipment are major factors that can be expected to affect the complication rates and final results of this type of surgery. The increasing availability of sophisticated cutting and coagulation equipment greatly facilitates these procedures, reducing the operating time and the need for blood transfusion. In future, the development of techniques for endoscopic-assisted flap dissection may help to accelerate the surgical procedure, while reducing scarring and postoperative morbidity.

## Breast-sparing reconstruction

The interrelationship between breast : tumour ratio, volume loss, cosmetic outcome and margins of clearance in breast cancer is a complex one, and the widespread popularity of breast-conserving surgery has focused attention on breast-sparing reconstruction. This approach can avoid the unacceptable cosmetic sequelae associated with very wide local excision, as a result of volume loss and unsightly scarring and distortion. Until now, there have been only two choices: breast-conserving surgery or mastectomy, depending on fairly well-defined indications.

Breast-sparing reconstruction provides a third option which can avoid the need for mastectomy in selected patients for a variety of reasons. First, it allows a very wide local excision of breast tissue without the risk of local deformity. Second, it extends the role of breast-conserving surgery to include patients where 10–20% or more of the breast volume needs to be removed, without compromising the adequacy of resection or the cosmetic outcome. Traditionally, this group of patients is treated by mastectomy. Third, volume replacement can be used after previous breast-conserving surgery and radiotherapy to correct unacceptable local deformity (Slavin *et al.* 1992), and may prevent the need for mastectomy in some cases of local recurrence when further local excision will result in considerable volume loss.

The choice of technique for breast-sparing reconstruction depends on a number of factors, including the extent of resection, the position of the tumour, the size of the breast, the timing of surgery, the experience of the surgeon and the expectations of the patient. Reconstruction at the same time as resection limits the surgical treatment to one episode, providing clear margins of resection can be assured at the time of primary surgery. As a general rule, it is much easier to prevent than to correct a deformity, as the sequelae of previous surgery, including dense scar tissue, fibrosis and skin changes do not have to be overcome.

Resection defects can be reconstructed in one of two ways. First, by volume replacement, importing volume from elsewhere to replace the amount of tissue resected (Noguchi *et al.* 1990; Raja *et al.* 1997; Rainbury & Paramanathan 1998). As a result, there is no net loss of volume and symmetry is maintained. Examples of this approach include the use of a myosubcutaneous flap or 'miniflap' of latissimus dorsi to reconstruct central and upper pole defects in the breast, or a myocutaneous flap of latissimus dorsi to reconstruct central and lower pole defects (Clough *et al.* 1999). Volume replacement techniques can restore the shape and size of the breast, achieving symmetry and excellent cosmetic results, without the need for contralateral surgery. These techniques require additional theatre time and may be complicated by donor site morbidity, flap loss and an extended convalescence.

The second approach is to use a volume displacement technique. This procedure combines resection with a variety of different conventional breast reduction procedures, according to the position of the tumour (Clough *et al.* 1999). This approach results in a net loss in volume of the breast, and frequently requires a contralateral procedure to achieve symmetry. Options include the superior pedicle technique for the resection of inferior pole tumours (Nos *et al.* 1998), the inferior pedicle or Grisotti technique for the resection of central tumours (Grisotti 1994), and the 'round block' or Benelli technique for the resection of peripheral tumours (Benelli 1990). These procedures may be complicated by necrosis of the dermoglandular flaps, and contralateral surgery is usually required to restore symmetry as volume loss is inevitable.

The timing of the reconstructive component of breast-sparing reconstruction is a 'hot topic'. If the operation is performed as a one-stage procedure, the patient needs to be informed of the need for a subsequent re-excision of the cavity wall or a mastectomy if the resection margins are positive. This is an uncommon event, as the technique allows for very wide local excision, which is reflected in the high resection weights and the low rates of local recurrence reported in the literature (Table 9.1). Alternatively, the procedure can be performed in two stages, with reconstruction of the resection defect (Dixon *et al.* 2002).

**Table 9.1** Outcomes associated with breast-sparing reconstruction: extent of resection and local control

|  | Number of cases | Specimen weight (g) | Local recurrence (%) | Follow up (yr) |
|---|---|---|---|---|
| Noguchi *et al.* 1990 | 50 | NS | 0 | 4 |
| Nos *et al.* 1998 | 87 | 270 | 6 | 5 |
| Rainsbury *et al.* 1998 | 103 | 165 | 3 | 5 |
| Dixon *et al.* 2002 | 25 | 94 | 0 | 2 |

NS, not stated

## Conclusion

Greater specialisation in breast surgery is leading to the emergence of a cohort of trainees with new skills and competencies, enabling greater patient choice and more appropriate care. Specialisation is increasing as a result of foreshortened training, greater demand and heightened trainee expectations, at the expense of general surgical skills. Ultimately, the skill base of today's breast surgeons will reflect personal preferences and professional networks, local needs and geographical constraints and future developments in advanced surgical training curricula. Modern training programmes are beginning to reflect these needs, supporting inter-professional, cross-specialty training, and encouraging professional development.

Over the past six years, a rolling programme for teaching breast reconstruction has been developed at several major UK teaching centres. This includes The Royal College of Surgeons of England, Manchester, Leeds and Glasgow, and incorporates in the programme a variety of different approaches, including demonstrations of reconstructive anatomy, small group tutorials and anatomical prosections. Moreover, course participants perform cadaver-based procedures reinforced by teaching videos and live operative demonstrations. There is an increasing interest in oncoplastic breast surgery among UK consultants and trainees, and in future novel modular assessment-based curricular training programmes will focus on the acquisition of appropriate competencies, including clinical, technical, interpersonal, team-based and knowledge-based skills.

## Acknowledgement

The author acknowledges the financial support provided by the Winchester Cancer Research Trust (charity no. 1003252).

## References

Benelli, L. (1990). A new periareolar mammoplasty: round block technique. *Aesthetic Plastic Surgery* **14**, 99–106.

Carlson, G. W., Bostwick, J., Styblo, T. M., Moore, V., Bried, J. T. & Murray, D. R. (1997). Skin-sparing mastectomy. oncologic and reconstructive considerations. *American Surgeon* **225**, 570–578.

Clough, K. B., Nos, C. & Fitoussi, A. (1999). Oncoplastic conservative surgery for breast cancer. *Operative Techniques in Plastic and Reconstructive Surgery* **6**, 50–60.

Dixon, J. M., Venizelos, B. & Chan, P. (2002). Latissimus dorsi miniflap: a new technique for extending breast conservation. *The Breast* **11**, 58–65.

Grisotti A. (1994). Immediate reconstruction after partial mastectomy. *Operative Techniques in Plastic and Reconstructive Surgery* **1**, 1–12.

Kroll, S. S., Shusterman, M. A., Tadjalli, H. E., Singletary, S. E., Ames, F. C. (1997). Risk of recurrence after treatment of early breast cancer with skin-sparing mastectomy. *Annals of Surgical Oncology* **4**, 193–197.

Kroll, S. S. & Khoo, A., Singletary, E. *et al.* (1999). Local recurrence risk after skin-sparing and conventional mastectomy: a 6-year follow-up. *Plastic and Reconstructive Surgery* **104**, 421–425.

Noguchi, M., Taniya, T., Miyasaki, I. & Saito, Y. (1990). Immediate transposition of a latissimus dorsi muscle for correcting a post quadrantectomy breast deformity in Japanese patients. *International Surgery* **75**, 166–170.

Nos, C., Fitoussi, A., Bourgeois, D. *et al.* (1998). Conservative treatment of lower pole breast cancer by bilateral mammoplasty and radiotherapy. *European Journal of Surgical Oncology* **24**, 508–541.

Peyser, P. M., Abel, J. A., Straker, V. F., Hall, V. L. & Rainsbury, R. M. (2000). Ultra-conservative skin sparing 'keyhole' mastectomy and immediate breast and areola reconstruction. *Annals of the Royal College of Surgeons of England* **82**, 227–235.

Rainsbury, R. M. & Paramanathan, N. (1998). Recent progress with breast-conserving volume replacement using latissimus dorsi miniflaps in UK patients. *Breast Cancer* **5**, 139–147.

Rainsbury, R. M. & Browne, J. P. (2001). Specialisation in breast surgery, opinions of UK higher surgical trainees. *Annals of the Royal College of Surgeons of England* (Suppl.) **83**, 298–301.

Raja, M. A. K., Straker, V. F. & Rainsbury, R. M. (1997). Extending the role of breast-conserving surgery by immediate volume replacement. *British Journal of Surgery* **84**, 101–105.

Rivadeneira, D. E, Simmons, R. M, Fish, S. K. *et al.* (2000). Skin-sparing mastectomy with immediate breast reconstruction: a critical analysis of local recurrence. *Cancer Journal* **6**, 331–335.

Slavin, S. A., Love, S. M. & Sadowsky, N. L. (1992). Reconstruction of the irradiated partial mastectomy defect with autogenous tissue. *Plastic and Reconstructive Surgery* **90**, 854–865.

Slavin, S. A., Schnitt, S. J. & Duda, R. B. *et al.* (1998). Skin-sparing mastectomy and immediate reconstruction: oncologic risks and aesthetic results in patients with early-stage breast cancer. *Plastic and Reconstructive Surgery* **102**, 49–62.

Chapter 10

# Neo-adjuvant therapy for operable breast cancer: current evidence and trends

*David A. Cameron*

## Introduction

The use of systemic drug therapy before surgery for operable breast cancer became more common in the latter half of the 1980s. There were three main arguments put forward to justify this approach. Once it had been clearly established that breast conservation was a safe and appropriate way to manage smaller cancers, it was felt that the reduction in tumour size achieved with drug therapy might allow more women to have successful breast conservation. Secondly, laboratory studies predicted that initiation of effective systemic therapy before removal of the primary tumour would result in improvements in metastasis-free survival for the patients. Thirdly, by observing possible tumour response to the therapy, the most appropriate post-surgical adjuvant therapy could be chosen. Several studies were done to address some or all of these questions. At the same time there were opponents to this approach, expressing concerns that delaying surgery, particularly in those patients whose tumours were not very responsive, might compromise operability, increase operative complications and possibly even long-term local control.

The published literature has addressed most of these issues, and it is clear that primary systemic therapy is not disadvantageous, but there are no data to support the theoretical arguments that it could give a survival advantage. This review will discuss the evidence relating to the above concerns, and then consider more recent data, some published only in abstract form, which suggest the direction of current research in this area.

## Breast conservation

The best evidence that primary systemic therapy can reduce the requirement for mastectomy comes from randomised trials in women whose optimum surgical treatment was clearly documented before randomisation to receive the same systemic therapy before or after surgery. Few published series give these data, but several report the actual rate of breast conservation in women given pre-operative and post-operative systemic therapy (see Table 10.1). The largest series is from the NSABP B-18 study, in which 1,523 women with operable breast cancer were randomised between surgery followed by four cycles of adriamycin-cyclophosphamide (AC) or the same chemotherapy followed by surgery. The two groups of women were well balanced in terms of tumour size, so that one can presume that similar rates of mastectomy would have occurred in the two arms in the absence of any pre-surgical tumour cyto-reduction. Certainly the data in the paper report that two-thirds of the women were felt suitable for conservative surgery at randomisation, although in fact only 60% in the conventional arm actually had a conservative procedure. Similar differences were seen in the study performed at the Royal Marsden Hospital, London, although the breast conservation rates were in general higher, despite having a lower proportion of T1 tumours (11% compared with 29% in the NSABP B-18 study), which is probably a reflection of different surgical practices.

However, a note of caution needs to be expressed. Firstly, in the NSABP study, although the rate of local recurrence was not significantly higher in the women treated with chemotherapy first (8% versus 6%), age was a significant risk factor for local recurrence, with women under 50 years having 8% recurrence in the conventional arm rising to 13% in those given pre-operative chemotherapy (Fisher *et al.* 1998). The evidence that this higher rate of local recurrence may be significant comes from a French study which had a different approach to loco-regional therapy. Patients were randomised to chemotherapy or not before radical radiotherapy, with surgery required for local recurrence and/or persistent disease. The women who did not receive the chemotherapy before surgery had a higher initial mastectomy rate (23% versus 18%), but this was no longer the case at 5 years, at which time point the rates were both 40% (Scholl *et al.* 1994). Another French study, in which all women in the control arm were to receive mastectomy, reported that among those women who had breast conservation after primary chemotherapy, 7% had breast recurrences within 3 years median follow-up, all but one of whom required a mastectomy. More importantly perhaps, after a median follow-up of almost 10 years, almost one-quarter had had a mastectomy for local recurrence (Avril *et al.* 1998). Finally, the European Organisation for Research and Treatment of Cancer (EORTC) randomised trial reported that those women randomised to the pre-operative chemotherapy arm, who would have needed a mastectomy at presentation but were able to have breast conservation after chemotherapy, had in fact a poorer survival than those women who could have had conservation at presentation (and were still able to do so after primary chemotherapy) (van der Hage *et al.* 2001). None of these data prove that surgical downsizing and permitting of breast conservation is detrimental, but they suggest that not only is there a proportion of cases that will require subsequent mastectomy for local recurrence, but that patients with enough tumour shrinkage to allow breast conservation remain at significant risk of local and systemic recurrence.

## Survival after pre- or post-operative systemic therapy

A total of seven randomised studies were identified that randomised patients to similar systemic therapy, to be given before or after loco-regional surgery. They are summarised in Table 10.1. However, two of them (Bordeaux and Edinburgh) used different criteria for selecting therapy in the two arms and cannot therefore be seen as

**Table 10.1** Randomised studies of pre- versus post-operative systemic therapy

| Study | Therapy | Number of patients | Improvement in outcome (pre vs post CT) | Increase in breast conservation rate? (pre vs post CT) |
|---|---|---|---|---|
| Bordeaux (Mauriac et al.1991) (Avril et al. 1998) | EVM → MTV (24% of control arm received none | 272 | 4-year OS 90% vs 75% 10-year 60% | 63% vs 0% @ 10 years 49% in pre-operative chemotherapy arm |
| NSABP B-18 (Fisher et al. 1998) | AC | 1,523 | NO – curves identical | 67% vs 60% (T1 79% → 81%; T3 9% → 33%) |
| Edinburgh (Cameron et al. 2002 | CAP or hormones if ER +ve tumour (CMF with different criteria in control arm) | 171 | 5 year OS 72% vs 62% (p < 0.1) | no clear data |
| Institut Curie (Scholl et al. 1994) | Radiotherapy ±FAC | 414 | 5 year OS 86% vs 78% NS @ longer follow-up (Scholl, Asselain et al. 1995) | Initial 82% vs 77% @ 5 year 61% in both |
| St Petersburg (Semiglazov et al.1994) | Radiotherapy ±TMF | 271 | DFS 72% → 81% OS 78% → 86% (NS) | None attempted |
| Royal Marsden (Powles et al. 1995) (Makris et al. 2001) | MM (m) + tamoxifen | 309 | NO – curves identical | 90% vs 78% (p < 0.003) |
| EORTC (van der Hage et al. 2001) | FEC | 698 | NO | 13% more patients had breast conservation than anticipated at trial entry |

EVM → MTV, epirubicin, vincristine, methotrexate, followed by mitomycin C, thiotepa, vindesine; AC, doxorubicin, cyclophosphamide; CAP, cyclophosphamide, doxorubicin, prednisolone; FAC, 5-fluorouracil, adriamycin, cyclophosphamide. TMF, thiotepa; MM (m), mitoxantrone, methotrexate (and mitomycin C also given to first 80 patients); FEC, 5-fluorouracil, epirubicin and cyclophosphamide; CMF, cyclophosphamide, methotrexate, 5-fluorouracil; CHOP, cyclophosphamide, doxorubicin, vincristine, prednisolone.

a pure test of the timing of the same systemic therapy. It is clear that there is no evidence of a survival detriment for delaying surgery, but it is equally clear that the published data strongly suggest that the effect of a particular systemic therapy is independent of its sequencing with surgery. One of the few studies to have reported a survival advantage for pre-operative systemic therapy found that it disappeared with longer follow-up: another did not give any chemotherapy to 24% of the control arm because of their better prognostic features.

## Predictors of benefit from neo-adjuvant chemotherapy

Many studies have attempted to define which tumours will respond well to neo-adjuvant chemotherapy. Although not all studies identify the same predictive factors, it is clear that a few are consistently reported. High grade/high proliferating tumours respond better (Foudraine *et al.* 1992; Fisher *et al.* 2002), but this does not predict for good long-term survival (Remvikos *et al.* 1993). The presence of oestrogen receptors lowers the response rate (Bélembaogo *et al.* 1992; Kuerer *et al.* 1999; Mauriac *et al.* 1991), as does the size of the tumour, with larger tumours less often manifesting a complete clinical or pathological response (Fisher *et al.* 1997). Several other factors have been studied, including Her2-neu, for which there are suggestions that tumours with higher levels of expression are more likely to respond to anthracyclines (Colleoni *et al.* 1999) although one study reported a lower response rate (Makris *et al.* 1997). This search for predictive markers of chemosensitivity is based on the perception that women whose tumours respond will have better outcomes, and that is certainly evidence based. Interestingly, as clinical experience in advanced disease might suggest, it is not only the degree of response that predicts for a better outcome, but also the speed, with tumours halving their volume in a shorter time having a better survival (Cameron *et al.* 1997).

Many studies have confirmed that a clinical complete response is associated with a survival advantage (Fisher *et al.* 1998; Scholl *et al.* 1996; Ellis *et al.* 1998; Wolmark *et al.* 2001; Eltahir *et al.* 1998), but the most consistent factor associated with good long-term outcome is the pathological response in the tumour and/or axillary nodes. The published data are summarised in Table 10.2. Although one can debate the relative importance of primary versus nodal response, it is well known that a lack of involvement of the axilla already confers a reasonable long-term prognosis. Confirmation that the post-therapy axillary node status may be the best predictor of long-term outcome comes from a retrospective analysis of patients treated with neo-adjuvant chemotherapy at the Institut Curie, Paris. The data were reviewed on 152 women who had fine needle aspirate proven involvement of the axilla before chemotherapy. They noted a higher rate of pathological clearance in the axilla than in the primary site. But more interestingly, they reported that the 5-year survival at 74% was almost the same for those women with post-therapy negative axillae as for those with a pathological complete response (pCR) at the primary site. However, the 14 women with no invasive disease in either the breast or axilla had the best outcome, at over 80%. In a multivariate analysis, axillary downstaging was significant, whereas clearance of the primary site was not. In the 9-year update of the original B-18 study, it was noted that pathological clearance at either the primary site or in the axillary nodes were independent predictors of a better outcome. However, the additional prognostic impact of negative node status over and above that of the primary tumour site was of much greater statistical significance than the reverse (Wolmark *et al.* 2001).

Based on these observations, current studies are now designed on the basis that a complete pathological response is a good surrogate. Although it is true that this link has not been confirmed for taxanes, it does seem a reasonable basis on which to explore cytotoxics. However, it is less certain that it will also be true for biological non-cytotoxic agents, because we do not even know what relationship a lack of a pathological complete response will have with outcome for primary endocrine therapy, because it has been much less well studied. Equally, not every patient with a poor pathological response after chemotherapy is doomed. Few studies have addressed this question, but data have been reported from the M. D. Anderson Cancer Center, Houston (Buchholz *et al.* 2001). They described 177 patients who achieved less than a partial response to neo-adjuvant chemotherapy, and found that the axillary node status remained a strong prognostic factor, with those women with a negative axilla having a 5-year survival of at least 75%. Outcome was generally better for those women whose tumours were oestrogen receptor (ER) positive, and the few women with primarily progressive disease had a very poor outcome, with only 19% alive at 5 years. Although it remains unclear whether it is the response to therapy or the underlying disease that is responsible for this latter group faring so badly, data from Aberdeen suggest that all is not lost. In this study, women who did not achieve at least a partial response to four cycles of doxorubicin-based chemotherapy (cyclophosphamide, doxorubicin, vincristine and prednisolone: CHOP) then had an additional four cycles of taxotere, whereas the responders were randomised to switch or continue with four more cycles of CHOP (Smith *et al.* 2002). Not only did the switch to taxotere improve the outcome for the responders, but in addition, the outcome for the non-responders does not appear worse than those women with a response but who continued with CHOP. Given that there is some non-cross resistance between anthracyclines and taxanes, these data suggest that the addition of taxotere will improve the outcome for patients irrespective of the response to anthracyclines.

Irrespective of the ideal neo-adjuvant chemotherapy regimen, it is clear that persistence of many involved axillary nodes is rarely accompanied by a good long-term outcome. Thus it may well be that the simplest predictor of long-term outcome after systemic therapy may turn out to be exactly the same as in women who have surgery first, namely the number of involved axillary nodes.

**Table 10.2** Studies reporting patient outcome by pathological status after neo-adjuvant systemic therapy

| Study | Therapy | Number of patients | Tumour pCR | Negative axilla |
|---|---|---|---|---|
| Instituto Tumori Milano (Bonadonna *et al.* 1998) | CMF and anthracycline based | 536 | 8 year disease-free survival 86% | 8 year disease-free survival 75% |
| NSABP B-18 (Fisher *et al.* 1998) | AC | 1,523 | 9 year disease-free survival 75% (Wolmark, Wang *et al.* 2001) | 9 year overall survival ~ 80% (Fisher, Wang *et al.* 2002) |
| Institut Curie (Pierga *et al.* 2000) | FAC | 488 | | 5 year disease-free survival 72%; 10 year disease-free survival 63% |
| Institut Curie (Rouzier *et al.* 2002) | FAC | 152 with FNA+ve axilla | 5 year disease-free survival 75% | 5 year disease-free survival 74% |
| EORTC (van der Hage *et al.* 2001) | FEC | 698 | HR 0.86 | No data |
| Royal Marsden (Ellis *et al.* 1998) | CMF, mitoxantrone or anthracycline | 120* | 5 year disease-free survival 73%† | 5 year disease-free survival 80%† (*n* = 76) |
| Edinburgh (Cameron *et al.* 1997) | CHOP or endocrine | 94 | 10 year overall survival 85% | 10 year overall survival 88% |
| M. D. Anderson (Valero *et al.* 2002) | Doxorubicin based | 772 (including T4) | 5 year overall survival 89% (Kuerer, Newman *et al.* 1999) | 10 year disease-free survival 75% |

*Does not include 39 patients with clinical complete recovery who electively had no surgery.
†Not statistically significant from those women with pathologically detected residual disease.

AC, doxorubicin, cyclophosphamide; FAC, 5-fluorouracil, adriamycin, cyclophosphamide; FEC, 5-fluorouracil, epirubicin and cyclophosphamide; CMF, cyclophosphamide, methotrexate, 5-fluorouracil; CHOP, cyclophosphamide, doxorubicin, vincristine, prednisolone.

## Choice of pre-operative systemic therapy

More recent phase III studies have attempted to identify better pre-operative regimens. Aside from a significant number of phase II studies, and the Aberdeen study discussed above, there are three other trials that suggest the addition of a taxane will be advantageous over non-taxane-containing regimens, although not all such studies are positive (Evans *et al.* 2002). The NSABP B-27 study looked at the addition of docetaxel after four cycles of doxorubicin, cyclophosphamide (AC) in the pre-operative setting. In one arm the docetaxel was given before surgery: in another afterwards. It was clear that as with the Aberdeen study, the addition of the docetaxel significantly increased the pathological complete response rate, rising from 9% in those given only AC to 19% for those also given taxotere. A similar high pCR rate with the addition of docetaxel was reported in another US study that actually focused on translational research questions (Minton *et al.* 2002), and in another multicentre study when the doxorubicin was combined with paclitaxel and followed by cyclophosphamide, methotrexate, 5-fluorouracil (CMF), all given pre-operatively (Gianni *et al.* 2002).

Most reported studies have focused on the use of chemotherapy, but there have been several studies that have looked at the use of endocrine agents. There are some that sought to avoid surgery in the elderly, but it is clear from the data that this is counter-productive: the outcome is worse for those women who were not given local therapy after primary tamoxifen (Dixon 1992; Mustacchi *et al.* 1994).

There are fewer studies that have defined the role of an endocrine agent vis-à-vis another systemic therapy, and none has randomised women between chemotherapy and endocrine therapy. The experience of the Edinburgh Breast Unit, pioneered by Professor Forrest, has been to give endocrine therapy to those women with ER-positive tumours, and only to give chemotherapy to those that did not respond, or had ER-negative disease. The data suggest that those who responded have not fared any worse than those with ER-poor tumours given chemotherapy (Cameron *et al.* 1997). However, this does not confirm that chemotherapy would not have improved their outcome had it also been given, for example, after their surgery: it merely confirms, of course, that tumours that respond to endocrine therapy do reasonably well.

Perhaps the most provocative results come from a study that randomised women between tamoxifen and letrozole for 4 months before surgery. It is clear from the data that the response rate was higher with the letrozole, whether assessed clinically or radiologically (Eiermann *et al.* 2001). A correlative science study has reported that letrozole was especially beneficial in those tumours with low levels of ER and/or over-expression of EGFR or HER2-neu (Ellis *et al.* 2001), tumours generally considered more suitable for chemotherapy. More recent data from Edinburgh suggest that letrozole may not be unique in this effect: in a series of phase II studies, the response rates to all the three available third-generation aromatase inhibitors (anastrazole, exemestane and letrozole) were significantly higher than for a historical group of women treated in the same centre with tamoxifen (Dixon *et al.* 2002a), and the response to anastrozole for the small group of women whose tumours co-expressed both ER and HER2 was not inferior to those found to be ER positive but HER2 negative (Dixon *et al.* 2002b).

These, and other, studies with endocrine agents also demonstrate that increased breast conservation is possible, with no data to suggest that there is a higher rate of local recurrence: if anything, indirect comparisons suggest that in these post-menopausal women treated with primary endocrine therapy, excellent local control is maintained despite the higher breast conservation rate (Dixon *et al.* 2002a).

## Choice of post-operative systemic therapy

Some studies have attempted to address this issue, but so far we have no clear idea about the optimal post-operative systemic therapy in women given several months' treatment before surgery. Most studies have given tamoxifen to women with ER and/or PgR-positive tumours, and few have given any chemotherapy afterwards, preferring to give it all beforehand. There are some exceptions to this rule, such as the trial from the Royal Marsden Hospital, which gave four cycles of mitoxantrone–methotrexate before and four after surgery in the experimental arm, and the trial from Edinburgh in which patients receiving four cycles of pre-operative cyclophosphamide, doxorubicin and prednisolone (CAP) also received an additional two further cycles after surgery. In both these studies, however, the response to the primary therapy was not taken into consideration when deciding upon post-operative systemic therapy.

No study has yet demonstrated that any particular post-operative approach improves outcome, although within the UK the Anglo-Celtic II trial did attempt this. Women with large operable or locally advanced breast cancer were randomised with either adriamycin–cyclophosphamide or adriamycin–taxotere as primary therapy, and then for those women with positive axillary nodes at surgery, there was a second randomisation between CMF and high-dose chemotherapy. However, the second part of the trial had to be closed because of poor accrual in the light of the discrediting of high-dose chemotherapy that occurred as phase III data became available at the end of the 1990s. The NSABP B-27 study may give some idea of the necessity for post-operative chemotherapy, in that there are two arms of the study which differ only as to whether the four cycles of taxotere are given either before or after the surgery.

At present therefore, there are differing practices, few of them evidence based: some clinicians and studies give no further chemotherapy, some give vinorelbine and 5-fluorouracil combined with radiation therapy (S. Scholl, personal communication) and others give CMF (based loosely on the adriamycin–CMF sequence data from Milan (Bonadonna *et al.* 1995)). UK practice indicates that taxanes are often given postoperatively after anthracycline–containing preoperative chemotherapy. It is clearly an area where hard data are needed but remain essentially lacking.

## Conclusion

Pre-operative chemotherapy has clearly come of age, and the published data are convincing that there is no survival detriment for delaying surgery. It is equally clear that those women whose tumours respond will live longer, and that it is the pathological rather than clinical response that best predicts for long-term outcome. Debate remains, however, about the optimal marker of pathological response, the best predictors of that benefit and the ideal regimen.

It is anticipated that with longer follow-up, the current generation of studies such as NSABP B-27, having demonstrated that the addition of taxanes increases the pathological complete response rate, will confirm that this in turn leads to better survival. This would validate the short-term pathological response as an evidence-based surrogate end-point for survival with post-operative adjuvant therapy. But the final word must be one of caution: at the San Antonio Breast Cancer conference in 2002, for example, there was a pair of abstracts that suggested that this may not always be the case. The pivotal CALGB 9741 adjuvant study reported that there was a significant survival benefit to be seen if the same chemotherapy was given in an accelerated fashion using the assistance of growth factors (Citron *et al.* 2002), whereas a German study suggested that a similar approach in the neo-adjuvant setting, albeit with a different regimen, resulted in a lower pathological complete response rate (Euler *et al.* 2002). CALGB 9741 suggests that eradication of micro-metastatic disease may be best achieved by accelerating the chemotherapy to reduce re-growth, but perhaps a longer, slower 'burn' is needed to clear the larger bulk of a primary cancer.

*References*

Avril, A., Faucher, A., Bussieres, E., Stockle, E., Durand, M., Mauriac, L., Bonichon, F., Dilhuydy, J. M. & Campo, M. L. (1998). Results of 10 years of a randomized trial of neoadjuvant chemotherapy in breast cancers larger than 3 cm. [In French.] *Chirurgie* **123**, 247–256.

Bélembaogo, E., Feillel, V., Chollet, P., Curé, H., Verrelle, P., Kwiatkowski, F., Achard, J. L., Le Bouëdec, G., Chassagne, J., Bignon, Y. J. *et al.* (1992). Neoadjuvant chemotherapy in 126 operable breast cancers, *European Journal of Cancer* **28A**, 896–900.

Bonadonna, G., Zambetti, M. & Valagussa, P. (1995). Sequential or alternating doxorubicin and CMF regimens in breast cancer with more than three positive nodes. Ten-year results. *Journal of the American Medical Association* **273**, 542–547.

Bonadonna, G. (1998). Primary chemotherapy in operable breast cancer: eight-year experience at the Milan Cancer Institute. *Journal of Clinical Oncology* **16**, 93–100.

Buchholz, T. A., Hill, B. S., Tucker, S. L., Frye, D. K., Kuerer, H. M., Buzdar, A. U., McNeese, M. D., Singletary, S. E., Ueno, N. T., Pusztai, L. *et al.* (2001). Factors predictive of outcome in patients with breast cancer refractory to neoadjuvant chemotherapy. *Cancer Journal* **7**, 413–420.

Cameron, D. A., Anderson, E. D., Levack, P., Hawkins, R. A., Anderson, T. J., Leonard, R. C., Forrest, A. P. & Chetty, U. (1997). Primary systemic therapy for operable breast cancer— 10-year survival data after chemotherapy and hormone therapy. *British Journal of Cancer* **76**, 1099–1105.

Cameron, D. A. (2002). Oestrogen receptor directed primary systemic therapy: a randomised trial compared with conventional therapy in operable breast cancer. *Breast Cancer Research and Treatment* **76**, abstract 157, p. S53.

Citron, M., Berry, D. A., Cirrincione, C., Hudis, C., Winer, E., Gradishar, W. J., Davidson, N. E., Ingle, J. N., Perez, E. A., Carpenter, J. *et al.* (2002). Superiority of dose-dense (DD) over conventional scheduling (CS) and equivalence of sequential (SC) vs. combination adjuvant chemotherapy (CC) for node-positive breast cancer (CALGB 9741, INT C9741). *Breast Cancer Research and Treatment* **76**, 32 (abstract 15).

Colleoni, M., Orvieto, E., Nole, F., Orlando, L., Minchella, I., Viale, G., Peruzzotti, G., Robertson, C., Noberasco, C., Galimberti, V. *et al.* (1999). Prediction of response to primary chemotherapy for operable breast cancer. *European Journal of Cancer* **35**, 574–579.

Dixon, J. M. (1992). Treatment of elderly patients with breast cancer. *British Medical Journal* **304**, 996–997.

Dixon, J. M., Anderson, T. J. & Miller, W. R. (2002a). Neoadjuvant endocrine therapy of breast cancer: a surgical perspective. *European Journal of Cancer* **38**, 2214–2221.

Dixon, J. M., Jackson, J., Hills, M., Renshaw, L., Cameron, D. A., Anderson, T. J., Miller, W. R. & Dowsett, M. (2002b). Anastrozole demonstrates clinical and biological effectiveness in erbB2 ER positive breast cancers. *Breast Cancer Research and Treatment* **76**, A 263.

Eiermann, W., Paepke, S., Appfelstaedt, J., Llombart-Cussac, A., Eremin, J., Vinholes, J., Mauriac, L., Ellis, M., Lassus, M., Chaudri-Ross, H. A. *et al.* (2001). Preoperative treatment of postmenopausal breast cancer patients with letrozole: a randomized double-blind multicenter study. *Annals of Oncology* **12**, 1527–1532.

Ellis, M. J., Coop, A., Singh, B., Mauriac, L., Llombert-Cussac, A., Janicke, F., Miller, W. R., Evans, D. B., Dugan, M., Brady, C. *et al.* (2001). Letrozole is more effective neoadjuvant endocrine therapy than tamoxifen for ERbB-1- and/or ErbB-2-positive, estrogen receptor-positive primary breast cancer: evidence from a phase III randomized trial. *Journal of Clinical Oncology* **19**, 3808–3816.

Ellis, P., Smith, I., Ashley, S., Walsh, G., Ebbs, S., Baum, M., Sacks, N. & McKinna, J. (1998). Clinical prognostic and predictive factors for primary chemotherapy in operable breast cancer. *Journal of Clinical Oncology* **16**, 107–114.

Eltahir, A., Heys, S. D., Hutcheon, A. W., Sarkar, T. K., Smith, I., Walker, L. G., Ah-See, A. & Eremin, O. (1998). Treatment of large and locally advanced breast cancers using neoadjuvant chemotherapy. *American Journal of Surgery* **175**, 127–132.

Euler, U., Dresel, V., Buhner, M., Volkholz, H. & Tulusan, A. H. T. (2002). Dose and time intensified epirubicin/cyclophosphamide (EC) as preoperative treatment in locally advanced breast cancer. *Breast Cancer Research and Treatment* **76**, abstract 154, p. S51.

Evans, T., Gould, A., Foster, E., Crown, J. P., Leonard, R. & Mansi, J. (2002). Phase III randomised trial of adriamycin (A) and docetaxel (D) versus A and cyclophosphamide (C) as primary medical therapy (PMT) in women with breast cancer: andACCOG study. *Proceedings of the American Society of Clinical Oncology* **21**, A 136, 35a.

Fisher, B., Brown, A., Mamounas, E., Wieand, S., Robidoux, A., Margolese, R. G., Cruz, A. B., J., Fisher, E. R., Wickerham, D. L., Wolmark, N. *et al.* (1997). Effect of preoperative chemotherapy on local–regional disease in women with operable breast cancer: findings from National Surgical Adjuvant Breast and Bowel Project B-18. *Journal of Clinical Oncology* **15**, 2483–2493.

Fisher, B., Bryant, J., Wolmark, N., Mamounas, E., Brown, A., Fisher, E. R., Wickerham, D. L., Begovic, M., DeCillis, A., Robidoux, A. *et al.* (1998). Effect of preoperative chemotherapy on the outcome of women with operable breast cancer. *Journal of Clinical Oncology* **16**, 2672–2685.

Fisher, E. R., Wang, J., Bryant, J., Fisher, B., Mamounas, E. & Wolmark, N. (2002). Pathobiology of preoperative chemotherapy: findings from the National Surgical Adjuvant Breast and Bowel (NSABP) protocol B-18. *Cancer* **95**, 681–695.

Foudraine, N. A., Verhoef, L. C. G. & Burghouts, J. T. M. (1992). Tamoxifen as sole therapy for primary breast cancer in the elderly patient. *European Journal of Cancer* **28A**, 900–903.

Gianni, L., Baselga, J., Eiermann, W., Guillem Porta, V., Semiglazov, V., Garcia-Conde, J., Zambetti, M., Valagussa, P. & Bonadonna, G. (2002). First Report of the European Cooperative Trial in operable breast cancer (ECTO): effects of primary systemic therapy (PST) on loco-regional disease. *Proceedings of the American Society of Clinical Oncology* **21**, A132, p. 34a.

Kuerer, H. M., Newman, L. A., Smith, T. L., Ames, F. C., Hunt, K. K., Dhingra, K., Theriault, R. L., Singh, G., Binkley, S. M. & Sneige, N. *et al.* (1999). Clinical course of breast cancer patients with complete pathologic primary tumor and axillary lymph node response to doxorubicin-based neoadjuvant chemotherapy. *Journal of Clinical Oncology* **17**, 460–469.

Makris, A. (1998). A reduction in the requirements for mastectomy in a randomized trial of neoadjuvant chemoendocrine therapy in primary breast cancer. *Annals of Oncology* **9**, 1179–1184.

Makris, A., Powles, T. J., Dowsett, M., Osborne, C. K., Trott, P. A., Fernando, I. N., Ashley, S. E., Ormerod, M. G., Titley, J. C., Gregory, R. K. *et al.* (1997). Prediction of response to neoadjuvant chemoendocrine therapy in primary breast carcinomas. *Clinical Cancer Research* **3**, 593–600.

Mauriac, L., Durand, M., Avril, A. & Dilhuydy, J-M. (1991). Effects of primary chemotherapy in conservative treatment of breast cancer patients with operable tumours larger than 3 cm. *Annals of Oncology* **2**, 347–354.

Minton, S. E., Muro-Cacho, C., Diaz, N., Bowman, T., Cox, C., Dupont, E., Shons, A., Fields, K., Dalton, W. & Sullivan, J. (2002). A phase III neoadjuvant tral of sequential doxorubicin and docetaxel for the treatment of stage III breast cancer measuring signal transducers and activators of transcription (STAT) activation of response to therapy. *Proceedings of the American Society of Clinical Oncology* **21**, A 125, p. 32a.

Mustacchi, G., Milani, S., Pluchinotta, A., De Matteis, A., Rubagotti, A. & Perrota, A. (1994). Tamoxifen or surgery plus tamoxifen as primary treatment for elderly patients with operable breast cancer: The G.R.E.T.A. trial. *Anticancer Research* **14**, 2197–2200.

Pierga, J. Y. (2000). Prognostic value of persistent node involvement after neoadjuvant chemotherapy in patients with operable breast cancer. *British Journal of Cancer* **83**, 1480–1487.

Powles, T. J. (1995). Randomized trial of chemoendocrine therapy started before or after surgery for treatment of primary breast cancer. *Journal of Clinical Oncology* **13**, 547–552.

Remvikos, Y., Mosseri, V., Zajdela, A., Fourquet, A., Durand, J. C., Pouillart, P. & Magdelenat, H. (1993). Prognostic value of the S-phase fraction of breast cancers treated by primary radiotherapy or neoadjuvant chemotherapy. *Annals of the New York Academy of Science* **698**, 193–203.

Rouzier, R. (2002). Incidence and prognostic significance of complete axillary downstaging after primary chemotherapy in breast cancer patients with T1 to T3 tumors and cytologically proven axillary metastatic lymph nodes. *Journal of Clinical Oncology* **20**, 1304–1310.

Scholl, S. M. (1995). Neoadjuvant versus adjuvant chemotherapy in premenopausal patients with tumours considered too large for conserving surgery: an update. *Anti-Cancer Drugs* **6** (Suppl. 2), 69 (abstract P48).

Scholl, S. M., Fourquet, A., Asselain, B., Pierga, J. Y., Vicoq, J. R., Durand, J. C., Dorval, T., Palangié, T., Jouve, M., Beuzeboc, P. *et al.* (1994). Neoadjuvant versus adjuvant chemotherapy in premenopausal patients with tumours considered too large for breast conserving surgery: preliminary results of a randomised trial: S6. *European Journal of Cancer* **30A**, 645–652.

Scholl, S. M., Pierga, J. Y., Asselain, B., Buezeboc, P., Dorval, T., Garcia-Giralt, E., Jouve, M., Palangié, T., Remvikos, Y., Durand, J. C. *et al.* (1996). Breast tumour response to primary chemotherapy predicts local and distant control as well as survival. *European Journal of Cancer* **31A**, 1969–1975.

Semiglazov, V. F. (1994). Primary (neoadjuvant) chemotherapy and radiotherapy compared with primary radiotherapy alone in stage IIb–IIIa breast cancer. *Annals of Oncology* **5**, 591–595.

Smith, I. C., Heys, S. D., Hutcheon, A. W., Miller, I. D., Payne, S., Gilbert, F. J., Ah-See, A. K., Eremin, O., Walker, L. G., Sarkar, T. K. *et al.* (2002). Neoadjuvant chemotherapy in breast cancer: significantly enhanced response with docetaxel. *Journal of Clinical Oncology* **20**, 1456–1466.

Valero, V. (2002). Pathologically involved axillary lymph nodes following primary chemotherapy (PCT) in locally advanced breast cancer (LABC) is an early biological prongostic factor of long-term outcome in LABC: The University of Texas M.D. Anderson Cancer Center experience. *European Journal of Cancer* **13**, 37 (abstract 132P).

van der Hage, J. A., van de Velde, C. J. H., Julien, J. P., Tubiana-Hulin, M., Vandervelden, C. & Duchateau, L. (2001). Preoperative chemotherapy in primary operable breast cancer: results from the European Organization for Research and Treatment of Cancer trial 10902. *Journal of Clinical Oncology* **19**, 4224–4237.

Wolmark, N., Wang, J., Mamounas, E., Bryant, J. & Fisher, B. (2001). Preoperative chemotherapy in patients with operable breast cancer: nine-year results from National Surgical Adjuvant Breast and Bowel Project B-18. *Journal of the National Cancer Institute Monographs* **30**, 96–102.

Chapter 11

# Can a 'low-risk' subgroup be identified in whom radiotherapy can be safely omitted after breast conservation surgery?

*Charlotte Westbury and John Yarnold*

## The contribution of postoperative radiotherapy to survival

The systematic overview of radiotherapy effects in more than 17,000 women with early breast cancer, published in 2000, combined results of mastectomy and postoperative radiotherapy, with approximately 6000 women randomised to radiotherapy after breast conservation surgery (Early Breast Cancer Trialists' Collaborative Group 2000). In this important subgroup, radiotherapy achieved a 14% (standard error or SE = 7) reduction in the annual odds of death from breast cancer, without any excess non-breast cancer mortality to date. Overall, the overview demonstrates that avoidance of 20 local recurrences by radiotherapy prevents 5 breast cancer deaths, a remarkably favourable 4:1 ratio. Radiotherapy after breast-conservation surgery and axillary dissection included the breast, but not the internal mammary chain or, in general, the axilla or supraclavicular fossa. This contrasts with patients entered into the post-mastectomy trials, most of whom received radiotherapy to all regional lymph node sites. In this respect, the two groups of patients may not be totally comparable in terms of estimating reductions in local recurrence and mortality risks. Nevertheless, it is absolutely clear that effective local–regional control is a determinant of cure in women with early stage breast cancer.

## Identification of 'low-risk' subgroups after breast-conservation surgery

An increasing proportion of women present via the screening programme with small, low-grade tumours, and the question arises as to whether a 'low-risk' group can be identified, in whom post-excision radiotherapy should be omitted. The definition of a 'low-risk' group is subjective, but some guidance can be obtained from current practice relating to adjuvant systemic therapies, e.g. international consensus guidelines suggest that adjuvant cytotoxic chemotherapy is considered for patients with an absolute survival gain of 2% or more at 10 years (Eifel *et al.* 2001; Goldhirsch *et al.* 2001). Taking this level of benefit as a reference point, the prevention of two breast cancer deaths involves the prevention of eight local recurrences. The subgroup with this level of benefit is one with a local recurrence risk of 10% at 10 years after optimal breast-conservation surgery. Can subgroups of women be reliably identified who have local recurrence risks significantly less than 10% after breast conservation surgery?

Risk factors for local recurrence after breast-conservation surgery identified in retrospective multivariate analyses include age under 40 years, surgical resection margin, lymph node status, the presence of lymphovascular invasion, increasing tumour size and grade, and the presence of an extensive intraductal component (Clemons *et al.* 2001). It is not certain that any combination of factors reliably identifies patients with a local recurrence risk that is significantly less than 10% at 10 years. However, a number of prospective trials have attempted to define low-risk patients, in whom omission of radiotherapy after breast-conserving surgery does not compromise local control, and they are reviewed below.

## Trials of breast-conserving surgery alone with or without radiotherapy

Several prospective studies have investigated whether radiotherapy can be safely omitted in well-defined 'low-risk' groups in whom adjuvant systemic therapy is not given (Table 11.1). These studies differ in terms of tumour features used to define low risk and also extent of surgery. Median follow-up varies from 2 to 20 years and overall local recurrence rates in patients not receiving radiotherapy are 16–36%.

Three studies involved women with unicentric tumours ≤ 2 cm and negative axillary lymph nodes. The Boston group (Schnitt *et al.* 1996) performed an observational study of tumour excision alone. All patients required re-excision to achieve clear margins. A breast recurrence rate of 16% was reported at a median follow-up of 56 months, and the trial was terminated early. An update at 86 months in abstract form (Lim *et al.* 1999) reported a risk of recurrence of approximately 2.8% per year. All other studies reviewed are randomised controlled trials of breast-conserving surgery alone or with postoperative radiotherapy. Holli *et al.* (2001) also strictly defined a subgroup by tumour size ≤ 2 cm and other favourable features. They showed that, after lumpectomy and axillary lymph node dissection, the 5-year actuarial local relapse rates were 6.3% in the group assigned to radiotherapy and 14.1% in the group not given radiotherapy.

The Uppsala–Orebro Breast Cancer Study Group (1990; Liljegren *et al.* 1994, 1999) investigated whether more extensive surgery resulted in better outcome for small tumours. They showed that, even in patients with tumours ≤ 2 cm undergoing sector resection and axillary lymph node dissection, surgery alone resulted in unacceptable rates of local failure, and that the addition of radiotherapy resulted in significantly improved outcome. They also showed the importance of longer follow-up for evaluation of local control. At a 10-year update they demonstrated significantly higher rates of local relapse than had been quoted in their initial report at an interim period of 30 months (Table 11.2). An update performed at 5 years showed that without radiotherapy the local recurrence rates approached 20% (Liljegren *et al.* 1994). At 10

**Table 11.1** Patient characteristics in trials of breast-conserving surgery alone with or without radiotherapy

| Trial | Design | Age | Tumour characteristics | Surgery/margins | Systemic therapy |
|---|---|---|---|---|---|
| Schnitt *et al.* (1996) Lim *et al.* update (1999) | Prospective one-arm trial ($n$ = 87) | None specified | ≤ 2 cm Infiltrating ductal, tubular or mucinous Unicentric EIC–ve, LVI–ve, LN–ve | BCS not specified Note: all patients had re-excision 1-cm margin | None |
| Holli *et al.* (2001) | RCT ($n$ = 152) | > 40 years old | < 2 cm visible on mammogram Unicentric EIC–ve Grade I–II PgR+ve LN–ve | Lumpectomy and axillary LN dissection 1-cm margin | None |
| Uppsala-Orebo (1990) Liljegren *et al.* update (1994, 1999) | RCT ($n$ = 381) | < 80 years old | ≤ 2 cm Visible on mammogram Unicentric LN–ve | Sector resection and axillary LN dissection Margin > 2 cm | None |
| Clark *et al.* (1992, 1996) | RCT ($n$ = 837) | No age criteria | ≤ 4 cm Unicentric LN–ve | Lumpectomy and axillary dissection Clear margins | None |
| Fisher *et al.* (2002) update (NSABP B-06) | RCT Three-arm (lumpectomy ± RT reviewed ($n$ = 1137) | No age criteria | ≤ 4 cm LN–ve or +ve | Lumpectomy and axillary dissection Clear margins | None in LN–ve (chemo-therapy in LN+ve) |

BCS, breast-conserving surgery; EIC, presence of extensive intraductal component; LN–ve, histologically negative axillary lymph nodes; LN+ve, histologically positive axillary lymph nodes; LVI, presence of lymphovascular invasion; PgR/ER +ve/–ve= positive or negative for progesterone/oestrogen receptors; RCT, randomised controlled trial; RT, radiotherapy.

years local recurrence was 24% in the group that did not receive radiotherapy, and was reduced by one-third to 8.5% in the group that did (Liljegren *et al.* 1999).

**Table 11.2** Results of Uppsala–Orebro group

| Trial | Follow-up | Local recurrence risk, BCS + no radiation (%)[a] | Local recurrence risk, BCS + radiation (%)[a] |
|---|---|---|---|
| Uppsala–Orebro (1990) | No radiation 27.5 months | 3 years 7.6 (3.0–12.3) | 3 years: 2.9 (0.1–5.8) |
| | Radiation 30.8 months | Estimated 5 years 10.2 | Estimated 5 years: 2.9 |
| Liljegren *et al.* (1994) (update) | 5 years | 18.4 (12.5–24.2) | 2.3 (0.1–4.3) |
| Liljegren *et al.* (1999) (update) | 10 years | 24.0 (17.6–30.4) | 8.5 (3.9–13.1) |

BCS, breast-conserving surgery.
[a]95% confidence intervals quoted.

The Uppsala–Orebro group further attempted to define a low-risk population by carrying out a multivariate analysis of risk factors for relapse. They defined a group of women older than 55 years and with favourable histological subtypes who made up 46% of the study population. Among these, the 10-year local recurrence risk without radiotherapy was 11%, which still remains above the working definition of 10% for 'low risk'.

Although greater tumour size has been shown to be a risk factor for local recurrence in some studies, other investigators have defined low-risk tumours using 4 cm as a cut-off for size. A group from Ontario (Clark *et al.* 1992, 1996) selected patients with tumours ≤ 4 cm and node-negative disease. They reported results at a median follow-up of 7.6 years; 11.3% patients developed local recurrence in the radiotherapy group compared with 35.2% in the no radiotherapy group. Using multivariate analysis, they were unable to define a low-risk group. Women with tumours ≤ 1 cm had a cumulative rate of local relapse of 28.5% without radiotherapy and, for patients who were 50 years or older with low-grade tumours, the rate was 24%.

Fisher *et al.* (2002) reported updated results from the NSABP-06 trial. Patients in this trial had tumours ≤ 4 cm, with positive or negative axillary disease. Women were randomised to undergo mastectomy, lumpectomy and radiotherapy or lumpectomy alone and did not receive systemic therapy if node negative. After 20 years, the cumulative incidence of ipsilateral breast recurrence in node-negative women was 36.2% in the group randomised to lumpectomy and was reduced to 17% in those receiving lumpectomy and radiotherapy. Subgroup analysis of patients with tumours ≤1 cm receiving lumpectomy alone showed unacceptable relapse rates of 25% at 8 years, and a benefit for using radiotherapy (Fisher *et al.* 1992).

The importance of longer follow-up for evaluation of outcome was also demonstrated in this study. For the surgery alone group, 26.8% of local recurrences occurred after 5 years and this rate was 60.3% in the group treated by surgery and radiotherapy.

## Trials of breast-conserving surgery and systemic therapy with or without radiotherapy

In the past few years the adjuvant use of tamoxifen and chemotherapy has become more widespread. Systemic therapy may contribute to reducing local recurrence but, in most women, it is unlikely to be sufficient to achieve a significant reduction without radiotherapy. Fisher *et al.* (2001) combined results from the National Surgical Adjuvant Breast and Bowel Project (NSABP) trials showing that the addition of chemotherapy to lumpectomy and radiotherapy further reduced the rate of locoregional recurrence in good prognosis tumours measuring < 1 cm. The reduction in recurrence in oestrogen receptor (ER)-negative patients treated with chemotherapy was from 8% to 4% and in ER-positive patients who received combined chemotherapy and tamoxifen 6% to 5%. Dalberg *et al.* (1998) also showed that, in postmenopausal women undergoing sector resection and radiotherapy, the 10-year cumulative risk of ipsilateral recurrence was reduced from 12% in those not receiving systemic therapy to 3% in those treated with tamoxifen.

Further trials have investigated whether systemic treatment combined with surgery alone is sufficient in preventing recurrence in good prognosis tumours (Table 11.3). The NSABP B-21 (Fisher *et al.* 2002) compared lumpectomy and axillary dissection with the addition of tamoxifen, radiotherapy or a combination of the two in women with node negative tumours of ≤1 cm. For patients taking tamoxifen, the 8 year cumulative incidence of local recurrence was 16.5% in the no radiation arm and reduced to 2.8% with radiotherapy.

The British Association of Surgical Oncology (BASO) II trial, presented in abstract form (Blamey *et al.* 2002), is also currently investigating the role of radiotherapy in patients with node negative tumours ≤2 cm who are receiving tamoxifen. Updated results at 35 months of median follow-up show recurrence rates of 1.2% per year in the no-radiotherapy arm. Interpretation is difficult because of short follow-up. The German Breast Cancer Study Group (Winzer *et al.* 2004) investigated the role of tamoxifen and radiotherapy in reducing local recurrence rates for women with similar tumour characteristics (≤2 cm and other favourable features). This study used a 2 × 2 factorial design comparing breast conserving surgery alone with surgery and radiotherapy, surgery and tamoxifen and the combination of all three treatments. The trial was small and there were too few events in the adjuvant therapy arms to establish the relative benefits of tamoxifen, radiotherapy or both in addition to surgery. Local recurrence appeared to be reduced in all adjuvant arms.

Fyles *et al.* (2001) investigated a group incorporating larger, node negative tumours (≤5 cm) in a subgroup of patients older than 50, taking tamoxifen. Local recurrence rates were reduced significantly with radiotherapy (6% to 0.3 % at 4 years), but again longer follow-up is required.

**Table 11.3** Patient characteristics in trials of breast-conserving surgery and systemic therapy with or without radiotherapy

| Trial | Design | Age (years) | Tumour characteristics | Surgery/ margins | Systemic therapy |
|---|---|---|---|---|---|
| Fisher *et al.* (2002) (NSABP B-21) | RCT, 3-arm (*n* = 1009) | none specified | ≤ 1 cm LN–ve | Lumpectomy and axillary dissection Clear margins | ± Tamoxifen |
| Blamey *et al.* (2002) (BASO II) | RCT (*n* = 1122) | < 70 | ≤ 2 cm Grade1 or special histological type LN–ve | Wide local excision Clear margins | Tamoxifen |
| Veronesi *et al.* (1993) Update (1995 and 2001) | RCT (*n* = 567) | ≤ 70 | < 2.5 cm LN+ve or –ve | Quadrantectomy and axillary dissection Clear margins | CMF and/or tamoxifen |
| Forrest *et al.* (1996) | RCT (*n* = 585) | < 70 | ≤ 4 cm Premenopausal LN–ve Postmenopausal LN+ve or –ve | Lumpectomy and axillary dissection 1-cm margin | CMF or tamoxifen |
| Hughes *et al.* (2001) (CALGB) | RCT (*n* = 647) | ≥ 70 | Stage I ER+ve | Lumpectomy | Tamoxifen |
| Fyles *et al.* (2001) | RCT (*n* = 769) | > 50 | ≤ 5 cm LN-ve | Not specified | Tamoxifen |
| Winzer *et al.* (2004) | RCT 2 x 2 factorial (*n* = 347) | 45–75 | ≤ 2 cm LN-ve Grade 1–2 LVI-ve EIC -ve Er +ve and/or PgR +ve | Not specified Clear margins | +/- Tamoxifen |
| Renton *et al.* (1996) | RCT (*n* = 418) | Not specified | ≤ 5 cm LN-ve or +ve | WLE Margin status categorised | CMF (ER-ve) Tamoxifen (ER+ve) |
| Malstrom *et al.* (2003) | RCT (*n* = 1187) | < 76 | ≤ 5 cm LN-ve | Sector resection and axillary dissection Clear margins | CMF (*n* = 24) Tamoxifen (*n* = 83) |

BASO, British Association of Surgical Oncology; BCS, breast-conserving surgery; CALGB, North American Cooperative Intergroup Cancer and Leukemia Group B; CMF, cyclophosphamide, methotrexate and 5-fluorouracil; LN–ve, histologically negative axillary lymph nodes; LN+ve, histologically positive axillary lymph nodes; LVI, presence of lymphovascular invasion; NSABP, National Surgical Adjuvant Breast and Bowel Project; PgR/ER +ve/–ve= positive or negative for progesterone/oestrogen receptors; RCT, randomised controlled trial.

Renton *et al.* (1996) performed a randomised trial of radiotherapy versus none after breast conservation in patients with tumours ≤5 cm, including those with node positive disease. All received systemic therapy. They demonstrated the importance of margin status in determining local recurrence risks and also showed unacceptable rates of recurrence of 22% in patients with clear margins not receiving radiotherapy. In patients receiving radiotherapy due to incomplete excision, recurrence rates were 17% compared with 12% in patients with clear margins. Of note, two-thirds of patients in this group had crossed over from the no radiation to radiotherapy arm because of positive margin status.

Forrest *et al.* (1996) looked at a subgroup of women with cancers measuring up to 4 cm. Premenopausal patients were required to have negative nodal status but postmenopausal women with node positive disease were eligible. All patients received systemic therapy with either tamoxifen or chemotherapy. Patients who did not receive radiotherapy had a significantly higher rate of local relapse of 24.5% at 5.7 years, reduced by radiotherapy to 5.8%.

The Milan group (Veronesi *et al.* 1993, 1995, 2001) performed a randomised trial of quadrantectomy and axillary node dissection with or without radiotherapy. Women had tumours < 2.5 cm in diameter and node-positive or -negative disease. The most recent update (Veronesi *et al.* 2001) showed that there was a significantly higher rate of local relapse in patients who did not undergo radiotherapy than those who did, with a 10-year cumulative incidence of 23.5% and 5.8% respectively (Table 11.4). Consistent with the Uppsala–Orebro group data, they concluded that more extensive surgery with quadrantectomy, combined with systemic therapy, was insufficient in this group of patients to provide acceptable local control rates. They also suggested that risk of local relapse without radiotherapy reduced with age and that the rate was more than halved in patients over 46 years of age compared with those younger than 45 years. In patients over 65 years of age, the rates of local recurrence were very low and were not reduced by radiotherapy. They proposed that women > 65 years formed a low-risk group in whom radiotherapy could be avoided. This was a retrospective subgroup analysis involving small numbers of events in patients > 65 years of age, useful for hypothesis generation about this age group but from which firm conclusions cannot be made.

Malstrom *et al.* (2003) investigated women from a screening population with node negative breast cancers in which a minority received systemic therapy. Sixty-five percent of women had tumours detected by screening. Radiotherapy reduced 5-year local recurrence rates from 14% to 4%. There appeared to be a lower risk of local recurrence after surgery in the screened population than in patients with clinically detected disease. This difference in local recurrence rates may be explained by more favourable tumours in the screened group, although the authors do not compare patient or tumour characteristics between the two groups.

**Table 11.4** Results of Milan III trial

| Trial | Follow-up | Local recurrence risk, BCS + no radiation (%) | Local recurrence risk, BCS + radiation (%) |
|---|---|---|---|
| Veronesi *et al.* (1993) | 39 months | 8.8 | 0.3 |
| Veronesi *et al.* (1995) (update) | No radiation 52 months [a]Radiation 82 months | 11.7 | [a]3.3 (*n* = 1006, Milan trials I–III) |
| Veronesi *et al.* (2001) (update) | 12 years | 23.5 (10-year cumulative) | 5.8 (10-year cumulative) |

BCS, breast-conserving surgery.
95% confidence intervals quoted
[a]BCS and radiation arm analysed for all patients in this arm in Milan I–III studies.

Observations made by the Milan group (Veronesi *et al.* 2001) and other authors (Liljegren *et al.* 1999) have led to the suggestion that local recurrence rates decline with age, independently of known prognostic factors. This has raised the question of whether radiotherapy can be omitted in a subset of elderly patients, but there is a paucity of data. The North American Cooperative Intergroup Cancer and Leukemia Group B (CALGB) (Hughes *et al.* 2001) have reported preliminary results of a trial of women aged 70 years or older with stage 1, ER-positive tumours treated with lumpectomy plus tamoxifen. At a follow-up of 28 months, they report a low recurrence risk in the group not receiving radiotherapy of 0.9% per year. The projected 10-year recurrence risk therefore approaches 10%. The actual 10-year figure may be higher than estimated here because local recurrence rates are always very low in the first year, and this leads to an underestimate of annual risk.

None of these prospective trials has therefore so far demonstrated a low-risk group in whom the risk of local recurrence with surgery alone is less than 10%. Definition of a low-risk subgroup is difficult even when a number of patient or tumour features that apparently confer good prognosis have been selected after multivariate analysis.

## Conclusion

None of the individual trials reviewed above was powered to detect a survival benefit. Recent data to support a survival benefit for radiotherapy comes from a pooled analysis of 13 trials of breast conserving surgery and radiotherapy (Vinh-Hung *et al.* 2004). This study demonstrated an 8.6% excess overall mortality risk for omission of radiotherapy (95% CI = 0.3–17.5%). Longer follow-up in many of these trials is necessary for accurate estimation of recurrence rates, to determine late side effects of radiotherapy beyond 10 years and to perform analysis estimating the magnitude of survival benefit. Based on the data reviewed above, it does not seem possible to make a reliable identification of patients in whom the risk of local recurrence is low enough to omit radiotherapy safely. This statement applies to tumours excised by quadrantectomy and to patients also treated with adjuvant systemic therapy, including cytotoxic chemotherapy and/or tamoxifen. This is not to say that very-low-risk subgroups do not exist. It is just that the planned omission of breast radiotherapy compromises cure prospects to a clinically significant degree. Ultimately, the issues of local control, breast cancer cure and radiotherapy morbidity need to be discussed with patients as part of a dialogue that establishes where the optimal balance of treatment lies.

## *References*

Blamey, R. W., Chetty, U., Mitchell, A. *et al.* (2002). The BASO II trial of adjuvant radiotherapy v none and tamoxifen v none in small node negative, grade I tumours. *European Journal of Cancer* **38**, S149 (abstract 413).

Clark, R. M., McCulloch, P. B., Levine, M. N. *et al.* (1992). Randomized trial to assess the effectiveness of breast irradiation following lumpectomy and axillary dissection for node-negative breast cancer. *Journal of the National Cancer Institute* **84**, 683–689.

Clark, R. M., Whelan, T., Levine, M. *et al.* (1996). Randomized clinical trial of breast irradiation following lumpectomy and axillary dissection for node-negative breast cancer: an update. *Journal of the National Cancer Institute* **88**, 1659–1664.

Clemons, M., Danson, S., Hamilton, T., Goss, P. (2001). Locoregionally recurrent breast cancer: incidence, risk factors and survival. *Cancer Treatment Reviews* **27**, 67–82.

Dalberg, K., Johansson, H., Johansson, U. *et al.* (1998). A randomized trial of long term adjuvant tamoxifen plus postoperative radiation therapy versus radiation therapy alone for patients with early stage breast carcinoma treated with breast-conserving surgery. *Cancer* **82**, 2204–2211.

Early Breast Cancer Trialists' Collaborative Group (2000). Favourable and unfavourable effects on long-term survival of radiotherapy for early breast cancer: an overview of the randomised trials. *The Lancet* **355**, 1757–1770.

Eifel, P., Axelson, J. A., Costa, J. *et al.* (2001). National Institutes of Health Consensus Development Conference Statement: Adjuvant therapy for breast cancer, November 1–3, 2000. *Journal of the National Cancer Institute* **93**, 979–989.

Fisher, B., Redmond, C. *et al.* (1992). Lumpectomy for breast cancer: an update of the NSABP experience. National Surgical Adjuvant Breast and Bowel Project. *Journal of the National Cancer Institute Monographs* **11**, 7–13.

Fisher, B., Anderson, S., Bryant, J. *et al.* (2002). Twenty-year follow-up of a randomized trial comparing total mastectomy, lumpectomy, and lumpectomy plus irradiation for the treatment of invasive breast cancer. *New England Journal of Medicine* **347**, 1233–1241.

Fisher, B., Bryant, J., Dignam, J. J. *et al.* (2002). Tamoxifen, radiation therapy, or both for prevention of ipsilateral breast tumor recurrence after lumpectomy in women with invasive breast cancers of one centimeter or less. *Journal of Clinical Oncology* **20**, 4141–4149.

Fisher, B., Dignam, J., Tan-Chiu, E. *et al.* (2001). Prognosis and treatment of patients with breast tumors of one centimeter or less and negative axillary lymph nodes. *Journal of the National Cancer Institute* **93**, 112–120.

Forrest, A. P., Stewart, H. J., Everington, D. *et al.* (1996). Randomised controlled trial of conservation therapy for breast cancer: 6 year analysis of the Scottish trial. *The Lancet* **348**, 708–713.

Fyles, A., McCready, D., Manchul, L. *et al.* (2001). Preliminary results of a randomized study of tamoxifen +/- breast radiation in T1/2 N0 disease in women over 50 years of age. *Proceedings of the American Society of Clinical Oncology* **24a**, (abstract 92).

Goldhirsch, A., Glick, J. H., Gelber, R. D. *et al.* (2001). Meeting highlights: International Consensus Panel on the Treatment of Primary Breast Cancer. Seventh International Conference on Adjuvant Therapy of Primary Breast Cancer. *Journal of Clinical Oncology* **19**, 3817–3827.

Holli, K., Saaristo, R., Isola, J. *et al.* (2001). Lumpectomy with or without postoperative radiotherapy for breast cancer with favourable prognostic features: results of a randomized study. *British Journal of Cancer* **84**, 164–169.

Hughes, K. S., Schnaper, L., Berry, D. *et al.* (2001). Comparison of lumpectomy plus tamoxifen with and without radiotherapy (RT) in women 70 years of age or older who have clinical stage I, estrogen receptor positive (ER+) breast carcinoma. *Proceedings of the American Society of Clinical Oncology* 24a, (abstract 93).

Liljegren, G., Holmberg, L., Adami, H-O. *et al.* (1994). Sector resection with or without postoperative radiotherapy for stage I breast cancer: five-year results of a randomised trial. *Journal of the National Cancer Institute* **86**, 717–722.

Liljegren, G., Holmberg, L., Bergh, J. *et al.* (1999). 10-year results after sector resection with or without postoperative radiotherapy for stage I breast cancer: A randomised trial. *Journal of Clinical Oncology* **17**, 2326–2333.

Lim, M., Nixon, A. J., Gelman, R. *et al.* (1999). A prospective study of conservative surgery (CS) alone without radiotherapy (RT) in selected patients with stage I breast cancer. *Breast Cancer Research and Treatment* **57**, 34.

Malmstrom, P., Holmberg, L., Anderson, H. *et al.* (2003). Breast conservation surgery, with and without radiotherapy, in women with lymph node-negative breast cancer: a randomised clinical trial in a population with access to public mammography screening. *European Journal of Cancer* **39**, 1690–1697.

Renton, S. C., Gazet, J. C., Ford, H. T. *et al.* (1996). The importance of the resection margin in conservative surgery for breast cancer. *European Journal of Surgical Oncology* **22**, 17–22.

Schnitt, S. J., Hayman, J., Gelman, R. *et al.* (1996). A prospective study of conservative surgery alone in the treatment of selected patients with stage I breast cancer. *Cancer* **77**, 1094–1100.

Uppsala–Orebro Breast Cancer Study Group (1990). Sector resection with or without postoperative radiotherapy for stage I breast cancer: A randomised trial. *Journal of the National Cancer Institute* **82**, 277–282.

Veronesi, U., Luini, A., del Vecchio, M. *et al.* (1993). Radiotherapy after breast-preserving surgery in women with localised cancer of the breast. *New England Journal of Medicine* **328**, 1587–1591.

Veronesi, U., Salvadori, B., Luini, A. *et al.* (1995). Breast conservation is a safe method in patients with small cancer of the breast. Long-term results of three randomised trials on 1,973 patients. *European Journal of Cancer* **31A**, 1574–1579.

Veronesi, U., Marubini, E., Mariani, L. *et al.* (2001). Radiotherapy after breast-conserving surgery in small breast carcinoma: Long-term results of a randomised trial. *Annals of Oncology* **12**, 997–1003.

Vinh-Hung, V., Verschraegen, C. *et al.* (2004). Breast-conserving surgery with or without radiotherapy: pooled-analysis for risks of ipsilateral breast tumor recurrence and mortality. *Journal of the National Cancer Institute* **96**, 115–121.

Winzer, K. J., Sauer, R., Sauerbrei, W. *et al.* (2004). Radiation therapy after breast-conserving surgery; first results of a randomised clinical trial in patients with low risk of recurrence. *European Journal of Cancer* **40**, 998–1005.

# Chapter 12

# Identification of high risk of recurrence in breast-cancer patients by DNA chip technology

*Thomas Karn, Andre Ahr, Uwe Holtrich and Manfred Kaufmann*

## Introduction

Breast cancer is a major cause of death among women aged 35–55 years, affecting about 10% in Western countries. Despite important advances in therapy, still more than half of the affected patients suffer from relapses (Ries *et al.* 2000). This is in part due to the highly heterogeneous nature of the disease; the various pathological breast cancer subclasses have markedly different clinical courses and treatment responses. In patients with breast cancer, assessment of axillary lymph nodes and status of steroid hormone receptors are the most important prognostic factors, because they can be used to predict disease-free and overall survival, and to direct adjuvant systemic therapy. At the moment, most patients with lymph-node-negative disease (i.e., with no evidence that cancer cells have spread beyond the primary tumour) can be effectively treated with surgery and local radiation. Patients with more aggressive disease can benefit from adjuvant chemotherapy or hormone therapy and are currently identified according to a combination of criteria (Eifel *et al.* 2001; Goldhirsch *et al.* 2001): age, the size of the tumour, axillary-node status, the histologic type and pathological grade of cancer, and hormone-receptor status as depicted in Table 12.1. For the outcome of an individual patient, the currently available prognostic factors are associated with a broad range of risk of recurrence. Thus, the ability of these criteria to predict individual disease progression and clinical outcome is imperfect. This uncertainty in forecasting outcome means that some patients who need adjuvant treatment do not receive it, whereas others are unnecessarily treated and as a result are exposed to the risk of side effects without good reason. Improved tools are clearly needed for the assessment of prognosis in breast cancer. A major goal, therefore, is the development of an individual risk-profile system with high accuracy and reproducibility to estimate patients' prognosis and best treatment.

**Table 12.1** Prognostic factors and guidelines for adjuvant therapy

| Prognostic factor | Low risk | High risk | |
|---|---|---|---|
| Lymph node status | Negative | negative and | positive or |
| Tumour stage | T < 1 cm | T 1–2 cm or | T > 2 cm or |
| Grading | 1 | 2–3 and | — |
| Hormone receptor | Positive | positive | negative or |
| Age | > 35 yrs | > 35 yrs | < 35 yrs |
| Adjuvant therapy (Goldhirsch *et al.* 2001) | nil or tamoxifen | tamoxifen +/- chemotherapy | chemotherapy + tamoxifen (if ER- or PR-positive) |

## DNA chip technology and expression profiling

The completion of the Human Genome Project and the development of new, high-performance screening techniques have revolutionised the ways in which researchers can study the pathogenesis of disease. Analysis of the levels of expression of thousands of genes in parallel with the use of DNA chips has shown distinct patterns in different kinds of tumour. Because the expression of the genes is measured, such analysis is mostly referred to as expression profiling. We can use these patterns to classify histologically similar tumours into specific subtypes (Alizadeh *et al.* 2001), a process that provides clinically relevant information. Studies on mammary carcinomas could already categorise several subtypes of breast cancer (Alizadeh *et al* 2000; Perou *et al.* 2000). However, these studies mostly lacked correlation with classic clinical variables and follow-up data. Global determination of cellular transcriptional activity is expected to identify gene expression signatures that predict clinical behaviour of tumours.

Figure 12.1 gives a representation of this new technology: a so-called DNA chip or microarray basically represents a glass slide, which carries probes for all human genes. The probes are spotted as a systematic array and the location of each probe is known to the investigator. An RNA sample from the tumour is now labelled and applied to this chip. Afterwards the chip is analysed with special equipment and the activity of each gene can be deduced from the intensity of the corresponding spot. The final result of a DNA chip analysis tells us the activity of all human genes in the cells of the corresponding sample. We can imagine this as if you are looking inside the cells and monitor the cellular program that is running there. The large amount of data from those analyses has to be analysed further by using mathematical methods to identify marker sets of interest. In addition, these multidimensional data mostly do not make immediate sense to the human eye. However, computational analyses can identify relationships in the data from different tumours and present them for example as tree-like structures or as scatter plots scaled in three dimensions.

## Identification of high-risk patients

In a previous study, we applied DNA chip analyses to identify differentially expressed

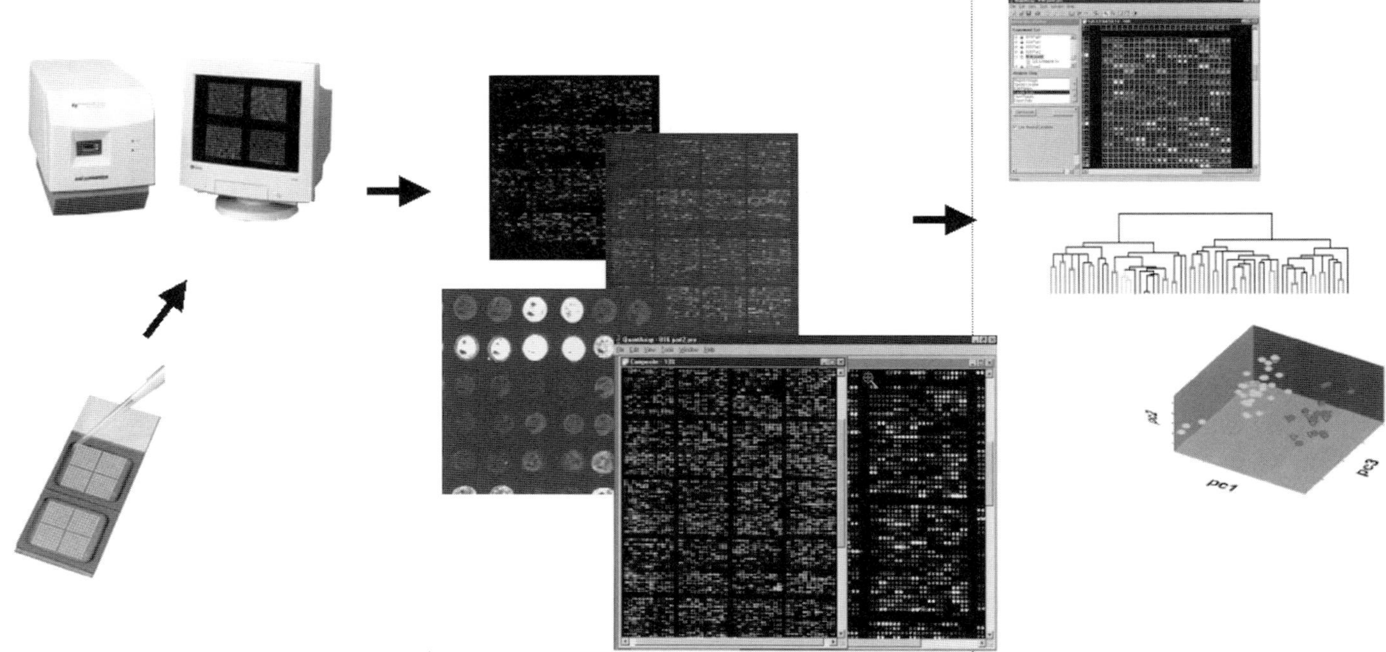

**Figure 12.1** Principle of the DNA chip technology. Left: labelled RNA from tumour samples is applied to the DNA chip and analysis is performed in a special fluorescence laser scanner. Middle: on the obtained electronic images each spot represents a probe for a individual human gene (note the microscopic spots in magnification) and the intensity of the spot correlates with the activity of this specific gene in the sample. A colour visualisation represents an array of thousands of those spots measuring the activity of thousands of different genes in the sample. Right: data are analysed by mathematical and statistical methods using special software; phenotypic relationships of different tumours can be graphically visualised. (A colour version of this diagram is available from the authors).

genes and to evaluate transcriptional diversity among human breast cancers (Ahr *et al.* 2001). The detected differentially expressed transcripts include several genes known from the literature, as well as previously unrecognised transcripts. We showed that class discovery analysis based on our gene expression profiling of 82 breast tissue specimens as well as some reference samples like cell lines identifies four main sample groups. A correlation of the cluster data with classical clinicopathological parameters revealed that one subgroup was characterised by a remarkably high number of node-positive tumours and a disproportionate number of patients who had already developed distant metastases at the time of diagnosis. These cluster analysis data suggested that the technique could help to define patients with an early onset of disease progression, providing a first step towards improved patient-adapted therapy.

Figure 12.2 shows a representation (available in colour from us) of the activity of 41 marker genes in 94 samples and as already mentioned, it is confusing for the human eye and difficult to find a structure in such data. However, computers can identify relationships between the tissue samples as represented by the tree-structure on the right. So we can analyse the resulting groups of patients according to their clinical data. Much easier to look at is the visualisation method in Figure 12.3, a principal component analysis (PCA) of the data from Figure 12.2, reducing the amount of information. From this we can clearly discriminate between two major tumour groups designated class A and non-A using this method. When one looks now at the clinical data of the patients, class A is characterised by many node-positive cases, suggesting a high risk of relapse for patients in this subgroup. This observation forced us to analyse the follow-up of the patients. And we found that nearly half of the patients in this group did suffer from a relapse in less than 2 years in contrast to only 11% in the other group (Ahr *et al.* 2002). Figure 12.4 shows the data for patients with available follow-up once more visualised by the tree like structure: The patients with a relapse are marked by red dots in the colour figure available from us; the clustering of those patients in class A, which is represented by red branches in this tree, is obvious. This accumulation cannot be explained by the number of lymph-node-positive patients, because these numbers are comparable in both groups. Strikingly, the high risk of patients in class A is further highlighted by the observation that three of the five node-negative patients in class A had a relapse in contrast to none of the 15 node-negative patients in class non-A.

Although validation studies with larger numbers need to be done, several lines of evidence support the suggestion that tumours of class A represent cancers with a high risk of recurrence. First, our initial clustering of the sample collective revealed an accumulation of tumours that had already developed distant metastases at diagnosis. Second, although class A and non-class-A contained similar numbers of node-positive tumours, progression was limited mainly to class A. Finally, we saw progression of node-negative tumours only in class A. Taken together, our cluster analysis identifies breast-cancer patients with a high risk of recurrence, and is a step towards the establishment of an individual risk-profile system. Future directions should combine

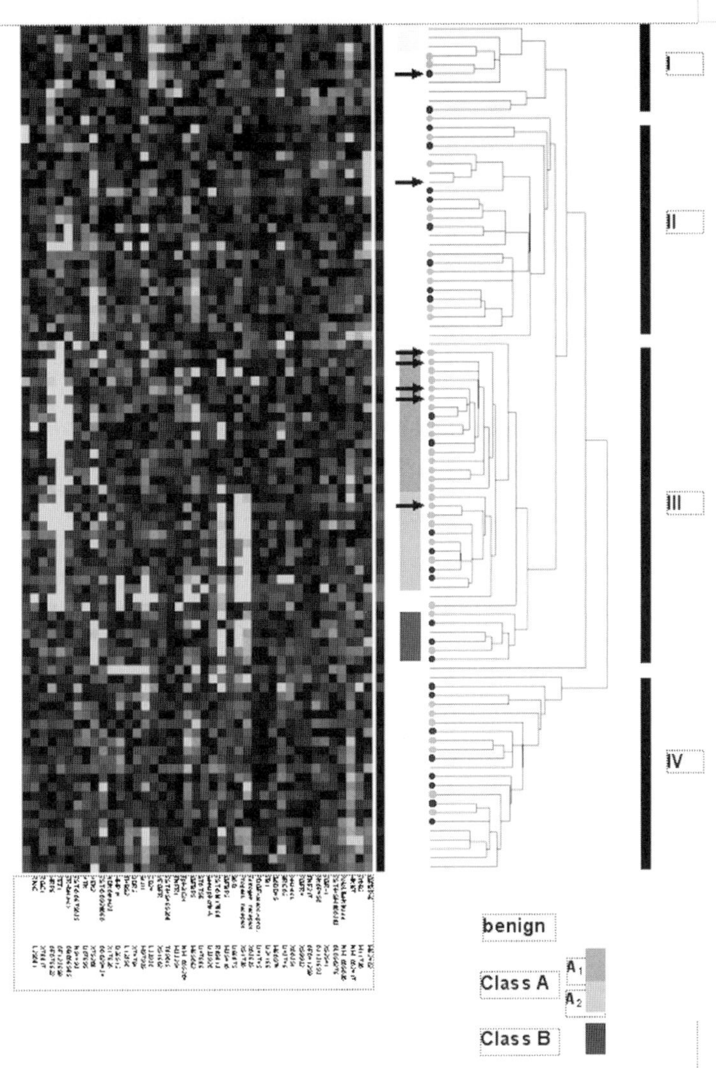


**Figure 12.2** Molecular classification of breast cancers. Genes repeatedly found to be differentially expressed in array analyses were applied in real-time polymerase chain reaction assays (TaqMan-technology) to perform a molecular tumour similarity classification of 82 normal and malignant breast specimens as well as reference samples. In the colour version of this diagram available from us, red indicates expression levels above median, green below. Each sample is represented by a horizontal line of the matrix. The columns refer to the analysed marker genes. The corresponding unrooted tree, where branch lengths represent distances (1, Pearson correlation coefficient) of samples as judged by their expression patterns, is depicted on the right. The four main sample groups (I–IV) are indicated by vertical bars on the right. For further information see Ahr *et al.* (2001) and online resources at http://www.kgu.de/zfg/dnachip.

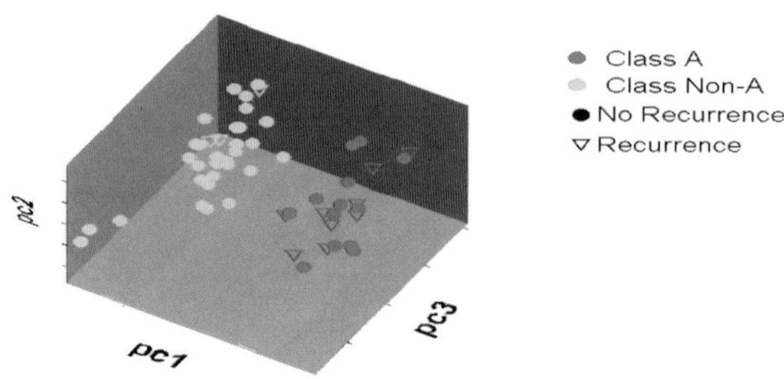


| follow up 23.5 months | class A | class Non-A | |
| --- | --- | --- | --- |
| relapses ( total ) | 9 ( 45% ) | 3 ( 11% ) | p = 0.016 |
| relapses ( N0 only ) | 3 of 5 | 0 of 15 | p = 0.009 |

Lancet 2002; 359: 131–32

**Figure 12.3** Discrimination of carcinoma classes. Fifty-five mammary carcinoma samples were characterised by expression profiling and the classification visualised by a principal component analysis. Tumours can be separated in two classes by using these methods: class A and class non-A (red and green symbols, respectively, in the colour version of this diagram available from the authors). The incidence of relapses is more than four times higher in class A, and recurrences in node-negative patients were only seen in class A. For further information see Ahr *et al.* (2002) and online resources at http://www.kgu.de/zfg/dnachip.

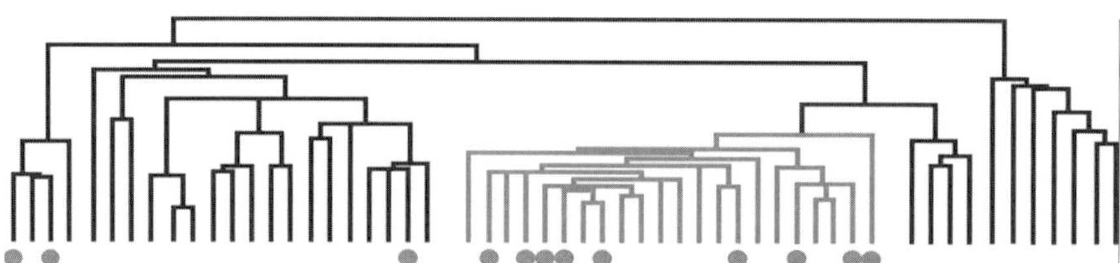

**Figure 12.4** Detection of high-risk patients. The 55 mammary carcinoma samples were grouped according to marker gene activity by hierarchical clustering with the Pearson correlation using the program CLUSTER (Stanford University, California, USA) Branch length represents similarity distances of samples as judged by their expression patterns. Class A breast cancers are represented by red branches. Tumour samples (T1–T3) of patients with recurrences during follow-up are marked by red dots. For further information see Ahr *et al.* (2002) and online resources at http://www.kgu.de/zfg/dnachip. (A colour version of this diagram is available from the authors).

these molecular methods with the standard tumour classification system to obtain improved patient-tailored therapies.

## Conclusions

Several studies on breast cancer have already been done using these novel techniques. In 2000, the pioneering microarray group from Stanford University categorised several new subtypes of breast cancer (Perou *et al.* 2000), and subsequently showed a correlation of these subtypes with survival data (Sorlie *et al.* 2001). In 2001, a group from the National Institutes of Health was able to distinguish hereditary cases of breast cancer (*BRCA1*, *BRCA2* and sporadic cases) according to their expression profiles (Hedenfalk *et al.* 2001). In January 2002, in addition to our results (Ahr *et al.* 2002), a group from The Netherlands Cancer Institute established a similar profiling system, allowing them the identification of those lower-risk patients who seem not to need an adjuvant treatment (van't Veer *et al.* 2002) and further progress continues to be made.

In summary, expression profiling can already distinguish known subtypes of breast cancer. In addition, however, novel subgroups have been identified using this technology, which differ in their clinical behaviour and which will have an impact on future treatment decisions. Finally, it is anticipated that further studies will supply us with profiles that allow the individual prediction of response to a specific therapy.


## *References*

Ahr, A., Holtrich, U., Solbach, C., Scharl, A., Strebhardt, K., Karn, T. & Kaufmann, M. (2001). Molecular classification of breast cancer patients by gene expression profiling. *Journal of Pathology* **195**, 312–320.

Ahr A., Karn T., Solbach C., Seiter T., Strebhardt K., Holtrich U. & Kaufmann M. (2002). Identification of high risk breast-cancer patients by gene expression profiling. *The Lancet* **359**, 131–132.

Alizadeh, A. A., Eisen, M. B., Davis, R. E. *et al.* (2000). Distinct types of diffuse large B-cell lymphoma identified by gene expression profiling. *Nature* **403**, 503–511.

Alizadeh, A. A., Ross, D. T., Perou, C. M. & van de Rijn, M. (2001). Towards a novel classification of human malignancies based on gene expression patterns. *Journal of Pathology* **195**, 41–52.

Eifel, P., Axelson, J. A. & Costa, J. *et al.* (2001). National Institutes of Health Consensus Development Conference Statement: adjuvant therapy for breast cancer, November 1–3, 2000. *Journal of the National Cancer Institute* **93**, 979–989.

Goldhirsch, A., Glick, J. H., Gelber, R. D., Coates, A. S., Senn, H. J. (2001). Meeting highlights: International Consensus Panel on the Treatment of Primary Breast Cancer: Seventh International Conference on Adjuvant Therapy of Primary Breast Cancer. *Journal of Clinical Oncology* **19**, 3817–3827.

Hedenfalk I, Duggan D, Chen Y, *et al.* (2001). Gene-expression profiles in hereditary breast cancer. *New England Journal of Medicine* **344**, 539–548.

Perou, C. M., Sorlie, T., Eisen, M. B. *et al.* (2000). Molecular portraits of human breast tumours. *Nature* **406**, 747–752.

Ries, L. A. G., Eisner, M. P., Kosary, C. L. *et al.* (eds) (2000). *SEER Cancer Statistics Review, 1973–1997*. Bethesda, Maryland: National Cancer Institute.

Sorlie, T., Perou, C. M., Tibshirani, R. *et al.* (2001). Gene expression patterns of breast carcinomas distinguish tumor subclasses with clinical implications. *Proceedings of the National Academy of Sciences of the United States of America* **98**, 10,869–10,874.

van 't Veer, L. J., Dai, H., van de Vijver, M. J., He, Y. D., Hart, A. A. M., Mao, M., Peterse, J. L., van der Kooy, K., Marton, M. J., Witteveen, A. T. *et al.* (2002). Gene expression profiling predicts clinical outcome of breast cancer. *Nature* **415**, 530–536.

***Online resources***

http://www.kgu.de/zfg/dnachip/

http://www.gene-chips.com/

# Radiotherapy and medical oncology

# Reducing radiotherapy dose in early breast cancer: the concept of conformal intra-operative brachytherapy

*Jeffrey S. Tobias, Jayant S. Vaidya and Michael Baum*

## Introduction

In *Time Magazine*'s extensively researched breast cancer issue published almost three years ago (10 June 2002), one particular quote had a special resonance for us. In the introduction to a remarkably comprehensive article, Dr Julie Gralow, an oncologist at the Fred Hutchinson Cancer Research Centre in Seattle, USA, stated 'We may be far overtreating our patients… We've now got women being diagnosed with tumours that would probably never have been treated if we didn't have mammography. They probably would have lived long, natural, healthy lives never knowing they had breast cancer' (see Gorman 2002).

For some years it has been apparent that for many patients, powerful treatment by surgery (even when limited to tumour excision with breast preservation) together with a six week programme of radiation therapy may be more than sufficient. We already know a good deal (though not enough, of course) about the profile of a typical breast cancer patient with low risk of local and distant recurrence: a small, low- or moderate-grade tumour, surgically completely excised, positive for oestrogen and/or progesterone receptors, negative for *HER2*, and with negative axillary nodes. Post-menopausal patients clearly have a lower incidence of local recurrence: for example, in the large study by Bartelink *et al.* (2001), patients over the age of 60 years had a rate of local recurrence after whole-breast radiation of 50 Gy of only 4% (without an additional boost), the rate reducing still further to 2.5% with an additional 16 Gy given by electron beam. For patients aged 41–50, the rates were 9.5% and 5.8%, respectively (median follow-up 5.1 years). What is more, an ever-increasing number of patients now present with small tumours (under 1 cm) identified on mammographic screening, of whom approximately three-quarters will have oestrogen receptor/progesterone receptor (ER/PR)-positive tumours, for which targeted hormone therapy with tamoxifen offers sustained long-term benefit, for both local and distant relapse (see Early Breast Cancer Trialists' Collaborative Group 1998a, b). Using a well tolerated oral aromatase inhibitor such as anastrazole reduces the risk still further (for both local and distant relapse), also, incidentally, reducing by three-quarters the risk of development of a contralateral primary breast cancer (ATAC Trialists Group 2002).

For all these reasons, we strongly support Gralow's view. Even in younger women known to be at higher risk of relapse, including those with axillary node positive disease, the use of systemic adjuvant cytotoxics sharply reduces the risk of recurrence (Early Breast Cancer Trialists' Collaborative Group 1992, 1998a, b). For hormone-receptor-positive patients, i.e. the large majority, adjuvant hormone therapy, surgical or medical oophorectomy all add further benefit (Early Breast Cancer Trialists' Collaborative Group 1992, 1998a,b; Bartelink *et al.* 2001).

What is the consequence of Gralow's observation? In the past, it has been regarded as mere flight of fancy to imagine that we can identify patients at such low risk of recurrence and that a less intensive form of treatment than local surgical excision followed by whole breast irradiation could be regarded as 'adequate'. In this sense, this general policy remains little different in principle from the equally compelling (in its day) policy of radical, then less damaging forms of mastectomy—though admittedly, using local excision, breast preservation and post operative radiotherapy is generally regarded as more 'humane' even though attempts at demonstrating an improved quality of life have been largely elusive (Fallowfield *et al.* 1986). Nonetheless, the evolving history of local treatment for early breast cancer has centred on an ever-increasing recognition of the importance of breast conservation for body image and cosmesis, an essential requirement for most women. This has largely been achieved by the increasing acceptance of breast conserving surgery with post-operative radiotherapy (Tobias 1986). Yet despite this ready acceptance, recent data from the world's largest ever randomised breast cancer study, with excellent quality control and a high level of expertise, confirm a mastectomy rate approaching 50% (ATAC Trialists Group unpublished data).

We believe that the time has come to move on. For many patients, particularly those presenting over the age of 50 years with small, low-grade, ER-positive, axillary-node-negative tumours, it is surely right to question the necessity of a lengthy and sometimes damaging course of radiation therapy. Radiation oncologists who are totally satisfied with their often excellent cosmetic results and low relapse rates after standard treatment should bear in mind the work of the Oxford-based Early Breast Cancer Trialists' Collaborative Group (EBCTCG): namely, that despite a lower breast cancer cause-specific death rate in irradiated patients, the increased mortality for other non-cancer causes wipes out this advantage (Early Breast Cancer Trialists' Group 2000). The assumption that the excess non-cancer related deaths in this large meta-analysis was due essentially to reliance on older outmoded radiation techniques may be correct—but it remains an assumption only, and considerable additional data attest to the cardiac, pulmonary and neurological dangers of whole-breast irradiation (Rutqvist and Johansson 1990; Lind *et al.* 1997; Royal College of Radiologists 1995). Moreover, the use of anthracycline-based chemotherapy regimens apparently increases some of these risks still further (Meinardi *et al.* 2001).

What about radiation dose and whole breast treatment? Most authorities recommend a standard dose of 50 Gy over a 5 week period with a boost for all patients, of up to

16 Gy (Bartelink *et al* 2000). However, in the much criticised randomised study performed in 1960s by the group from Guy's Hospital, even a low radiation dose to the whole breast, considered 'inadequate' by today's standards, seemed to be sufficient for patients with axillary node-negative disease, i.e. with a low risk of local recurrence (Atkins *et al.* 1972). This was probably the earliest of prospectively randomised breast cancer studies comparing mastectomy (in this study, radical mastectomy was still the standard surgical procedure, with a formal axillary dissection) with wide local excision (often quadrantectomy) followed by radiation therapy. It was clear that for axillary-node-positive patients, the low dose of radiation employed (38 Gy to the breast but only 27 Gy to the axilla) was insufficient; the overall survival was clearly worse in this group, for patients treated by a breast conserving surgical technique. However, in an important result often overlooked, the stage 1 patients (node negative) had an equally good survival prognosis whether subjected to radical mastectomy or treated by breast conserving surgery with low dose radiation therapy.

The use of single fraction intra-operative irradiation, at the time of initial surgical excision, is attracting considerable interest. Not only the article and associated reporting in *Time Magazine* but more importantly, the Istituto Nazionale Milan, have recognised it as an important potential step forward, reducing the otherwise inevitable treatment delay between surgery and radiation therapy that patients (and staff in radiotherapy departments) find so unsettling. In Milan, use of electron beam intra-operative radiation therapy (ELIOT) uses a substantial electron generating linear accelerator brought in a dedicated fashion to the operating room (Orecchia & Veronesi 2002; Veronesi 2002; Veronesi *et al.* 2001), but other techniques have also been employed. This group is now formally testing the intra-operative technique against conventional external beam radiation therapy in a prospective randomised study (Veronesi *et al.* 2002).

Our own approach has been to use the intrabeam device, essentially a miniaturised low-energy photon generator, brought to the operating theatre at the time of surgery. The technique has been fully described (Vaidya *et al.* 2001a, 2002a) and can be used both in conjunction with surgery or alternatively, for frail patients whose general medical condition precludes either a general anaesthetic or major surgical procedure (Vaidya *et al.* 2002b). As part of the rationale for treating low-risk patients with intra-operative irradiation (without added external beam therapy), it is important to recall that most in-breast local recurrences after breast-conserving surgery occur within the index quadrant, despite the fact many breasts are known to harbour foci of other malignant sites (usually non-invasive) (Vaidya *et al.* 1996, 2001a, b).

## Methodology

### The new radiotherapy technique

*Targeted intra-operative radiotherapy (Targit)*

We have previously published the pilot study performed at University College London Hospitals. A novel method of radiotherapy was used to deliver therapeutic radiation to the tissues around the primary tumour immediately after excision, with a degree of precision impossible with an external beam. The photon radiosurgery system (PRS), developed by the Photoelectron Corporation in Massachusetts, USA, is a simple and ingenious device, in essence a miniature electron-beam-driven X-ray source providing a point source of low energy X-rays (50 kV maximum). The unit is connected, through a low-voltage cable, to a control box housing a rechargeable NiCd battery. Within the unit itself, electrons are produced and accelerated to the desired energy by a multi-stage anode, and directed down a 10 cm long, 3.2 mm diameter evacuated drift tube towards a thin-film hemispherical gold target at its tip. The radiation source can be inserted into the area of interest, to provide intra-operative interstitial irradiation. The physics, dosimetry and early clinical applications of this soft X-ray device have been well studied and the probe has already been used for treatment of malignant brain tumours in man (Douglas *et al.* 1996; Cosgrove *et al.* 1997), though treatment of breast cancer had not previously been attempted.

We regard this as a form of intra-operative conformal brachytherapy. For use in breast, the radiation source is surrounded by a conical sheath with a sphere at the tip (see Figures 13.1–13.3). The sphere is specially designed to produce an accurately calculated uniform dose rate at its surface, enabling delivery of a uniform dose of radiation to a prescribed depth, with rapid attenuation of the beam to reduce the dose to more distant tissues. Depending upon the size of the surgical cavity, various sizes of applicator sphere are available and for each size, the radiation received is proportional to the time the machine is switched on and left *in situ*. The precise dose rate depends on the diameter of the applicator and the energy of the beam, both of which may be varied to optimise the radiation treatment. The radiation dose at various distances from the cavity margin varies as shown for the simulated assembly in Table 13.1. For example, a dose of about 5 Gy can be delivered in about 20 min at 1 cm from the margins of a 3.5 cm cavity after wide local excision of the tumour. The whole assembly is small and lightweight (mass: 1.8 kg; dimensions: X-ray generator body 7× cm × 11× cm × 14 cm; applicator: 16 cm long conical applicator sheath with a 2–5 cm applicator sphere at the tip) and hangs dependently from a mobile gantry in perfect balance, remaining steady wherever it is positioned. If necessary, the chest wall and skin can be protected (95% shielding) by radio-opaque tungsten-filled polyurethane caps which can be cut to size on the operation table, another advantage of using soft X-rays. With this elegant approach the pliable breast tissue around the cavity of surgical excision wraps around the radiotherapy source, i.e. the target is 'conformed' to the source. This feature of the methodology represents a fundamental

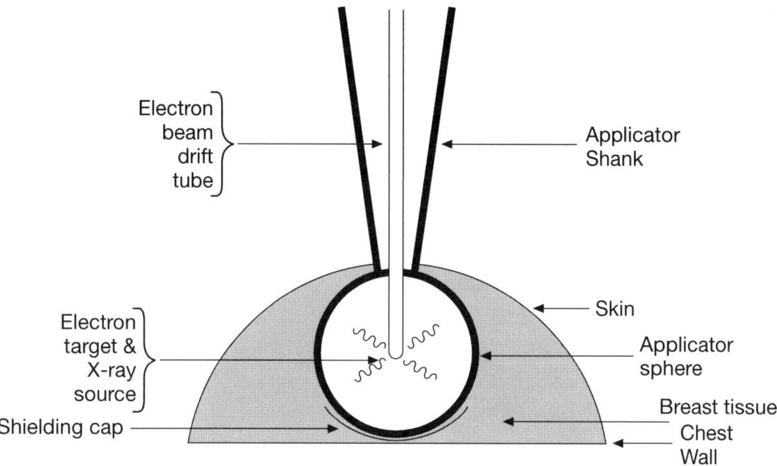


**Figure 13.1** The photon-radiosurgery system (PRS). The electrons are generated and accelerated in the main unit (seen in Figure 13.3) and travel through the electron beam drift tube which is surrounded by the conical applicator sheath such that its tip lies at the epicentre of the applicator sphere. Once the electrons hit the inner surface of the hemisphere at the tip, X-rays are generated. Thus, a uniform radiation dose rate is available at the surface of the applicator sphere. There is a small very high dose region close to the applicator which attenuates quickly $(a \times 1/r^3)$.

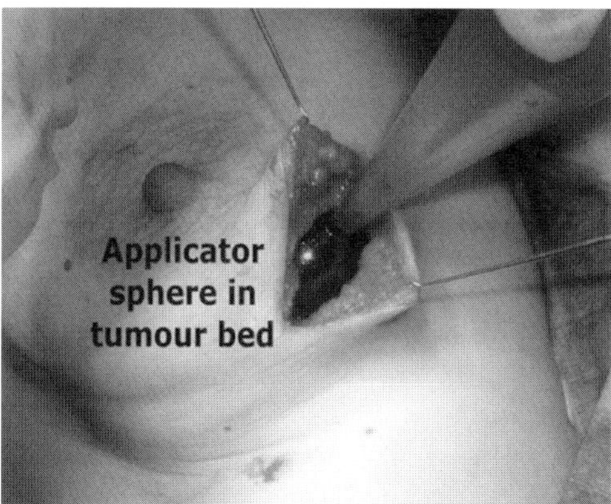


**Figure 13.2** The applicator being placed in the tumour bed, immediately after the excision of the tumour.

shift from more traditional forms of brachytherapy with wires, hairpins or radioactive seeds.

It also avoids the demanding complexity and attention to meticulous radiation protection of using interstitial of radioactive wires to provide high-dose radiotherapy,

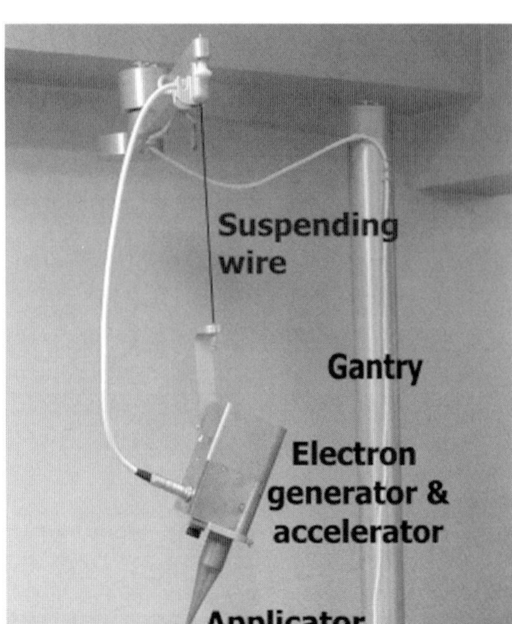


**Figure 13.3** The PRS assembly. The whole assembly is suspended on a counter-balance system so that the position of the applicator remains steady irrespective of the respiratory movements. Once the applicator is positioned, the electron beam drift tube with the electron generator and accelerator is inserted in the applicator and maintained by a spring-loaded system.

**Table 13.1** Standard dosimetry table. (Calculations for a 3.5 cm diameter spherical diameter and a period of irradiation of 21 min as measured from the periphery of the sphere in a breast phantom (PRS operating parameters: 50 kV). Radial doses are stated for a treatment prescription on 5 Gy at 1 cm.)

| Distance from the surface of the applicator | PE probe (Gy) | | External beam radiotherapy | | Whole breast radiotherapy tumour bed boost | |
|---|---|---|---|---|---|---|
| | Physical X-ray dose (Gy) | BED | Physical X-ray dose (Gy) | BED | Physical X-ray Dose (Gy) | BED |
| 0.1 cm | 15 | 165 | 10 | 12 | 50 | 60 |
| 0.2 cm | 12.5 | 121 | 10 | 12 | 50 | 60 |
| 0.5 cm | 8.75 | 59 | 10 | 12 | 50 | 60 |
| 1 cm | 5.0 | 21.7 | 10 | 12 | 50 | 60 |

Biologically effective dose (BED) is given by the equation (Dale 1985): $BED = D \times (1 + (d/(a/b)))$ where $D$ is the total physical dose, $d$ is the physical dose per fraction and $a/b$ is the biological coefficient, which is 10 for early and tumour effects for tumour tissues when the radiotherapy is delivered in fractions of about 2 Gy. For the single dose we have assumed the value of $a/b$ to be equal to 1.5.

or the equally challenging technique of conformal radiotherapy by external beams from a linear accelerator. The steep attenuation of the radiation dose allows the treatment to be carried out in unmodified operating theatres, whose walls usually incorporate adequate shielding for microwave radiation from electronic equipment such as mobile phones, thus providing sufficient staff protection for the present purpose.

## Results

We began the pilot study on 2 July 1998 in appropriately selected patients. They all had early operable breast cancer, suitable for breast conserving surgery. The ages ranged from 30–80 years (mean 51.5 years). The pathological tumour size ranged from 0.42 cm to 4.0 cm. Twenty-two tumours were infiltrating duct carcinomas (four grade 1, seven grade 2 and 11 grade 3); one was the tubular variant and three were invasive lobular carcinomas (two grade 1, and one grade 2).

Twenty-two patients had axillary node dissection and three had sentinel node biopsy only. All sentinel nodes were negative and three patients had involved lymph nodes (1, 2 and 1 each). The applicator size was 3.5 cm in 13 cases, 4 cm and 4.5 cm in four cases each, 3 cm in three cases and 2.5 cm in one case. In all except the first case, the operating voltage was 50 kV at 40 μA. The mean treatment time required to treat the prescribed dose of 5 Gy at 1 cm was 26.5 min (95% confidence interval (CI): 24.3–28.8) The total mean operation time for the wide local excision, axillary clearance and intraoperative radiotherapy was 1 h 57 min (95% CI: 1 h 47 min – 2 h 7 min). In the first case, we used a 40 kV voltage and took 36.8 min. Three patients received intra-operative radiotherapy as the only form of radiotherapy. One patient was blind, 80 years old, and keen to avoid daily post-operative visits for external beam radiotherapy. In a joint decision, she was prescribed 7.5 Gy (150% of the usual dose) at 1 cm, effectively giving about 23 Gy to the cavity margin as the only radiotherapy. Another patient had a contralateral breast cancer treated 14 years before, on that occasion with an interstitial iridium wire boost and whole-breast radiotherapy. So as not to overlap radiation beams in the mid-line, she was prescribed 6 Gy at 1 cm, giving 20 Gy to the cavity margin as the only radiotherapy. The third patient (patient 21 in the pilot study) fully understood the rationale of our subsequent randomised study and chose not to undergo the five-week course of whole breast radiotherapy, although we had not yet started the randomised trial to test this approach. All other patients received the routine external beam radiotherapy to the whole breast (50 Gy over 5 weeks). None has had major operative or post-operative complications either in general or for the wound. Two patients had a delay in wound healing, and one had wound infection. We believe that one of these was due to excessive radiation and radionecrosis. This was our third patient as mentioned before, who had radionecrosis of a 1 cm area of skin close to the applicator. The skin breakdown occurred three months after an initial good healing and resulted in delayed healing by secondary intention. In the 80-year-old blind patient, both the axillary (unirradiated site) and primary wound had delayed healing. Both these patients were very satisfied with the final appearance and/or texture of the breast. In the patient who developed a wound infection, the wound healed satisfactorily within two weeks without delay to her adjuvant treatment. Some short-term erythema around the scar was seen in three patients.

The longest follow up is 35 months, with a median of 24 months and a minimum of 16 months. No patient has had a local recurrence. None of the patients who were eligible (essentially all those who were suitable for breast conserving therapy) have refused to participate in the study. Many found the technique appealing and logical, and could immediately see the practical advantage of fewer visits to the radiotherapy department. The concept of giving the radiotherapy to the tumour bed 'there and then' was also very attractive. The actual score of appearance of breast and texture of breast, as judged by the patients themselves, either matched or exceeded their expected score in 21 out of 25 patients. At 12–16 months after surgery, the satisfaction index (observed/expected score) was 1.2 (95% CI: 1.1–1.4) for breast appearance, and 1.2 (95% CI: 1.0–1.4) for breast texture.

Updating these data, the UK pilot study has been encouraging: at a median follow-up of 34 months, there are no recurrences among the 25 patients initially studied and cosmetic appearances have been satisfactory. In addition, centres in the USA and Australia have now treated larger patient numbers in local feasibility studies (D. Joseph and B. S. Hilaris, personal communication).

We have embarked upon a multi-centre randomised trial to test this novel approach and several centres in the USA, UK, Europe, India and Australasia have expressed interest and developed local expertise with the technique.

## Discussion

For a variety of reasons, many hospitals in the UK and elsewhere are currently experiencing lengthening delays for patients who require radiotherapy. It is far from unusual for patients to be told that treatment cannot begin for three or four months or even longer. For younger women, either with positive axillary nodes or other features indicating a high risk of recurrence, initial treatment is likely to be with chemotherapy—in which case, the patient can be sensibly booked in for radiotherapy at the outset of the programme, undergoing the radiotherapy itself at the appropriate time, after chemotherapy has been completed, typically four or five months after the first cycle.

Most patients, however, fall into the low risk category, or for other reasons cannot justifiably be recommended to undergo chemotherapy. This will include most post-menopausal patients who, after all, still comprise 75% of all women we see. What of these? No scientifically justifiable treatment can be recommended between surgical excision (usually conservative, with breast preservation) and radiation therapy, though many are started during the interim period on adjuvant hormone therapy. For this large group, the use of immediate intra-operative conformal brachytherapy is especially attractive.

We recognise that the follow-up of the pilot study is relatively short (median 24 months, longest 35 months) for assessing local recurrence rates, but this was a phase II pilot study mainly assessing the feasibility, safety and acceptability of the technique and not local control, which will be tested in the next phase of the randomised study. We have already received ethics approval and in March 2000 began the randomised trial (entitled *Targit*: *Tar*geted *i*ntraoperative radio*t*herapy), comparing conventional radiotherapy with radiotherapy delivered to the index quadrant alone, using the intrabeam device (protocol site http://www.thelancet.com/info/info.isa?n1= authorinfo&n2=Protocol+review&uid=9920). This is a pragmatic multicentre trial, in which patients suitable for breast-conserving therapy undergoing wide local excision and axillary clearance are randomised to receive either the intra-operative radiotherapy only, or the conventional extended course of post-operative radiotherapy. If, on final histopathology, the tumour is found to be lobular cancer or harbouring extensive intraductal component, patients receive additional post-operative whole breast radiotherapy, excluding an additional tumour bed boost. In the pilot study we had only one patient with a positive margin: the deep margin. Because this was the blind patient who had received the higher (7.5 Gy at 1 cm) dose of radiotherapy, the area adjacent to the tumour bed would have received about 23 Gy, which was thought to be adequate. A decision to give no further treatment was taken jointly in our multidisciplinary meeting and with the patient, and she has not recurred. In the randomised trial, the protocol includes a provision to re-excise the tumour in patients with grossly positive margins, and to re-irradiate the revised tumour bed if they were randomised to the intra-operative radiotherapy arm. Previous intra-operative radiotherapy should not contraindicate, because the previously irradiated area would have been excised in the re-excision.

Clearly, a substantial multi-centre randomised study is the only means of confirming whether or not this exciting new treatment will prove adequate, but the many potential advantages make such a trial essential. These include: immediate treatment with radiotherapy at the time of surgery; accuracy of locating the radiation at the site of the tumour bed (currently guesswork for most patients, using conventional external boosts (see, for example, Doleckova 2001), elimination of a lengthy treatment programme for a large proportion of women with breast cancer; and a freeing up of precious resources in oncology departments, thereby allowing general waiting lists for other urgent indications to fall sharply. Furthermore, many patients still have little access to breast preserving treatment because of the demands of such lengthy radiation programmes, not only in developing countries, but even closer to home. Patients most likely to benefit and prove suitable include those diagnosed in the post-menopausal age group with small-, low- or moderate-grade ER-positive tumours with only a small risk of local recurrence. These comprise a substantial proportion of the patients we see. We urgently need to know if Dr Gralow is right in her contention that many patients with breast cancer are grossly overtreated, but we think she is indeed correct. The medical and economic implications deriving from this insight are considerable because treatment of breast carcinoma often represents one-third or more of the total case-load of radiotherapy units worldwide. Many women from the developing world and remote areas of the developed world (e.g. distant rural areas of Australia or India) cannot benefit from breast-conserving therapy because of the large distances between their home and radiotherapy centre. All too frequently they have to choose mastectomy because they cannot stay in or travel daily to the metropolis for the six weeks of post-operative radiotherapy.

If proven equal to the standard approach, the novel technique would allow these women to have breast-conserving therapy at one sitting. In terms of operational expenses the novel technique needs about three man–hours and 45 min each of operation theatre time and patient time. The conventional six-week course of post-operative radiotherapy on the other hand, costs about nine man–hours, six hours of radiotherapy room time and 30–60 h of patient time. If the cost of conventional radiotherapy is of the order of £5,000, then considering only the 66% saving of man–hours, the novel technique would save £3,750 per patient. Furthermore, if we assume that 60% of the 27,000 breast cancer patients diagnosed every year in the UK could be treated by conservative surgery, the novel technique might potentially save over £60 million (0.60 × 27,000 × 3,750) per year for the NHS. In addition, the saving of expensive resource time on linear accelerators would be very substantial.

## Acknowledgements

We thank Mr Michael Douek for comments on the manuscript and Ms Vardhini Vijay for helping with illustrations. The project is funded by the University College London Hospitals Trust and the Photoelectron Corporation. An edited version of this chapter was published with permission as a Commentary in the *British Journal of Radiology* **77**, 279–284.

## *References*

ATAC (Arimidex, Tamoxifen alone or in Combination) Trialists' Group (2002). Anastrozole alone or in combination with tamoxifen versus tamoxifen alone for adjuvant treatment of postmenopausal women with early breast cancer: first results of the ATAC randomised trial. *The Lancet* **359**, 2131–2139.

Atkins, H., Hayward, J. L., Klugman, D. J. & Wayte, A. B. (1972). Treatment for early breast cancer: a report after ten years of a clinical trial. *British Medical Journal* **ii**, 423.

Bartelink, H., Horiot, J.-C., Poortmans, P. *et al.* (2001). Recurrence rates after treatment of breast cancer with standard radiotherapy with or without additional radiation. *New England Journal of Medicine* **345**, 1378–1387.

Baum, M., Vaidya, J. S. & Mittra, I. (1997). Multicentricity and recurrence of breast cancer. *The Lancet* **349**, 208.

Cosgrove, G. R., Hochberg, F. H., Pardo, F. S. *et al.* (1997). Interstitial irradiation of brain tumors using a miniature radiosurgery device: Initial experience. *Neurosurgery* **40**, 518–525.

Dale, R. G. (1985). The application of the linear quadratic dose effect equation to fractionated and protracted radiotherapy. *British Journal of Radiology* **58**, 515–528.

Dale, R. G., Jones, B. & Price, P. (1997). Comments on inadequacy of iridium implant as sole radiation treatment for operable breast cancer, Fentiman *et al. Eur J Cancer* 1996; **32A**: 608–611. *European Journal of Cancer* **33**, 1707–1708.

Deng, G., Lu, Y., Zlotnikov, G. *et al.* (1996). Loss of heterozygosity in normal tissue adjacent to breast carcinomas. *Science* **274**, 2057–2059.

Doleckova, M. (2001). The problem of the planning of electron boost in breast cancer. Presented at ISRO 2001, Melbourne, Australia.

Douglas, R.M., Beatty, J., Gall, K. *et al.* (1996). Dosimetric results from a feasibility study of a novel radiosurgical source for irradiation of intracranial metastases. *International Journal of Radiation Oncology, Biology, Physics* **36**, 443–450.

Early Breast Cancer Trialists' Collaborative Group (1995). Effects of radiotherapy and surgery in early breast cancer. An overview of the randomized trials. *New England Journal of Medicine* **333**, 1444–1455.

Early Breast Cancer Trialists' Collaborative Group (1992). Systemic treatment of early breast cancer by hormonal, cytotoxic or immune therapy: 133 randomised trials involving 31,000 recurrences and 24,000 deaths among 75,000 women (part I). *The Lancet* **339**, 1–15.

Early Breast Cancer Trialists' Collaborative Group (1998a). Polychemotherapy for early breast cancer: an overview of the randomised trial. *The Lancet* **351**, 1451–1467.

Early Breast Cancer Trialists' Collaborative Group (1998b). Tamoxifen for breast cancer: an overview of the randomised trials. *The Lancet* **352**, 930–942.

Early Breast Cancer Trialists' Collaborative Group (2000). Favourable and unfavourable effects on long-term survival radiotherapy for early breast cancer: an overview of the randomised trials. *The Lancet* **355**, 1757–1770.

Fallowfield, L. J., Baum, M. & Maguire, G. P. (1986). Effects of breast conservation on psychological morbidity associate with diagnosis and treatment of breast cancer. *British Medical Journal* **293**, 1331–1334.

Fentiman, I. S., Poole, C., Tong, D. *et al.* (1996). Inadequacy of iridium implant as sole radiation treatment for operable breast cancer. *European Journal of Cancer* **32A**, 608–611.

Fisher, E. R., Anderson, S., Redmond, C., Fisher, B. (1992). Ipsilateral breast tumor recurrence and survival following lumpectomy and irradiation: Pathological findings from NSABP protocol B-06. *Seminars in Surgical Oncology* **8**, 161–166.

Gorman, C. (2002). Rethinking breast cancer. *Time Magazine* **159**, 46–54.

Lind, P. A., Gagliardi, G., Wennberg, B. & Fornander, T. (1997). A descriptive study of pulmonary complications after post-operative radiation therapy in node-positive stage II breast cancer. *Acta Oncologica* **36**, 509–515.

Meinardi, M. T., van Veldhuisen, D. J., Gietema, J. A *et al.* (2001). Prospective evaluation of early cardiac damage induced by epirubicin containing adjuvant chemotherapy and locoregional radiotherapy in breast cancer patients. *Journal of Clinical Oncology* **19**, 2746–2753.

Orecchia, R. & Veronesi, U. (2002). The Milan Trial. 3rd European Breast Cancer Conference, Barcelona, March 2002. *European Journal of Cancer* **38** (Suppl. 3), abstract 193, S90.

Ribeiro, G. G., Magee, B., Swindell, R. *et al.* (1993). The Christie Hospital breast conservation trial: an update at eight years from inception. *Clinical Oncology (Royal College of Radiologists)* **5**, 278–283.

Royal College of Radiologists (1995). Report of the independent review commissioned by The Royal College of Radiologists into brachial plexus neuropathy following radiotherapy for breast carcinoma (ed. T. Bates & R. G. B. Evans). London: Royal College of Radiologists. (ISBN 1 872599 18 4.)

Rutqvist, L. E. & Johansson, H. (1990). Mortality by laterality of the primary tumour among 55,000 breast cancer patients from the Swedish Cancer Registry. *British Journal of Cancer* **61**, 866–868.

Tobias, J. S. (1986). Radiotherapy and breast conservation. *British Journal of Radiology* **59**, 653–666.

Vaidya, J. S., Vyas, J. J., Chinoy, R. F. *et al.* (1996). Multicentricity of breast cancer: whole organ analysis and clinical implications. *British Journal of Cancer* **74**, 820–824.

Vaidya, J. S. & Baum, M. (1998). Clinical and biological implications of the Milan Breast conservation trials. *European Journal of Cancer* **34**, 1143–1144.

Vaidya, J. S., Baum, M., Tobias, J. S. *et al.* (2001a). Targeted intra-operative radiotherapy (Targit). *Annals of Oncology* **12**, 1–6.

Vaidya, J. S., Baum, M., Tobias, J. S. *et al.* (2001b). Targeted intraoperative radiotherapy for breast cancer (Targit) – a randomised trial. *Breast Cancer Research and Treatment* **69**, 145.

Vaidya, J. S., Baum, M., Tobias, J. S. *et al.* (2002a). The novel technique of delivering targeted intra-operative radiotherapy (Targit) for early breast cancer. *European Journal of Surgical Oncology* **28**, 447–454.

Vaidya, J. S., Hall-Craggs, M., Baum, M., Tobias, J. S. *et al.* (2002b). Percutaneous minimally invasive stereotactic primary radiotherapy for breast cancer. *The Lancet Oncology* **3**, 252–253.

Veronesi, U. (2002). Intraoperative radiotherapy: rationale, techniques, results. Proceedings, 3rd European Breast Cancer Conference, Barcelona, March 2002. *European Journal of Cancer* **38** (Suppl. 3), abstract 190, S89.

Veronesi, U., Orecchia, R., Luini, A. *et al.* (2001). A preliminary report of intraoperative radiotherapy (IORT) in limited-stage breast cancers that are conservatively treated. *European Journal of Cancer* **37**, 2178–2183.

Veronesi, U., Vicini, F. & Orecchia, R. (2002). Highlights of surgery and radiotherapy. *The Breast* **11**, 194–195.

Chapter 14

# Current thinking on the role of radiotherapy in metastatic disease

*Sandra M. de Canha and Peter J. Hoskin*

The incidence of female breast cancer in the UK is one of the highest in the world with approximately 38,000 cases per year. Although less than 10% of women present with disseminated disease, 40–70% will develop metastases in the course of their lives. Once patients develop symptomatic distant metastases, the median life expectancy is 2 years. It is important that, in the remainder of their lives, treatments should be aimed at symptom relief and maintaining quality of life, and this is where radiotherapy has an important role to play.

## Bone metastases

In the UK about 9000 women with breast cancer develop bone metastases each year, making metastatic bone pain one of the most common symptoms in disseminated breast cancer. Breast tumours are responsible for 40% of all painful bony metastases. Interestingly, the clinical incidence of bone metastases is significantly higher with steroid receptor-positive tumours and those that are well differentiated (Breast Specialty Group of the British Association of Surgical Oncology [BASO] 1999).

Up to one-fifth of patients with bone metastases will be alive at 5 years, and therefore it is important that palliation is effective and durable.

The morbidity of bone metastases includes pain, impaired mobility, hypercalcaemia, pathological fracture, spinal cord or nerve root compression, and bone marrow infiltration. The aims of treatment of bone metastases are to relieve pain, prevent development of pathological fractures and other complications, and to improve mobility and function. Localised pain should be treated by radiotherapy, as a single direct field or parallel opposed fields, which is successful in over 80% of patients (Royal College of Radiologists [RCR] 1999).

By 1990, several prospective randomised trials had tested radiation schedules delivering fewer, larger fractions against conventional schedules. More has been learned in the past 10 years, and the results have been summarised in a consensus statement on behalf of the participants of the Second Workshop on Palliative Radiotherapy and Symptom Control (Hoskin *et al.* 2001).

Altogether, 10 randomised trials have used prospective patient self-assessments to test the efficacy of fewer fractions in more than 3500 patients. Six of these studies have tested a single fraction (usually 8 Gy) against 20 Gy in 5 fractions or 30 Gy in

10 fractions in more than 2000 patients. A meta-analysis presented at the workshop and awaiting publication shows a difference of 0.9% in favour of the single fraction (95% confidence interval = −3% to +5%), constituting level 1a evidence for the efficacy of the single fraction (SM Bentzen, unpublished observation). This leads to a grade A recommendation that, for the large majority of patients requiring local radiotherapy for metastatic skeletal pain unassociated with spinal cord compression or pathological fracture of a long bone, a single fraction of 8 Gy tumour dose is effective and appropriate treatment. The use of single fraction schedules has the added benefits of patient convenience, reducing the radiotherapy work load and allowing re-treatment in the case of recurrent pain.

There is an alternative view that the results of higher-dose fractionated schedules are 'much better' on the basis that none of the single-dose trials has shown a frequency or duration of benefit comparable with the conventional fractionated schedules used in one of the earliest fractionation trials undertaken in the USA by the Radiation Therapy Oncology Group (RTOG), the RTOG 74-02 trial. There are, however, serious criticisms of this trial, perhaps the most important of which is that physician scores of pain were used as end-points that are likely to correlate poorly with patient self-assessments and will usually systematically over-estimate the effect (Ingham and Portenoy 1998). Furthermore, to compare the levels of pain relief achieved in different trials is notoriously unreliable.

Specific areas of clinical uncertainty that remain include: the relative efficacy of an 8-Gy single fraction compared with conventional multi-fraction treatment for pain relief and bone healing beyond 12 months; the response of neuropathic pain to single-fraction radiotherapy, a question being addressed by an ongoing Trans Tasman Radiation Oncology Group (TROG) randomised trial; the role of postoperative radiotherapy in pathological fracture of a long bone and the optimal dose fractionation in this setting; and the optimal dose regimen for patients with spinal cord compression.

Interesting questions have been raised about the relationships of pain relief, bone healing and tumour response after radiotherapy. The relatively short tumour growth delay expected after an 8-Gy single fraction, possibly only a few weeks, is inconsistent with the durable pain responses after 8 Gy now demonstrated at 1 year after treatment. This raises the possibility that radiosensitive host cells, including macrophages and osteoclasts, may be therapeutic targets. Cells of the macrophage series produce chemical mediators of pain, and osteoclasts are chiefly responsible for generating pain via bone breakdown products. Both cell types are radiosensitive, possibly responding to low doses of ionising radiation by apoptosis, although little is known about re-population after low-dose radiotherapy. Recent data suggest that the response to radiotherapy may relate to markers of osteoclast activity (Hoskin *et al.* 2001). This hypothesis is further supported by the increasing role of bisphosphonates as chemical osteoclast inhibitors in the management of painful bone metastases.

## Pathological fracture

Before administering radiotherapy, it is important to obtain an orthopaedic opinion when there is a likelihood of an imminent fracture, in which setting surgical fixation will be the initial treatment of choice. Wherever 50% of the cortex has been destroyed, there is a high risk of pathological fracture and prophylactic fixation should be performed before radiotherapy. Where there is less than 50% cortical erosion, radiotherapy may be administered; the exception is the femoral neck where any degree of cortical erosion should be considered as an indication for prophylactic fixation (BASO 1999). Other high-risk scenarios include diffuse lytic changes in a long bone and a single lytic lesion larger than 3 cm in the proximal femur (Harrington 1986).

Spinal instability is likely to occur when more than 50% of the vertebral body is destroyed (RCR 1999) and is reported to occur in 10% of cancer patients. It is a cause of excruciating back pain on movement. As the pain is mechanical in origin, radiotherapy will not help and the only solution is stabilisation of the spine (Coleman 1998). This should be followed by postoperative radiotherapy (RCR 1999), as soon as the wound is healed.

## Palliation of diffuse bone pain

An important development in the past decade has been the increasing use of radioisotope therapy for scattered metastatic bone pain using isotopes that are concentrated at sites of bone damage and remineralisation as a result of the osteoblastic response. These include strontium-89 and samarium-192 complexed in a phosphonate compound (Sm–ethylenediaminetetramethylene phosphonic acid (EDTMP)). This treatment has been shown to reduce pain. The isotopes imitate calcium in vivo and therefore localise in bone mineral. Strontium is preferentially concentrated in areas of osteoblastic activity and delivers a small dose of radiation to the bone marrow, with only minimal haematological toxicity as a result. Studies have demonstrated a rapid washout from healthy bone (Baziotis *et al.* 1998). It is retained at sites of osteoblastic bone metastases for up to 100 days and, taking strontium's half-life of 50.5 days, the result is the delivery of high localised irradiation dose (Hoskin 1988). It has been shown to achieve an absorbed dose in bone lesions of between 2 and 20 Gy (Baziotis *et al.* 1998).

The onset of pain relief with strontium occurs within 10–21 days and peaks around 6 weeks. By 3 months about 22% of patients achieve complete pain relief and an overall response rate of about 60% is expected when strontium is used for breast bone metastases. Granulocytopenia and thrombocytopenia are seen within a month (with a 30–40% drop in counts at nadir) and usually resolves by 6 months. An initial pain flare-up occurs in 10–20% of patients and usually lasts 2–4 days (Salazar *et al.* 2001).

Strontium is relatively easy to administer, requiring a single outpatient intravenous injection, and has mild toxicity, but is infrequently used because of increasing costs. With increasing experience it is becoming clear that it is important to select patients for this treatment: those with advanced disease and a short life expectancy rarely benefit from it, and ideally it will be selected for patients early in the presentation of metastatic bone pain (Hoskin *et al.* 2001).

Another way of giving 'systemic' radiotherapy for diffuse bone pain is the use of hemibody irradiation (HBI). HBI involves radiation in a single or multiple fractions to a large tissue volume (upper half body, lower half body or mid-body). The dose is 6 Gy administered in one fraction to the upper half body or 8 Gy in one fraction to the mid-body or lower half body. Single-dose HBI achieves pain relief faster than strontium, but it does cause more acute, but transitory gastrointestinal toxicity. This toxicity can be minimised with the use of premedication. HBI also has the added advantage of being able to deliver treatment to lymph node-bearing and gross tumour areas, outside of bone, which may be causing pain (Salazar *et al.* 2001).

A prospective trial of HBI (RTOG 78-10) demonstrated that single-dose HBI gives effective pain relief and patients with primary breast cancer demonstrated a response rate of almost 90%, with nearly 30% achieving complete pain relief. Nearly 50% of responders were noted to experience relief within 48 hours and 80% within 1 week (Salazar *et al.* 1986).

Fractionating HBI reduces the need for premedication or close patient monitoring and also allows for an increase in the total dose delivered.

It has similar toxicity and response rates to single-dose HBI, but more durable palliation has been suggested from one study (Ciezki *et al.* 2000).

In a randomised phase III trial, Salazar *et al.* (2001) demonstrated that delivering two daily doses of 3 Gy each on 2 consecutive days appears to be as effective and efficient as delivering a single daily dose of 3 Gy on 5 consecutive days, although no direct comparison between this and a single dose has been undertaken.

## Spinal cord compression

Spinal cord compression is an oncological emergency. All patients with suspected or proven cord compression should be started immediately on dexamethasone to relieve local oedema, which contributes to the cord damage.

Both surgery and radiotherapy are effective in the relief of pain and reversal of neurological dysfunction and should be started within 12 hours of the first symptoms. The decision on treatment will depend on many factors, including the site and number of levels, whether the compression is partial or complete, fixability, duration, performance status and predicted survival.

Radiotherapy is the treatment of choice in patients with spinal cord compression. Indications for surgery are spinal instability or compression by bone and failure to respond to radiotherapy, and in patients who have received previous radiotherapy. Anterior decompression with mechanical stabilisation has replaced laminectomy as the main surgical treatment for epidural metastases arising from the vertebral body (Fuller *et al.* 2001).

Outcome, especially preservation of motor function, depends on how early treatment is initiated. Patients who are paraplegic for longer than 24 hours rarely recover ambulatory function. Studies have shown that, once paraplegia occurs, less than 10% of patients will ever walk again. Some small series have shown that patients who were ambulatory on presentation maintained ambulation 96% of the time, but only 45% of those patients who were non-ambulatory before therapy regained ambulation (Hill *et al.* 1993). Overall survival could also be predicted by whether patients regained ambulatory function or remained non-ambulatory – the 1-year survival rates were 66% and 10% respectively (Cha *et al.* 1999).

For irradiation of the lumbar, cervical or thoracic spine, a direct posterior field is used, giving 20 Gy in five fractions. For cervical spine irradiation, paired lateral portals can be used, which largely avoids irradiation of the mouth, oropharynx and other soft tissues. It is important to remember that the cord and cauda equina may be at a significant depth, unless the patient is very thin (with a separation < 21 cm), and on occasions it may be more appropriate to treat with parallel opposed fields to ensure that a reasonable percentage depth dose to the spinal cord is achieved.

## Brain metastases

Breast cancer is the second most common cause of metastatic brain tumour, accounting for approximately 20% of all patients with brain metastases. The median survival of untreated patients with multiple metastases is usually 1–2 months, but after radiotherapy an increase in survival is reported in the range of 3–6 months. In one randomised trial, it was shown that patients with brain metastases from primary breast cancer had a better prognosis than those with other primary sites (Table 14.1) (Priestman *et al.* 1996).

**Table 14.1** Multivariate analysis of risk factors for survival from brain metastases (based on Priestman *et al.* 1996)

| Factor | Grouping | Risk ratio | p value |
| --- | --- | --- | --- |
| Performance status | 0, 1, 2 vs 3 | 1.49 | 0.0001 |
| Primary tumour | Breast vs rest | 1.38 | 0.006 |
| Dexamethasone (mg) | ≤ 8 vs > 8 | 1.33 | 0.004 |
| Age (years) | ≤ 60 vs > 60 | 1.22 | 0.037 |

Gaspar *et al.* (1997) did a retrospective analysis of RTOG trials and demonstrated the following good prognostic features: < 65 years with a Karnofsky performance status (KPS) of ≥ 70 (WHO 0 or 1), a controlled primary tumour and no systemic

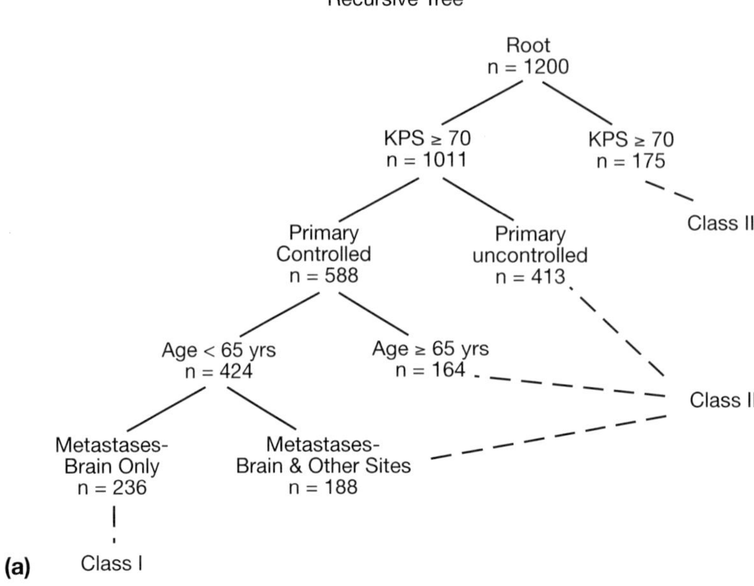


**(a)**

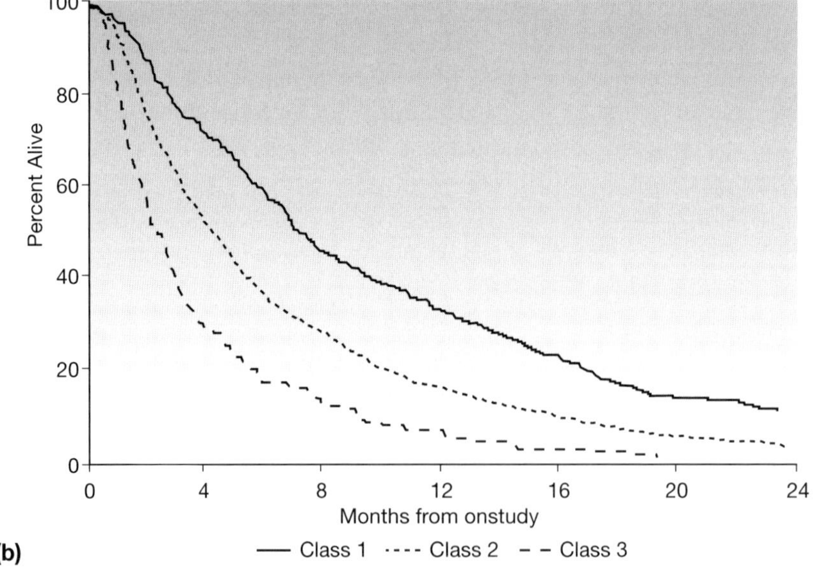


**(b)**

**Figure 14.1** Survival after brain metastases: (a) recursive analysis tree; (b) survival curves for class I, II, III (Gaspar *et al.* 1997). (Reproduced with permission of the publishers.)

metastases (median survival of over 7 months), compared with patients with a KPS of < 70 who had a median survival of only 2.3 months (Figure 14.1).

Radiation is an excellent palliation for patients with symptomatic brain metastases. Relief of symptoms is seen in 70–93% of patients depending on the symptoms at presentation (Coia *et al.* 1992), although this may not be permanent. It has been noted that 20% of patients with an initial response will develop recurrence of symptoms by 6 months and 35% by 1 year (Coia *et al.* 1991). Radiotherapy produces a general improvement in neurological function in 40–70% of patients with primary breast cancer (RCR 1999).

Initial management will involve corticosteroids and, in those patients presenting with a fit, anticonvulsants. There is no proven difference between the use of dexamethasone or prednisolone in this setting. The standard recommendation is to use dexamethasone 16 mg daily and then to taper the dose. However, one small study has shown no benefit in quality of life between patients receiving 4 mg, 8 mg or 16 g dexamethasone, with more frequent toxic effects in the 16 mg group (Vecht *et al.* 1994).

There has always been debate as to whether the steroid response should be used as a predictor for further management, because it is commonly believed that patients who do not respond to steroids are also unlikely to respond to radiotherapy; however, it has been reported that a radiotherapy response is as likely to be seen in responders and non-responders to steroids (Bezjak *et al.* 2002). The consensus is that this probably should not be taken into account when considering patients for radiotherapy (Hoskin and Brada 2001).

## Solitary brain metastases

Patients with a solitary brain metastasis should be considered for either primary surgical excision or radiosurgery.

Stereotactic radiosurgery is a non-invasive technique that delivers a single large fraction of radiation to a well-defined target volume with a very sharp peripheral dose fall-off, resulting in minimal exposure to the normal surrounding brain. Two types of device are used: the cobalt-60 'Gamma Knife' (Figure 14.2a) or a modified linear accelerator fitted with a special narrow beam collimator (Figure 14.2b). Radiosurgery is limited by the size of the metastasis, with a limit of 4.0–4.5 cm maximum diameter. No consensus on dose for radiosurgery has been reached and single doses of 15–25 Gy have been used.

Brachytherapy is not used widely and no advantages over external beam radiosurgery techniques have been noted.

Surgery is limited by the accessibility and proximity to functionally critical structures; in addition to resection it should also be considered for the relief of obstructive hydrocephalus. Surgery for operable lesions and radiosurgery is considered to be equivalent in the treatment of solitary brain metastases, but there are no

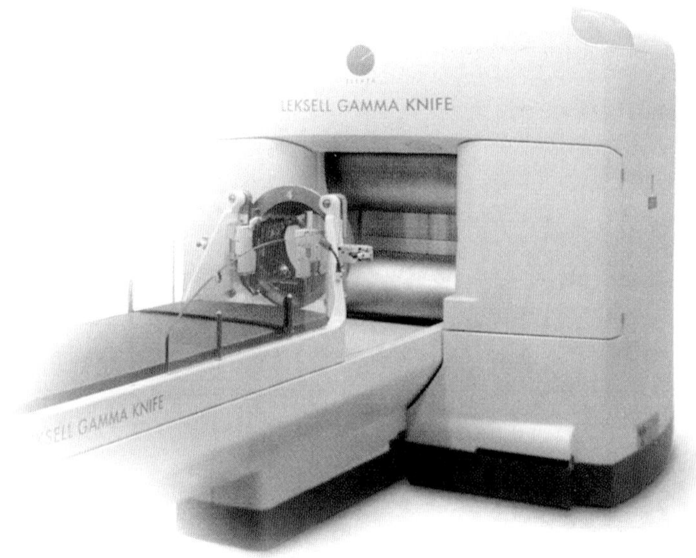


(a)

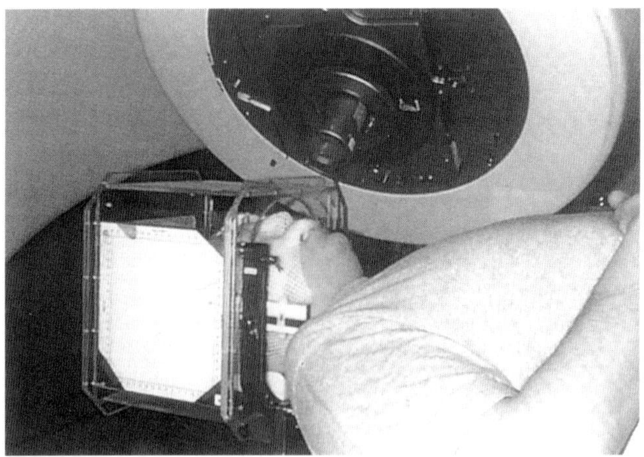

(b)

**Figure 14.2** Stereotactic radiosurgery devices: (a) Leksell Gamma Knife – Elekta Oncology systems (Elekta 1999); (b) patient in treatment position on the linac couch with the target positioner box mounted on the stereotactic frame; a shaped collimator is mounted on the accessory tray of the linac – BrainLAB (Clark and McKenzie 1999). (Reproduced with permission of the publishers.)

randomised data to confirm this. The overall 12-month local progression-free survival rate for surgery or radiosurgery is 60–80%. A survival advantage is obtained only if there is no active extracranial disease.

The addition of whole-brain irradiation to surgery has been addressed in one randomised controlled trial. Patchell *et al.* (1998) demonstrated a statistically significant reduction in 'neurological deaths' with the addition of radiation, but no effect on overall survival. The lack of survival benefit was attributed to the high incidence of deaths from progressive systemic disease. The optimum radiotherapy dose has not been explored in this setting and doses of 30–50.4 Gy in 10–28 fractions have been described in the literature.

The role of whole-brain irradiation in addition to radiosurgery has not been evaluated in randomised trials and remains uncertain; retrospective data suggest that it may add no extra survival benefit over radiosurgery alone. The addition of whole-brain irradiation may improve intracranial tumour control, but there may be an increased risk of radiation damage at the radiosurgery site.

## Multiple brain metastases

Whole brain radiotherapy is indicated in patients with good prognostic features, as noted earlier. The large randomised trials carried out by the RTOG showed no disadvantage for short commonly used schedules of 20 Gy in 5 fractions or 30 Gy in 10 fractions compared with more protracted fractionation schedules. In the trial by the Royal College of Radiologists of the UK (Priestman *et al.* 1996), 544 patients were randomised to receive 30 Gy in 10 fractions or 12 Gy in 2 fractions. They demonstrated a small survival advantage for the 30-Gy arm of 84 days compared with 77 days; the magnitude of this difference was greater in the favourable prognosis group (Figure 14.3). Overall this difference in survival is not considered clinically significant and 30 Gy in 10 fractions, 20 Gy in 5 fractions and 12 Gy in 2 fractions can all be recommended as appropriate treatment for whole brain irradiation in patients with brain metastases, with the longer schedules reserved for patients with good prognostic features.

Figure 14.4 shows an overall strategy for the management of brain metastases, based on the international consensus statement (Hoskin and Brada 2001), with the different levels of evidence for each decision arm.

## **Meningeal metastases**

Direct tumour involvement of the leptomeninges is a less common manifestation of metastatic breast cancer. In patients with untreated meningeal metastases, survival is approximately 6 weeks. Local irradiation to specific sites of spinal nerve involvement and cranial irradiation for distressing cranial nerve abnormalities may be combined with intrathecal administration of methotrexate to achieve palliation. With irradiation and intrathecal treatment, 65% of patients will show a response and survival can be in the order of 4–7 months (Wilson and Cox 1995; Cha *et al.* 1999).

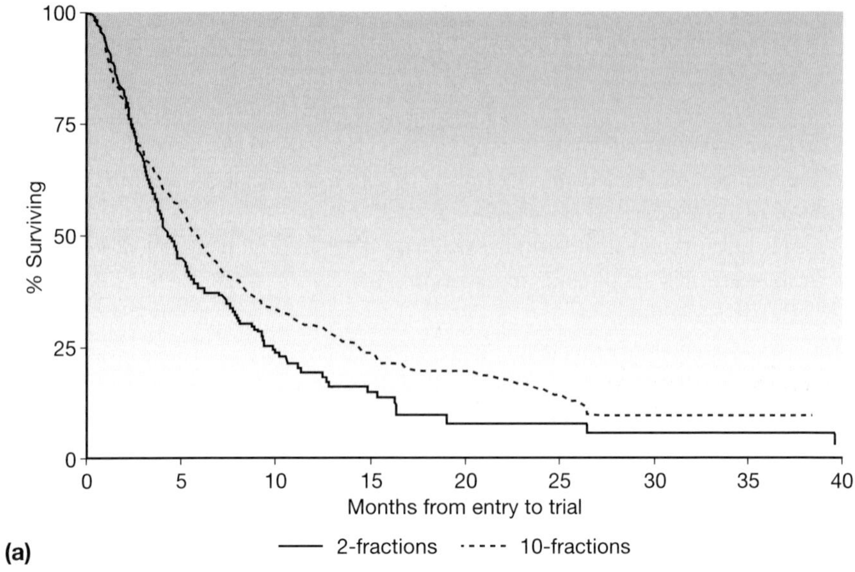


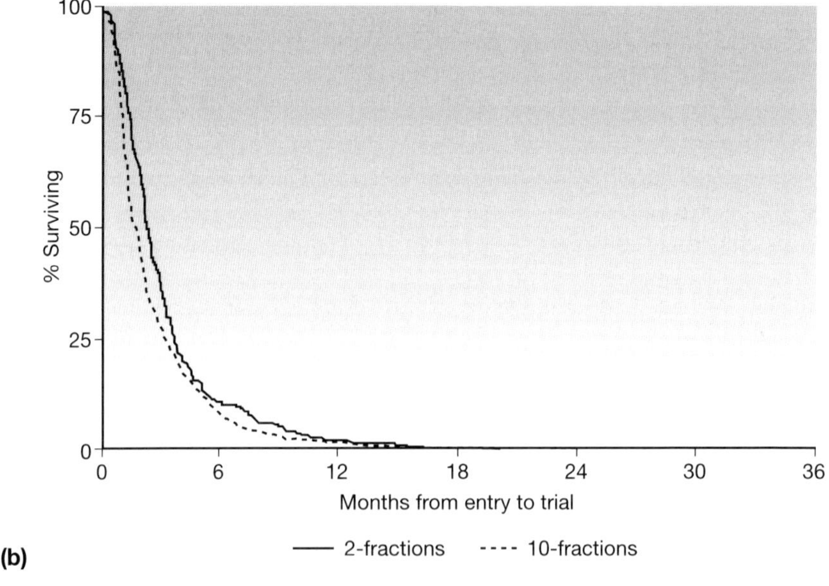


**Figure 14.3** Predicted survival curves for patients with brain metastases: (a) for the good prognostic group; (b) for the poor prognostic group (Priestman *et al.* 1996). (Reproduced with permission of the publishers.)

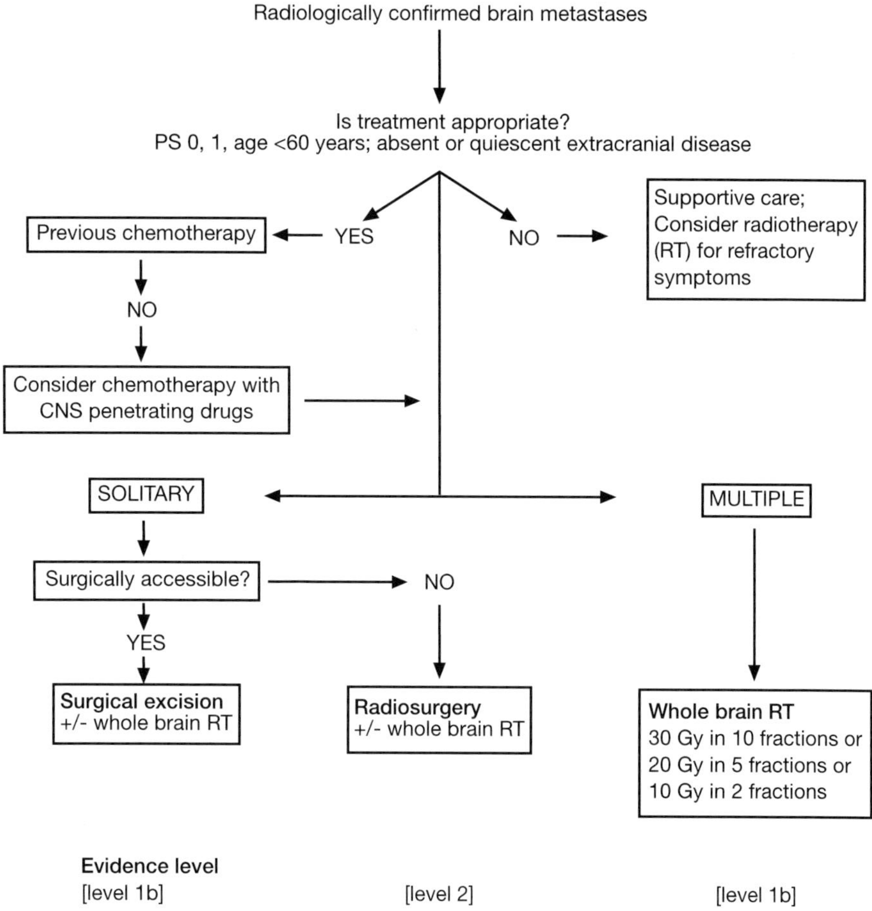


**Figure 14.4**  Decision tree for the management of brain metastases (based on Hoskin and Brada 2001).

## Ocular metastases

Metastatic lesions to the eye have a tendency to involve the uvea, with the choroid being the most common site, as a result of its vascular nature. Choroidal metastases may present as deteriorating vision and produce a poor quality of life, with reported median survival of 9 months after diagnosis.

Radiotherapy is the treatment of choice, with 60–70% of patients benefiting (RCR 1999). It can successfully restore or preserve useful vision and it should be given promptly to achieve the best outcome. A multivariate analysis by Rudoler *et al.* (1997) reported that the presence of retinal detachment did not preclude a good response to radiotherapy, as was previously thought (Figure 14.5).

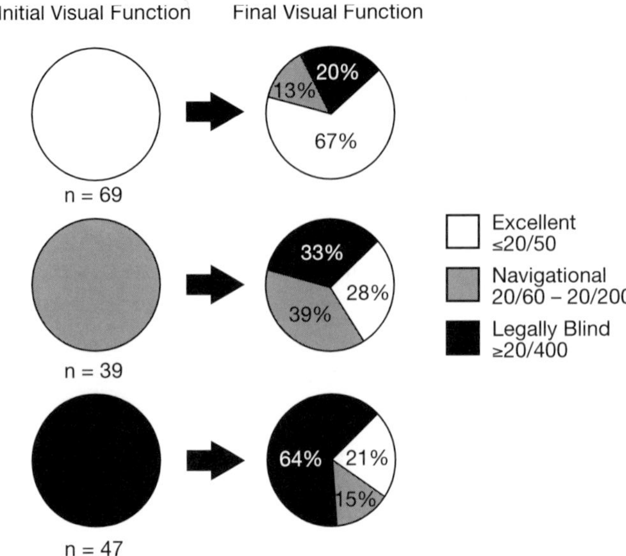


**Figure 14.5** Multivariate analysis of final visual function to radiotherapy (Rudoler *et al.* 1997).

Radiotherapy should not be withheld from patients with poor vision because, even if maximal visual response is not achieved, 98% of patients can avoid enucleation for intractable pain caused by angle-closure glaucoma.

The following characteristics have proved to be predictive of a good radiation response: excellent vision before radiotherapy, age < 55 years and tumours < 15 mm (Rudoler *et al.* 1997).

To minimise visual morbidity, a short radiotherapy course (i.e. 30 Gy in 10 fractions) using a lens-sparing technique, should be given to the involved eye (Amichetti *et al.* 2000).

## Liver metastases

The radiation tolerance of the liver limits the dose that can be given for palliation. There is a marked increase in the incidence of radiation hepatitis observed with doses exceeding 35 Gy. Despite this, several studies have confirmed that hepatic irradiation with doses of 20–30 Gy effectively palliates symptoms 60–80% of the time (Borgelt *et al.* 1981; Hoegler *et al.* 1997; Cha *et al.* 1999), particularly pain resulting from stretching of the capsule of the liver. Less benefit is derived from irradiation for abnormal liver function or hepatomegaly.

## Lymphatic involvement

Lymph node involvement is present in 70% of patients with advanced breast cancer (Hoskin and Makin 1998). Nodal groups involved include: axillary, supraclavicular, cervical and internal mammary. Secondary mediastinal involvement can lead to hoarseness, dysphagia and superior vena caval obstruction (SVCO), although there may be reluctance to re-irradiate through an area of previous chest wall irradiation. Each of these symptoms can be palliated with mediastinal irradiation. Radiotherapy usually delivers relief in patients with SVCO within 2 weeks in approximately 70% of patients (Ciezki *et al.* 2000).

## Locoregional recurrences

With locoregional recurrences, ulceration, bleeding, severe pain and watching a tumour grow at the surface of the body can cause severe suffering. Good palliation can be achieved with radiotherapy. Sometimes a 'toilet' mastectomy is possible after a good response to irradiation of the breast. When irradiating the chest wall for local recurrences, the peripheral lymphatics should also be irradiated because this practice is associated with an improved long-term survival (Wilson and Cox 1995). In locally advanced breast cancer, systemic treatment, in the form of chemotherapy or hormonal treatment, also plays an important role.

In the case of a recurrent tumour within a previously irradiated area, further radiation can be given using low doses of 10–20 Gy for growth delay and palliation with superficial low energy X-ray or electron beams. Re-irradiation may also be combined with hyperthermia to enhance its effect. The International Collaborative Hyperthermia Group (1996) demonstrated encouraging results when local hyperthermia was combined with re-irradiation. Further studies of the use of hyperthermia are indicated.

## Conclusions

Radiotherapy provides effective palliation for nearly all sites to which breast cancer can metastasise. Patient selection is as important for palliative radiotherapy as radical treatment, with greatest benefit being obtained in those with a good performance status and limited metastatic disease. Simple, short, hypofractionated treatment schedules are the ideal in the palliative setting.


*References*

Amichetti, M., Caffo, O., Minatel, E. *et al.* (2000). Ocular metastases from breast carcinoma: A multicentric retrospective study. *Oncology Reports* **7**, 761–765.

Baziotis, N., Yakoumakis, E., Zissimopoulos, A. *et al.* (1998). Strontium-89 chloride in the treatment of bone metastases from breast cancer. *Oncology* **55**, 377–381.

Bezjak, A., Adam, J., Barton, R., Panzarella, T., Laperriere, N., Wong, C. S. *et al.* (2002). Symptom response after palliative radiotherapy for patients with brain metastases. *European Journal of Cancer* **38**, 487–496.

Borgelt, B. B., Gelber, R., Brady, L. W. *et al.* (1987). The palliation of hepatic metastases. Results of the Radiation Therapy Oncology Group pilot study. *International Journal of Radiation Oncology Biology and Physics* **7**, 587–591.

Breast Specialty Group of the British Association of Surgical Oncology (1999). The management of metastatic bone disease in the United Kingdom. *European Journal of Surgical Oncology* **25**, 3–23.

Ciezki, J. P., Komurcu, S., Macklis, R. M. (2000). Palliative radiotherapy. *Seminars in Oncology* **27**, 90–93.

Cha, C. H., Kennedy, G. D., Niederhuber, J. E. (1999). Metastatic breast cancer. *Surgical Clinics of North America* **79**, 1117–1143.

Clark, B., McKenzie, M. (1999). Conformal stereotactic radiotherapy at Vancouver, British Columbia. Clinical Application Paper, BC Cancer Agency, 1–3.

Coia, L. R., Aaronson, N., Linggood, R. *et al.* (1992). A report of the consensus workshop panel on the treatment of brain metastases. *International Journal of Radiation Oncology Biology and Physics* **23**, 223–227.

Coleman, R. E. (1998). How can we improve the treatment of bone metastases further? *Current Opinion in Oncology* **10**, S7–S13.

Elekta (1999). IMRT technique enhances efficiency and homogeneity for breast treatments. *Wavelength* **3**, 1–11.

Fuller, B. G., Heiss, J. D., Oldfield, E. H. (2001). Spinal cord compression. In: DeVita, V. T., Hellman, S., Rosenberg, S. A. (eds), *Cancer – Principles and Practise of Oncology*, 6th edn.. Lippincott Williams & Wilkins, pp. 2617–2633.

Gaspar, L., Scott, C., Rotman, M. *et al.* (1997). Recursive partitioning analysis (RPA) of prognostic factors in three Radiation Therapy Oncology Group (RTOG) brain metastases trials. *International Journal of Radiation Oncology, Biology and Physics* **37**, 745–751.

Harrington, K. D. (1986). Impending pathologic fractures from metastatic malignancy: evaluation and management. *American Academy of Orthopaedic Surgeons* **35**, 357–381.

Hill, M. E., Richards, M. A., Gregory, W. M. *et al.* (1993). Spinal cord compression in breast cancer: a critical review of 70 cases. *British Journal of Cancer* **68**, 969–973.

Hoegler, D. (1997). Radiotherapy for palliation of symptoms in incurable cancer. *Current problems in Cancer* **21**, 129–183.

Hoskin, P. J., Brada, M. (2001). Consensus statement. Radiotherapy for brain metastases. *Clinical Oncology* **13**, 91–94.

Hoskin, P. J. (1988). Scientific and clinical aspects of radiotherapy in the relief of bone pain. *Cancer Surveys* **7**, 69–86.

Hoskin, P. J., Makin, W. (1998). Breast cancer. In: *Oncology for Palliative Medicine*. Oxford: Oxford University Press, pp 68–70.

Hoskin, P. J., Yarnold, J. R., Roos, D. R. *et al.* (2001). Consensus Statement. Radiotherapy for bone metastases. *Clinical Oncology* **13**, 88–90.

Ingham, J., Portenoy, R. K. (1998). The measurement of pain and other symptoms. In: Doyle, D., Hanks, G. W. C., MacDonald, N. (eds), *Oxford Textbook of Palliative Medicine*, 2nd edn. Oxford: Oxford University Press, pp 203–219.

International Collaborative Hyperthermia Group (1996). Hyperthermia in the treatment of superficial localized primary and recurrent breast cancer – results from five randomized controlled trials. *International Journal of Radiation Oncology Biology and Physics* **35**, 731–744.

Patchell, R. A., Tibbs, P. A., Regine, W. F. *et al.* (1998). Postoperative radiotherapy in the treatment of single metastases to the brain: a randomized trial. *Journal of the American Medical Association* **280**, 1485–1489.

Priestman, T. J., Dunn, J., Brada, M. *et al.* (1996). Final results of the Royal College of Radiologists' trial comparing two different radiotherapy schedules in the treatment of cerebral metastases. *Clinical Oncology* **8**, 308–315.

Royal College of Radiologists (1999). Clinical Oncology Information Network. Guidelines on the non-surgical management of breast cancer. *Clinical Oncology* **11**, S96–S97, S120–S124.

Rudoler, S. B., Shields, C. L., Corn, B. W. *et al.* (1997). Functional vision is improved in the majority of patients treated with external beam radiotherapy for choroids metastases: A multivariate analysis of 188 patients. *Journal of Clinical Oncology* **15**, 1244–1251.

Salazar, O. M., Rubin, P., Hendrickson, F. R. *et al.* (1986). Single-dose half-body irradiation for palliation of multiple bone metastases from solid tumors. Final Radiation Therapy Oncology Group report. *Cancer* **58**, 29–36.

Salazar, O. M., Sandhu, T., da Motta, N. W. *et al.* (2001). Fractionated half-body irradiation (HBI) for the rapid palliation of widespread, symptomatic, metastatic bone disease: A randomized phase III trial of the International Atomic Energy Agency (IAEA). *International Journal of Radiation Oncology Biology and Physics* **50**, 765–775.

Wilson, J. F., Cox, J. D. (1995). Palliative radiation therapy for mammary cancer. In: Donegan, W. L., Spratt, J. S. (eds), *Cancer of the Breast*, 4th edn. Philadelphia: W. B. Saunders Co., pp 511–518.

Vecht, C. J., Hovestadt, A., Verbiest, H. B. *et al.* (1994). Dose–effect relationship of dexamethasone on Karnofsky performance in metastatic brain tumours: a randomized study of doses 4, 8 and 16mg per day. *Neurology* **44**, 675–680.

# Chapter 15

# Evidence and opinion for the adjuvant use of taxoids in early breast cancer

*Richard Adams, Peter Barrett-Lee and Paul Ellis*

## Introduction

Breast cancer remains the most common malignancy in women. It accounts for 31% of all female cancers, and in the UK each year alone 38,000 are newly diagnosed and nearly 13,000 die of the disease (Cancer Research Campaign (CRC) 2001). Despite ongoing advances in the management of early breast cancer, there are still continuing major clinical problems, including considerable mortality and morbidity and an ever-increasing demand on limited health resources.

Slowly but surely we are seeing increasing evidence to suggest that we are making inroads into this disease and influencing breast cancer mortality. Within the UK this is evidenced by work such as that of Beral *et al.* (1995) who demonstrated a fall in death rates in England and Wales despite an increase in incidence. This is still the beginning; vast quantities of research energy continue in an attempt to push further through the boundaries of this disease. It remains the small incremental steps that appear to be so important in this process.

## Adjuvant therapy in early breast cancer

Breast cancer is frequently described as a systemic disease at the outset, rather than simply a local disease that sometimes becomes metastatic. This theory adds impetus to the advancement of adjuvant systemic therapy. Both hormone therapy and systemic chemotherapy have now been demonstrated as showing a clear benefit. The recent overview from the Early Breast Cancer Trialists' Collaborative Group (EBCTCG) has confirmed a benefit from adjuvant chemotherapy to most groups of patients regardless of menopausal, nodal or hormonal status. Evidence suggests that there is a reduction in the odds of recurrence of 24% and the odds of death of 15%; with subgroup analysis confirming a higher benefit for node positive women less than 50 years of age (36% and 25% respectively). Most clinical trials so far have used a cyclophosphamide, methotrexate and 5-fluorouracil (CMF)-based regimen, but there is now good evidence to suggest that an anthracycline-based regimen provides more of a gold standard. The 2000 EBTCG overview demonstrated a clear advantage in the use of anthracycline-based chemotherapy (Early Breast Cancer Trialists' Collaborative Group 2000). In addition to those results, evidence has now accumulated to support a further 'move of the goalposts' with the addition of taxanes to the adjuvant setting.

## High dose chemotherapy

Several clinical trials have tested high-dose chemotherapy (HDC) with bone marrow transplant (BMT) or stem cell support in women with more than 10 positive lymph nodes and in women with 4 to 9 positive lymph nodes. One of these trials demonstrated a non-statistically significant ($p = 0.09$) relapse-free survival advantage to HDC in a preliminary analysis (Rodenhuis *et al.* 2003). Another five trials comparing conventional chemotherapy to HDC with BMT or stem cell support in high risk patients in the adjuvant setting indicate no overall or event-free survival benefit from the HDC (Tallman *et al.* 2003; Bergh *et al.* 2000; Hortogyi *et al.* 2000; Schrama *et al.* 2002). This was confirmed in the Anglo-Celtic I study, where the event-free survival for the HDC group at 5 years was 51% whereas for the group treated with doxorubicin followed by CMF chemotherapy the event-free survival was 54%. The overall survival rates at 5 years were 63% and 62%, respectively (Crown *et al.* 2002). In contrast, the adjuvant PEGASE 01 trial showed a significantly better 3-year disease-free survival for the HDC arm, but with an unchanged overall survival rate. The ongoing Phase III 06 trial is studying a higher dose regimen (Roche *et al.* 2003). While further follow-up of these studies is required to resolve the role of high dose consolidation therapy in this setting, this information to date does not support the use of HDC outside of the context of randomised controlled trials.

## The taxanes: experience and effectiveness in breast cancer

The taxanes have a unique mechanism of action, causing increased polymerisation of nuclear microtubules and thereby disrupting mitosis and replication (Diaz *et al.* 1993). The first of these drugs to be developed, paclitaxel (Taxol®, Bristol-Myers Squibb) has been licensed for use in metastatic breast cancer, ovarian cancer and non-small-cell lung cancer. The second and chemically distinct taxoid, docetaxel (Taxotere®) is a semi-synthetic product from the needles of the European yew tree, *Taxus baccata*, and is manufactured in the UK (Aventis). Docetaxel has a licence in combination with doxorubicin for initial chemotherapy of advanced or metastatic breast cancer; or as a single agent in advanced or metastatic breast cancer where adjuvant cytotoxic chemotherapy has failed (it is also licensed for use in non-small-cell lung cancer).

## The metastatic setting

As with most systemic therapies entering adjuvant trials and usage, there has been evidence of activity within the metastatic setting initially. Both drugs have been shown to be very effective in patients with metastatic breast cancer resistant to anthracyclines, with response rates around 40–50% (Gianni *et al.* 1994; O'Brien *et al.* 1999). Superior activity has been shown by docetaxel used in patients who have failed or progressed on anthracyclines: Nabholtz *et al.* (1999a) showed that docetaxel was superior to MV (mitomycin, vinblastine) and Chan *et al.* (1999) demonstrated superiority for docetaxel over doxorubicin. In the first-line metastatic setting, Nabholtz *et al.* (1999b, 2001) showed docetaxel in combination to be superior with AT (doxorubicin, docetaxel) versus AC (doxorubicin, cyclophosphamide) and later with TAC (docetaxel, doxorubicin, cyclophosphamide) versus FAC (5-fluorouracil, doxorubicin, cyclophosphamide).

## The neo-adjuvant setting

Can we extrapolate information from the neoadjuvant setting, for use in the adjuvant setting? Credence is lent to this idea, as postulated by Hackshaw *et al.* (2002) who stated; 'there is a relationship between surrogate markers and survival in women receiving first-line chemotherapy for advanced breast cancer'. Their analysis illustrated that time to disease progression (TTP) and overall response (OR) can be used as surrogate markers for survival in patients with metastatic breast cancer; from this one might postulate a greater efficacy in the adjuvant setting. Neoadjuvant clinical trials that have led to this theory include NSABP B-27 and Tax 301. The larger NSABP B-27 trial randomised 2,210 patients with operable breast cancer to three arms; all had AC ×4 pre-operatively, arm 2 had docetaxel ×4 sequentially pre-operatively and arm 3 had docetaxel ×4 post-operatively. The interim results were presented at a San Antonio Breast Cancer Symposium (SABCS 2001): 25.6% of those receiving docetaxel sequentially with AC pre-operatively, had a pathological complete response (pCR) compared with 13.7% of those receiving AC only ($p <$ 0.001); this in turn was highly correlated with an increase in overall survival (OS). However, it has been argued that in the face of an extra four cycles of chemotherapy pre-operatively it is not surprising that the docetaxel arm did better. Tax 301 a recently published study used docetaxel as primary (neo-adjuvant) therapy before surgery. This study enrolled 158 patients. All patients received four cycles of cyclophosphamide 1000 mg/m$^2$ doxorubicin 50 mg/m$^2$ plus vincristine and prednisolone (CVAP) at 3-weekly intervals. One hundred and four patients had a clinical response to this therapy after four cycles and were then randomised to either a further four cycles of CVAP or four cycles of docetaxel at 100 mg/m$^2$ every 3 weeks. In this small study there was a significant difference in both clinical and pathological response in the docetaxel arm. This has translated into a significant overall survival at 3 years of 97% versus 84% ($p = 0.05$). (Smith *et al.* 2002; Hutcheon *et al.* 2000, 2001, 2003).

Evidence for the use of taxanes in the adjuvant setting thus comes from trials revealing high activity in metastatic breast cancer, high pCR rates in the neoadjuvant setting and a lack of cross resistance with the, so far, most important and proven chemotherapy agent in breast cancer; the anthracycline.

It has therefore been postulated that sequential or concomitant administration of these non-cross resistant taxanes to proven breast cancer chemotherapy combinations may be superior to standard combination chemotherapy in the adjuvant setting.

## Taxanes as adjuvant therapy for early breast cancer: evidence from clinical trials

This idea was initially reinforced by the first presentation of the data from the North American Cooperative Intergroup Cancer and Leukaemia Group B study 9344 (CALGB 9344). A total of 3,170 women with node-positive breast cancer were randomised to receive AC with doxorubicin at one of three dose levels (60 mg/m$^2$, 75 mg/m$^2$, or 90 mg/m$^2$) and then to receive paclitaxel or not. With a median follow-up of only 30 months this study did not confirm any benefit for dose escalation of doxorubicin but identified significant improvements in disease-free (90% versus 86%) and overall (97% versus 95%) survival (Henderson *et al.* 1998). If these benefits were maintained with longer follow-up they would translate into a reduction in the odds of recurrence of 22% and in the odds of death of 26%—a significant advance. Much of these data led to the US Federal Drugs Administration granting a license for the use of paclitaxel in the adjuvant therapy of breast cancer in 1999. However, in the National Institutes of Health Consensus Conference (NIH 2000) on adjuvant therapy in Breast Cancer, at 52 months median follow-up there appears to have been substantial weakening of the benefits for paclitaxel. While remaining statistically significant, the latest results show a reduction in odds of recurrence now of 13% ($p < 0.05$), and death 14% (not significant at this stage) (Table 15.1). This represented an actuarial absolute survival benefit of only 3% (84% versus 81%). Another caveat to this study is that the benefits of paclitaxel were confined to oestrogen receptor (ER)-negative patients, with no discernible benefits to over 2,000 women with ER positive disease (Retrospective analysis).

**Table 15.1** The CALGB 9344 trial: three interim analyses

| Date of analysis: | May 1998 | April 1999 | November 2000 |
|---|---|---|---|
| Initially presented | ASCO | sNDA | NIH CDC |
| Reduction in the odds of recurrence. | 22%* | 22%* | 13%* |
| Reduction in the odds of death | 26%* | 26%* | 14% |

The benefit of paclitaxel is still only seen in ER-negative patients. No difference in ER-positive patients. (Retrospective analysis.) *$p < 0.05$.

The design of this trial has also been criticised: i.e. whether four cycles of AC was insufficient therapy for these node positive patients. Also, whether the comparison of four cycles of chemotherapy versus eight cycles (in the paclitaxel arm) was appropriate and whether the addition of paclitaxel would provide a similar degree of benefit for high-risk node-negative patients.

A similarly designed trial from the National Surgical Adjuvant Breast and Bowel Project in the US (NSABP B-28) randomised 3,060 patients with lymph-node-positive breast cancer to four cycles of AC ($60/600mg/m^2$), with or without four cycles of paclitaxel at a dose of 225 $mg/m^2$ as a 3-hour infusion every 21 days. The first presentation of interim results from this trial were also presented at NIH Consensus Conference (2000): after 34 months median follow-up there are no significant differences in disease-free (81%) or overall survival (AC: 92%; AC-T 90%; $p = 0.98$) for the two arms of the trial (NIH 2000).

The M. D. Anderson Cancer Centre (Buzdar *et al.* 2002) has also performed a smaller trial using paclitaxel as adjuvant therapy. This randomised 524 patients between eight cycles of 5-fluorouracil at 500 $mg/m^2$ on days 1 and 4, doxorubicin at 50 $mg/m^2$ by continuous infusion over 72 hours and cyclophosphamide at 500 $mg/m^2$ on day 1 (FAC) or to four cycles of paclitaxel at 250 $mg/m^2$ over 24 hours every 3 weeks followed by four cycles of FAC. One-third of patients had neo-adjuvant chemotherapy and two-thirds received adjuvant chemotherapy after surgery. After median follow-up of 60 months the disease-free survival is 83% in the FAC arm and 86% in the FAC-paclitaxel arm ($p = 0.09$; not statistically significant at this time).

The one published adjuvant trial using docetaxel differs not only in which taxane was used but also in its concomitant as opposed to sequential usage. Breast Cancer International Research Group (BCIRG) 001 randomised 1,491 node-positive patients to FAC ×6 versus docetaxel plus AC (TAC) ×6; the interim results were presented at ASCO 2002 (Nabholtz *et al.* 2002). These showed that at 33 months median follow-up, TAC gave a 32% reduction in relapse overall but when stratified by nodal status; 1–3 nodes-positive patients (N1–3) had a 50% reduction in relapse compared with FAC ($p = 0.0002$) whereas 4+ nodes (N4+) showed no difference. Interestingly, and in contrast to the CALGB 9344 study, ER-positive and negative patients showed 32% and 38% reduction in relapse rate, respectively compared with the FAC arm. The secondary endpoint of overall survival showed a 24% relative reduction for TAC compared with FAC, which was not statistically different except when looking at the subgroup of N1–3 patients whereby an absolute reduction in mortality of 7% was seen, translating into a relative reduction of 54% ($p = 0.006$) (see Figure 15.1). See Tables 15.2 and 15.3 for comparisons between the major trials.

## Docetaxel or paclitaxel in the adjuvant setting

If one is to believe that data from the metastatic setting can be extrapolated to the adjuvant setting as far as drug efficacy is concerned, then studies such as Paridaens *et al.* (2000) and Sledge *et al.* (1997) using paclitaxel in the first-line metastatic setting have suggested that monotherapy with paclitaxel is very much on a level playing field with doxorubicin. However, there is some evidence to suggest that docetaxel has activity in breast cancer that is the equal of or possibly better than paclitaxel (Sledge *et al.* 1997).

Of the adjuvant taxane trials that have reported, in at least a preliminary fashion so far, there are currently three phase III trials with almost 7,000 patients using

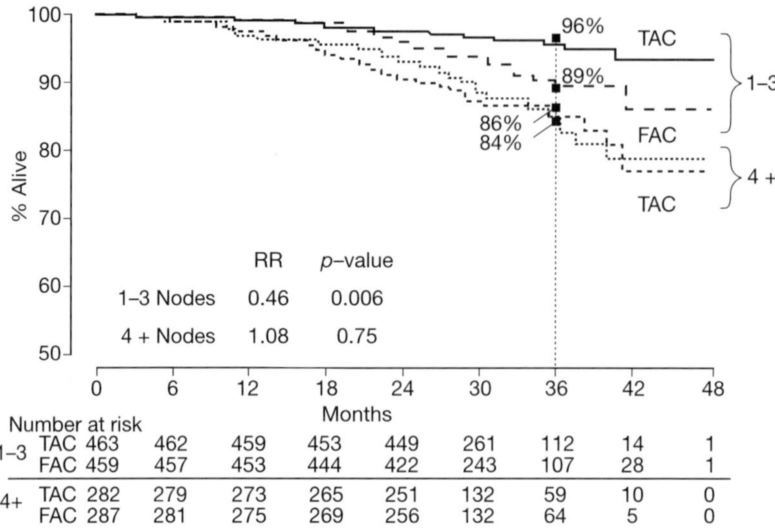


| | | 0 | 6 | 12 | 18 | 24 | 30 | 36 | 42 | 48 |
|---|---|---|---|---|---|---|---|---|---|---|
| 1–3 | TAC | 463 | 462 | 459 | 453 | 449 | 261 | 112 | 14 | 1 |
| | FAC | 459 | 457 | 453 | 444 | 422 | 243 | 107 | 28 | 1 |
| 4+ | TAC | 282 | 279 | 273 | 265 | 251 | 132 | 59 | 10 | 0 |
| | FAC | 287 | 281 | 275 | 269 | 256 | 132 | 64 | 5 | 0 |

**Figure 15.1** Overall survival by Nodal Status (Nabholtz *et al.* ASCO 2002)

paclitaxel in the adjuvant setting and only one with almost 1,500 patients using docetaxel.

**Table 15.2** A Comparison of the three largest Adjuvant Taxane Trials: Absolute Differences Disease-Free and Overall Survival; All patients

| | *Per cent patients disease-Free* | *Per cent patients alive* |
|---|---|---|
| CALGB 9344 3-year | | |
| 3120 patients | | |
|     AC+T(P) | 79 | 88 |
|     AC | 74 | 85 |
|     Per cent difference | 5 | 3 |
| | | |
| NSABP B-28 3-year | | |
| 3060 patients | | |
|     AC+T(P) | 82 | 91 |
|     AC | 82 | 91 |
|     Per cent difference | 0 | 0 |
| | | |
| BCIRG 001 3-year | | |
| 1491 patients | | |
|     T(D)AC | 82 | 92 |
|     FAC | 74 | 87 |
|     % Difference | 8 | 5 |

A, doxorubicin; C, cyclophophamide; T(P), paclitaxel (Taxol); F, 5- fluorouracil; T(D), docetaxel (Taxotere).

**Table 15.3** Comparative efficacy of adjuvant systemic therapies (Riva ASCO 2002)

| *Therapies of:* | | *Per cent risk reduction in annual odds* | | |
| --- | --- | --- | --- | --- |
| | n | *Follow up* | *Recurrence* | *Death* |
| CT versus no CT (EBCTCG 1995) | ~10,000 | 15 years | 23.5 $p < 0.00001$ | 17 $p < 0.00001$ |
| Doxorubicin versus no doxorubicin (ECBCTCG 2000) | ~7,000 | 10 years | 10.8 $p = 0.0055$ | 15.7 $p < 0.00001$ |
| Paclitaxel versus no paclitaxel (CALGB 9344) | ~3,000 | 52 months | 13.0 $p = 0.032$ | 14.0 $p = 0.074$ |
| Docetaxel versus no docetaxel (BCIRG 001) | 1,491 | 33 months | 32.0 $p = 0.0011$ | 24.0 $p = 0.11$ |
| One to three lymph nodes docetaxel versus no docetaxel (BCIRG 001) | ~1,000 | 33 months | 50.0 $p = 0.0002$ | 54.0 $p = 0.006$ |

There is at least one study (ECOG E-1199) with four arms (see Table 15.4), recently to have completed recruitment, which directly compares paclitaxel and docetaxel in the adjuvant setting. This trial with a taxane in all arms assumes that the role of taxanes is already established but its comparative role should certainly help identify the leading taxane in the adjuvant setting.

It is particularly important, when current opinion and evidence place anthracyclines as a core component to any adjuvant chemotherapy regimen, to consider what the use of a taxane will add and what difficulties will arise. It is widely believed that, because of the lack of cross resistance between anthracyclines and taxanes, this combination has greater theoretical value, for cell kill. However, because of the possible future prospects of the taxanes in the adjuvant setting it becomes increasingly important to look at the toxic and long-term side effects of any adjuvant regimens. There is evidence from some phase I/II studies in metastatic or advanced breast cancer that have suggested excellent anti-tumour activity in combinations of paclitaxel with doxorubicin, but this has been complicated by a high rate of cardiotoxicity when paclitaxel was given as a 3-hour infusion close to doxorubicin administration. Gianni *et al.* (1995, 1997) reported an overall response rate of 94% in 32 patients. However, simultaneously 21% of patients developed congestive heart failure. Similar studies with doxorubicin and docetaxel have not shown such problems in the doses and combinations used while retaining response rates of up to 81% (Misset *et al.* 1999). Further, studies are ongoing using epirubicin in combination with the taxanes in place of doxorubicin and looking at sequential, rather than concomitant, administration of taxanes. One can therefore see from Table 15.4 that

**Table 15.4** Recent/current trials incorporating taxanes as adjuvant systemic therapy for breast cancer

| Co-ordinating group | Trial code | Eligible patient types | Numbers of patients | Comparative regimens | Main outcome measures |
|---|---|---|---|---|---|
| CALGB | 9344 | Node positive early breast cancer | 3120 | AC × 4 versus AC × 4 then T(P) × 4 (3 weekly) Study closed | DFS, OS |
| NSABP | B-28 | Node positive early breast cancer | 3060 | AC × 4 versus AC × 4 then T(P) × 4 (3 weekly) Study closed | DFS, OS |
| MD Andersen Cancer Centre Trial | | Early Breast Cancer | 524 | FAC × 8 versus T(P) × 4 then FAC × 4 (3 weekly) 1/3 received neo-adjuvant chemotherapy. Study closed | DFS, OS |
| ECOG, NCCTG, SWOG, CALGB | E-1199 | Stage IIA, IIB, IIIA (including high-risk node negative | 5000 | AC × 4 then T(P) × 12 (weekly) versus AC × 4 then T(P) × 4 (3 weekly) versus AC × 4 then T(D) × 12 (weekly) versus AC × 4 then T(D) × 4 (3 weekly) Study closed | DFS, OS |
| International Collaborative Cancer Group | ICCG-C 14/96 | Post-menopausal node positive | 850 | E days 1 and 8 × 6 (4 weekly) versus E days 1 and 8 × 3 (4 weekly) then T(D) × 3 (3 weekly) | DFS, OS |
| CRC/ UKCCCR | TACT | Early breast cancer | 3300 | FEC × 8 (or E × 4 then CMF × 4) versus FEC × 4 then T(D) × 4 (3 weekly) | DFS, OS |
| Federation Nationale des Centres de Lutte Contre le Cancer | FRE- FNCLCC- PACS-01 | Node positive early breast cancer | 1600 | FEC × 6 (3weekly) versus FEC × 3 then T(D) × 3 (3 weekly). Study closed | DFS, OS |

contd . . .

A, doxorubicin; C, cyclophosphamide; E, epirubicin; F, 5-fluorouracil; M, methotrexate; T(P), paclitaxel; T(D), docetaxel; G-CSF, granulocyte colony stimulating factor. Numbers in bold represent final patient recruitment and studies discussed in the text. DFS, disease-free survival; OS, overall survival; ER, oestrogen receptor; PR, progestogen receptor.

**Table 15.4** contd

| Co-ordinating group | Trial code | Eligible patient types | Numbers of patients | Comparative regimens | Main outcome measures |
|---|---|---|---|---|---|
| Breast Cancer International Research Group | 001/ TAX 316 | Node positive | 1491 | FAC × 6 (3weekly) versus T(D)AC × 6 (3weekly). Study closed. (Interim results ASCO 2002) | DFS, OS |
| Instituto Nazionale per la Ricerca sul Cancro | GONO-MIG-5 | Stage IIA, IIB, III | 1000 | E T(P) × 4 (3 weekly) versus FEC × 6 Study closed | DFS, OS |
| ECOG | E -2197 | One to three nodes positive or high-risk node negative breast cancer | 2778 | AT(D) × 4 (3 weekly) versus AC × 4 (3 weekly) Study closed | DFS, OS |
| ECOG, NCCTG, SWOG, CALGB | CLB-9741 | Node positive; stage II or IIIA | 2000 | A × 4 then T(P) × 4 then C × 4 (3weekly) versus A × 4 then T(P) × 4 then C × 4 (2 weekly with G-CSF) versus AC × 4 then T(P) × 4 (3 weekly) versus AC × 4 then T(P) × 4 (2 weekly with GCSF) Study closed | DFS, OS |
| European Breast International Intergroup | EBII Adjuvant Study | Node positive | 2200 | AT(D) × 4 then CMF × 3 (3 weekly) versus AC × 4 then CMF × 3 (3 weekly) versus A × 4 then CMF × 3 (3 weekly) versus A × 3 then T(D) × 3 then CMF × 3 (3 weekly) | DFS, OS |

*contd* . . .

A, doxorubicin; C, cyclophosphamide; E, epirubicin; F, 5-fluorouracil; M, methotrexate; T(P), paclitaxel; T(D), docetaxel; G-CSF, granulocyte colony stimulating factor. Numbers in bold represent final patient recruitment and studies discussed in the text. DFS, disease-free survival; OS, overall survival; ER, oestrogen receptor; PR, progestogen receptor.

**Table 15.4** contd

| Co-ordinating group | Trial code | Eligible patient types | Numbers of patients | Comparative regimens | Main outcome measures |
|---|---|---|---|---|---|
| Breast International Group | BIG-2-98 | Node positive | 2200 | A × 4 then CMF × 3 (3 weekly) versus AC × 4 then CMF × 3 (3 weekly) versus A × 3 then T(D) × 3 then CMF × 3 (3 weekly) versus AT(D) × 4 then CMF × 3 (3 weekly) | DFS, OS |
| NCIC Clinical Trials Group | MA21 | Node positive or high-risk node negative. | 1500 | EF days 1 and 8 C  days 1-14 × 6 (4 weekly) versus EC × 6 (2 weekly with G-CSF and epoetin alpha) then T(P) × 4 (3 weekly with G-CSF) versus AC × 4 then T(P) × 4 (3 weekly with G-CSF) | DFS, OS |
| NSABP | B-30 | Node positive | 4000 | AC × 4 then T(D) × 4 (3 weekly) versus AT(D) (3 weekly with G-CSF) versus T(D)AC × 4 (3 weekly with G-CSF) | DFS, OS |
| NSABP | B-31 | Node positive N1 and HER-2 strongly positive | 2700 | AC × 4 then T(P) × 4 (3 weekly) versus as arm one but then from day 1 of T(P), trastuzumab is given weekly for 51 weeks. | Cardio-toxicity DFS, OS |
| CRC/UKCCCR | tAnGO | Early stage, ER/PR poor | 3000 | EC × 4 (3weekly) then T(P) × 4 (3weekly) versus EC × 4 (3weekly) then T(P) and Gemcitabine (days1 and 8) × 4 (3weekly). | DFS, OS |
| BCIRG | 005 | Node positive, HER-2 negative. | 3130 | AC × 4 then T(D) × 4 versus T(D)AC × 6 | DFS, OS |

contd . . .

A, doxorubicin; C, cyclophosphamide; E, epirubicin; F, 5-fluorouracil; M, methotrexate; T(P), paclitaxel; T(D), docetaxel; G-CSF, granulocyte colony stimulating factor.  Numbers in bold represent final patient recruitment and studies discussed in the text. DFS, disease-free survival; OS, overall survival; ER, oestrogen receptor; PR, progestogen receptor.

**Table 15.4** contd

| Co-ordinating group | Trial code | Eligible patient types | Numbers of patients | Comparative regimens | Main outcome measures |
|---|---|---|---|---|---|
| BCIRG | 006 | Node positive, HER-2 positive | 3150 | AC × 4 then T(D) × 4 versus T(D) Carboplatin × 6 plus Herceptin concomitantly and then for one year after versus AC × 4 then T(D) plus Herceptin concomitantly with T(D) and for one year after. | DFS, OS |

A, doxorubicin; C, cyclophosphamide; E, epirubicin; F, 5-fluorouracil; M, methotrexate; T(P), paclitaxel; T(D), docetaxel; G-CSF, granulocyte colony stimulating factor. Numbers in bold represent final patient recruitment and studies discussed in the text. DFS, disease-free survival; OS, overall survival; ER, oestrogen receptor; PR, progestogen receptor.

paclitaxel is now used as a sequential agent wherever it is part of a doxorubicin-containing regimen, whereas docetaxel is continuing assessment in combination and sequence with doxorubicin.

## Ongoing trials and awaited results

The adjuvant trials can already be divided into those in which both or all arms contain a taxane and those still comparing an anthracycline based regimen with or without a taxane. In the UK the TACT trial is looking at the adjuvant use of eight cycles of cyclophosphamide, epirubicin, 5-fluorouracil (FEC) or epirubicin plus CMF versus four cycles of docetaxel followed by four cycles of FEC. There are even trials directly comparing the two taxanes: docetaxel and paclitaxel in the adjuvant setting (ECOG E-1199). More recent trials have added in newer agents, i.e. trastuzumab (Herceptin®) therapy, and this has also led to a scare of increased cardiotoxicity; this resulted in a temporary stoppage to recruitment in one trial while toxicity was assessed, although this trial has recently restarted. Some of these trials and brief descriptions are shown in Table 15.4.

## Conclusions

The taxanes paclitaxel and docetaxel have shown tremendous promise and generated great interest over the past decade. Their activity in the breast cancer setting is now such that they are established cytotoxic agents in the treatment of metastatic breast cancer. The positive results have quite reasonably led to trials attempting to seek a role and gain experience in the adjuvant setting for breast cancer. There are now data available on over 8,000 patients, in the adjuvant setting, with median follow-up of between 60 and 34 months. From trials in progress (i.e. ECOG E-1199, tAnGO) some investigators feel that the place for taxanes in the adjuvant setting is already proven and should be used routinely in this setting. Yet again we find the difficulty of obtaining a consensus on a standard of treatment for chemotherapy regimen. Currently, the data for the use of paclitaxel appear to get weaker, though still positive, as these trials mature. The one adjuvant trial with docetaxel shows promise but has yet to prove itself through the test of time. The trials reported so far still leave many questions to be answered, and well-respected research groups and organisations are now conducting further trials in thousands of patients worldwide. There are now at least nine trials containing over 15,000 women that have completed recruitment and closed. These trials compare a variety of standard anthracycline-containing regimens with these same regimens with the addition of a taxane, concomitantly or sequentially. More than 4,500 women will have received paclitaxel in this setting and over 3,000 women will have received docetaxel. Over the next few years the role of taxanes (and which taxane) in the adjuvant setting will be better defined. We await the results with interest and look forward to the meta-analyses of such data.

## *References*

Beral, V. *et al.* (1995). Sudden fall in breast cancer death rates in England and Wales. *The Lancet* **345**, 1642–1643.

Bergh, J., Wiklund, T., Erikstein, B. *et al.* (2000). Tailored flourouracil, epirubicin and cyclophosphamide compared with marrow-supported high-dose chemotherapy as adjuvant treatment for high-risk breast cancer: a randomised trial. Scandinavian Breast Group 9401 study. *The Lancet* **356**(9239), 1384–1391.

Buzdar, A. U. *et al.* (2002). Evaluation of paclitaxel in adjuvant chemotherapy for patients with operable breast cancer: preliminary data of a prospective randomized trial. *Clinical Cancer Research* **8**, 1073–1079.

Chan S. *et al.* (1999). Prospective randomized trial of docetaxel versus doxorubicin in patients with metastatic breast cancer. *Journal of Clinical Oncology* **17**, 2341–2354.

CRC (2001). Cancer statistics. See www.crc.org.uk/cancer

Crown, J. P., Lind, M., Gould, A. *et al.* (2002). High-dose chemotherapy with autograft is not superior to cyclophosphamide, methotrexate and 5-FU following doxorubicin induction in patients with breast cancer and four or more involved axillary lymph nodes: the Anglo-Celtic 1 Study. *Proceedings of the American Society of Clinical Oncology* Abstract 166.

Diaz, J. F. *et al.* (1993). Assembly of purified GDP-tubulin into microtubules induced by taxol and taxotere: reversibility, ligand stoichiometry, and competition. *Biochemistry* **32**, 2747–2755.

Peto, R. EBCTCG (2000). EBCTCG – updated results from September 2000 worldwide overview. *European Journal of Cancer* **36**(Suppl. 5), abstract 13, S47.

Gianni, L., Capri, G., Munzone, E. *et al.* (1994). Paclitaxel (Taxol) efficacy in patients with advanced breast cancer resistant to anthracyclines. *Seminars in Surgical Oncolology* **21**(Suppl. 8), 29–33.

Gianni, L., Munzone, E., Capri, G. *et al.* (1995). Paclitaxel by 3-hour infusion in combination with bolus doxorubicin in women with untreated metastatic breast cancer: High antitumour activity and cardiac effect in a dose finding and sequence finding study. *Journal of Clinical Oncology* **13**, 2668–2699.

Gianni, L. *et al.* (1997). Human pharmacokinetic characterization and in vitro study of the interaction between doxorubicin and paclitaxel in patients with breast cancer. *Journal of Clinical Oncology* **15**, 1906–1915.

Hackshaw, A., Barret-Lee, P., Leonard, R., Knight, J. (2000). The relationship between surrogate markers and survival in women receiving first-line chemotherapy for advanced breast cancer. *Proceedings of the American Society of Clinical Oncology* **21** (abstract 224).

Hortogyi, G. N., Buzdar, A. U., Theriault, R. L. *et al.* (2002). Randomised trial of high-dose chemotherapy and blood cell autografts for high-risk primary breast carcinoma. *Journal of the National Cancer Institute* **92**(3), 225–233.

Hutcheon, A., Ogston, K., Heys, S. *et al.* (2000). Primary chemotherapy in the treatment of breast cancer: significantly enhanced clinical and pathological response with docetaxel. *Proceedings of the American Society of Clinical Oncology* **19**, 83a. abstract 317.

Hutcheon, A. W., Heys, S. D. & Sarkar, T. K. (2003). Neoadjuvant docetaxel in locally advanced breast cancer. *Breast Cancer Research and Treatment* **79**(Suppl. 1), S19–S24.

Misset, J. L., Dieras, V., Gueruia, G. *et al.* (1999). Dose finding study of docetaxel and doxorubicin in first-line treatment of patients with metastatic breast cancer. *Annals of Oncology* **10**, 553–560.

Nabholtz, J. M. *et al.* (1999a). Prospective randomized trial of docetaxel versus mitomycin plus vinblastine in patients with metastatic breast cancer progressing despite previous anthracycline-containing chemotherapy. *Journal of Clinical Oncology* **17**, 1413–1424.

Nabholtz, J., Falkson, G., Campos, D. *et al.* (1999b). A Phase III Trial Comparing Doxorubicin (A) and Docetaxel (T) (AT) to Doxorubicin and Cyclophosphamide (AC) as First Line Chemotherapy for MBC. (Meeting abstract). *Proceedings of the American Society of Clinical Oncology* **36** *(*abstract 485).

Nabholtz, J., Paterson, A., Drix, L. *et al.* (2001). A Phase III Randomized Trial Comparing Docetaxel (T), Doxorubicin (A) and Cyclophosphamide (C) (TAC) to FAC as First Line Chemotherapy (CT) for Patients (Pts) with Metastatic Breast Cancer (MBC). *Proceedings of the American Society of Clinical Oncology* **37** (abstract 83).

Nabholtz, J., Pienkowski, T., Mackey, J. *et al.* (2002). Phase III trial comparing TAC (docetaxel, doxorubicin, cyclophosphamide) with FAC (5-fluorouracil, doxorubicin, cyclophosphamide) in the adjuvant treatment of node positive breast cancer (BC) patients: interim analysis of the BCIRG 001 study. *Proceedings of the American Society of Clinical Oncology* **38** (abstract 141).

NIH (2000). Adjuvant therapy for breast cancer. NIH consensus statement. *Online 2000* **17**(4), 1–23 (CALGB).

O'Brien, M. E. R., Leonard, R. C., Barrett-Lee, P. J., Eggleton, P. H. & Bizzari, J-P. (1999) Docetaxel in the community setting: An analysis of 377 breast cancer patients treated with docetaxel (Taxotere) in the UK. *Annals of Oncology* **10**, 205–210.

Paridaens, R., Biganzoli, L., Bruning, P. *et al.* (2000). Paclitaxel versus doxorubicin as first-line single-agent chemotherapy for metastatic breast cancer; A European Organisation for Research and Treatment of Cancer randomised study with cross-over. *Journal of Clinical Oncology* **18**, 724–733.

Roche, H., Viens, P., Biron, P. *et al.* (2003). High-dose chemotherapy for breast cancer: the French PEEASE experience. *Cancer Control* **10**(1), 42–47.

Rodenhuis, S., Bontenbal, M., Beex, L. V. *et al.* (2003). High-dose chemotherapy with hematopoietic stem-cell rescue for high-risk breast cancer. *New England Journal of Medicine* **349**(1), 7–16.

Riva, A. (2002). Taxanes in adjuvant treatment of breast cancer. Presented at 'Kick-off' meeting, ASCO 2002.

Schrama, J. G., Faneyte, I. F., Schomagel, J. H. *et al.* (2002). Randomised trial of high-dose chemotherapy and hematopoietic progenitor-cell support in operable breast cancer with extensive lymph node involvement: final analysis with 7 years of follow-up. *Annals of Oncology* **13**(5), 689–698.

Sledge, G. W., Neuberg, D., Ingle, J. *et al.* (1997). Phase III trial of doxorubicin vs paclitaxel vs doxorubicin plus paclitaxel as first line therapy for metastatic breast cancer: an intergroup trial. *Proceedings of the American Society for Clinical Oncology* **16**, (abstract 2) 1a.

Smith, I. C., Heys, S. D., Hutcheon, A. W., Miller, I. D., Payne, S., Gilbert F. J., Ah-See, A. K., Eremin O., Walker, L. G., Sarkar, T. K. *et al.* (2002). Neoadjuvant chemotherapy in breast cancer: significantly enhanced response with docetaxel. *Journal of Clinical Oncology* **20**,1456–1466.

Tallman, M. S., Eastern Cooperative Oncology Group. NCI High Priority Clinical Trial – Phase III randomised study of adjuvant CAF (cyclophosphamide/doxorubicin/fluorouracil) vs adjuvant CAF followed by intensification with high-dose cyclophosphamide/thiotepa plus autologous stem cell rescue in women with stage II/III breast cancer at high risk of recurrence. (Summary last modified 12/98), EST-2190, Clinical trial, closed.

Tallman, M. S., Gray, R., Robert, N. J. *et al.* (2003). Conventional adjuvant chemotherapy with or without high-dose chemotherapy and autologous stem-cell transplantation in high-risk breast cancer. *New England Journal of Medicine* **349**(1), 17–26.

Chapter 16

# Developing the evidence base for the management of advanced breast cancer: current clinical trials

*Andreas Polychronis and Robert Leonard*

Breast cancer is the most common malignancy and the second most common cause of cancer-related deaths in Western European and North American women. About 40% of the 38,000 women presenting each year in the UK with potentially curable breast cancer will subsequently relapse and a large proportion of those will be candidates for further systemic therapy to palliate their disease-related symptoms and hopefully extend their survival. Although the incidence of breast cancer is increasing, the mortality rates from breast cancer have decreased approximately 1.9% per year since 1990 in the United States. This is most likely due to earlier diagnosis through mammographic screening and the increased use of adjuvant systemic therapy (Esteva *et al.* 1999). However, when breast cancer cells metastasise to distant organs, the disease is essentially incurable by conventional treatments (hormone therapy and chemotherapy). Therefore when considering the treatment options for such patients, a balance needs to be achieved between the goals of the treating clinician and the patient. For many patients, a reduction in detectable tumour is the primary goal of therapy. This is commonly interpreted by patients as an indicator of prolongation of their life expectancy. For symptomatic patients, however, palliation of symptoms is the commonest aim of therapy. Sutherland *et al.* (1990) interviewed breast cancer patients in order to determine the importance of 28 items concerned with general health or with disease and treatment. The group reported that general health items, notably self-care, mobility, and physical activity, appetite, sleep, and family relationships were ranked in the upper quartile of the group of items rated, but surprisingly, items concerned directly with the common side-effects of chemotherapy were given lower rankings. The ratings were shown to be reproducible. This clearly demonstrates that the use of quality of life instruments, however well-validated, risk missing issues that are of major importance to patients.

A variety of cytotoxic and hormonal agents provide significant palliation for patients with metastatic breast cancer. The role of cytotoxic chemotherapy is well established for patients with life-threatening disease that requires rapid tumour control. Chemotherapy is also the treatment of choice for patients with hormone-resistant breast cancer. The most active cytotoxic agents include alkylating drugs, antimetabolites, vinca alkaloids, anthracyclines, and taxanes. Used as single agents, these various cytotoxics produce major objective responses in 20–80% of patients with metastatic breast cancer (Henderson 1991, Ellis *et al.* 2000, Hortobagyi *et al.* 1998). However, complete responses (CR) are rare and less than 20% of patients who achieve a CR maintain that status beyond 5 years (Greenberg *et al.* 1996). A variety of systemic treatments have been used, either as a single agent or in combination, in an attempt to re-induce remission in patients for whom initial chemotherapy has failed. However, the response rates (RR) in these programmes have been considerably lower than those for initial chemotherapy, and the durations of response and survival have been shorter. Achieving a balance between toxicity and anti-cancer benefit has long concerned physicians managing advanced breast cancer. Interestingly two widely quoted trials suggest that maintaining dose and schedule may be beneficial in terms of quality of life, despite potential toxicity. A trial by Coates in Australia indicated that treatment given on time and on schedule produced a better quality of life as compared to "on demand" treatment (Coates *et al.* 1987). A second by Tannock and colleagues showed that a higher dose intensity of CMF (cyclophosphamide, methotrexate, 5-fluorouracil) produced a better quality of life compared to low dose CMF (Tannock *et al.* 1988). For patients the goals of treatment are to maintain a good quality of life and prolong survival.

## Anthracyclines

For decades, the systemic treatment of patients with metastatic breast cancer has been based on hormonal manipulations and the rational use of cytotoxic agents. These include DNA alkylators, antimetabolites, antitumor antibiotics, and tubulin inhibitors (Greenspan 1965). The chemotherapy regimens most commonly used in the late 1960s consisted of cyclophosphamide, methotrexate, 5-fluorouracil (5-FU), prednisolone, and vincristine combinations (CMF, CMFP, CMFVP). These regimens produced objective RR in 50–60% of patients, including a 5–10% CR rate. The duration of response ranged from 6 to 9 months and the overall survival rate was 15–18 months (Henderson 1991). It is likely that the criteria for reporting response rates were less stringent in the 1960's than they are currently.

The 1970s were marked by the clinical development of doxorubicin and epirubicin. Regimens that included an anthracycline were superior to regimens that did not, at the expense of higher toxicity. Single-agent doxorubicin produced RR of 35–50% when given as first-line therapy. In patients previously treated with alkylating agent-based chemotherapy, RR were 25–30%. Doxorubicin-containing combinations produced overall responses in the range of 50–80% (Henderson 1991). The duration of response was 8–15 months, and the median survival following a doxorubicin-alkylating agent combination was reported in the range of 17–25 months. The most commonly used doxorubicin-based combinations are AC (doxorubicin, cyclophosphamide), and FAC (5-fluorouracil, doxorubicin, cyclophosphamide) (Hortobagyi *et al.* 1979). Several randomised clinical trials showed superior RR and improvements in disease-free survival for patients treated with FAC compared to CMF (A'Hern *et al.* 1993, Bull *et al.* 1978, Smalley *et al.* 1977, Muss *et al.* 1978, Tormey *et al.* 1984, Aisner *et al.* 1987). Other studies showed equivalence between these regimens. However, no randomised study has demonstrated superior results with FAC over CMF. Although more efficacious in the metastatic setting, doxorubicin-containing regimens are more toxic than CMF-type regimens. Almost all patients treated with doxorubicin develop alopecia, and some degree of nausea and vomiting; approximately 2–4% of patients develop congestive heart failure (CHF). The degree of myelosuppression is similar for CMF and FAC regimens.

Epirubicin is a doxorubicin analogue that has been shown to have similar efficacy and arguably less toxicity than doxorubicin at equipotent therapeutic doses (Camaggi *et al.* 1993). Both agents bind DNA and inhibit RNA and protein synthesis. They also generate cytotoxic-free radicals, block DNA cleavage by topo-isomerase II, inhibit helicase activity, and interfere with DNA replication and transcription. It has been suggested that the pharmacokinetic characteristics of doxorubicin and epirubicin are responsible for their different toxicity profiles. A randomised clinical trial compared FAC with FEC at equimolar doses of doxorubicin and epirubicin ($50$ mg/m$^2$) (French Epirubicin Study Group 1988). In this study, the FEC regimen was as effective as FAC in terms of RR, time to progression, and survival. The FEC regimen was associated with less gastrointestinal, haematological, and cardiac toxicity. However, the optimal dose of epirubicin is not established. Another randomised trial compared single-agent epirubicin with FEC-75 (epirubicin $75$ mg/m$^2$) and FEC-50 (epirubicin $50$ mg/m$^2$) (French Epirubicin Study Group 1991). In this study FEC was superior to single-agent epirubicin, and FEC-75 produced higher RR than FEC-50. Survival was better for FEC-75 ($p = 0.006$). Another area of interest is the optimal duration of chemotherapy for patients with metastatic breast cancer. A large randomised clinical trial evaluated the duration of FEC therapy. Patients were randomised to FEC-75 for 11 cycles; FEC-100 for four cycles followed by eight cycles of FEC-50; or to four cycles of FEC-100. Patients randomised to the latter group were treated with the same regimen (FEC-100) at the time of progression. Although the RR was higher using the FEC-100 regimen, the overall survival rate was similar for the three groups (French Epirubicin Study Group 2000).

## Taxanes

The introduction of paclitaxel and docetaxel in the 1990s followed a 15-year period of little progress in the development of new drugs for breast cancer. Both agents bind reversibly to the beta subunit of tubulin and induce tubulin polymerisation (Schiff *et al.* 1979). Normal microtubules need to maintain a balance between polymerisation and depolymerisation. The taxanes disrupt this balance, leading to arrest at the $G_2/M$ phase of the cell cycle. In addition, the taxanes inactivate the bcl-2 protein and induce apoptosis in breast cancer cells in vitro (Haldar *et al.* 1997).

## Paclitaxel

Paclitaxel is a natural product isolated from the bark of the Pacific yew tree, *Taxus brevifolia* (Wani *et al.* 1971). In patients with anthracycline-resistant metastatic breast cancer, paclitaxel produced RR of 6% to 48%. As first-line therapy in patients not previously exposed to chemotherapy, the RR ranged between 32% and 62% (Holmes *et al.* 1991, Holmes FA *et al.* 1993, Seidman *et al.* 1995, Abrams *et al.* 1995, Nabholtz *et al.* 1996). Several different doses and schedules of paclitaxel have been investigated and the optimal administration regimen has yet to be determined. The recommended doses for single-agent paclitaxel are 135 mg/m$^2$ to 175 mg/m$^2$ given over 3 hours. Higher doses and longer schedules of administration are safe, but none have been shown to be definitely superior to the "standard" 175 mg/m$^2$ given as a 3-hour infusion (Nabholtz *et al.* 1996, Smith *et al.* 1999, Winer *et al.* 1998). A randomised study showed that paclitaxel (200 mg/m$^2$ over 3 hours) was as effective as a combination of cyclophosphamide, methotrexate, fluorouracil, and prednisone (CMFP) in untreated metastatic breast cancer patients. Although RR were similar, the quality of life was improved for patients treated with paclitaxel (Bishop *et al.* 1999). The median time to progression was longer with CMFP (6.4 months versus 5.5 months), but median survival was higher with paclitaxel (16.5 months versus 11.3 months). Two large randomised trials have compared paclitaxel to doxorubicin as front-line therapy for patients with metastatic breast cancer. A multi-centre trial conducted by the European Organization for Research and Treatment of Cancer (EORTC) randomised patients to paclitaxel (200 mg/m$^2$ over 3 hours) versus doxorubicin (75 mg/m$^2$ bolus) Paridaens *et al.* 2000). In this study, which allowed cross-over to the alternate therapy, RR and median progression-free survival were significantly better with doxorubicin (RR = 41%) compared with paclitaxel (RR = 25%). In another large randomised study conducted by the Eastern Cooperative Oncology Group (ECOG), doxorubicin (60 mg/m$^2$ as a bolus) was directly compared with paclitaxel (175 mg/m$^2$ over 24 hours) and the combination of the two agents (doxorubicin 50 mg/m$^2$ and paclitaxel 150 mg/m$^2$ over 24 hours) (Sledge *et al.* 1997). In this three-arm trial, RR were similar between the doxorubicin (RR = 34%) and the paclitaxel (RR = 33%) arms of the study. Median time to treatment failure and median overall survival were not significantly different between the two single-agent arms of the study. Patients on the single-agent arms of this study were crossed over to the other agent upon progression. This limits the ability to detect differences in overall survival between the groups. However, according to the available data, paclitaxel and doxorubicin appear to have similar anti-tumour activity. Partial responses (PR) were seen in 20% of patients who crossed over from doxorubicin to paclitaxel and in 14% of patients who crossed over from doxorubicin to paclitaxel (20%), and from paclitaxel to doxorubicin (14%).

## Docetaxel

Docetaxel is a second-generation taxane, derived from the needles of the European yew tree, *Taxus baccata* (Verweij *et al.* 1994). Docetaxel has been recommended for breast cancer at doses ranging from 60–100 mg/m$^2$ administered as a 1-hour infusion. It is a highly effective agent for metastatic breast cancer. In previously untreated patients, RR range from 40–68%, better than any other single-agent chemotherapy (Valero 1997, Cortes *et al.* 1995). Docetaxel is particularly active in patients with anthracycline-resistant breast cancer. In two studies published simultaneously, the objective RR to docetaxel in patients with breast cancer resistant to anthracyclines were 53% and 57%, respectively (Ravdin *et al.* 1995, Valero *et al.* 1995). This excellent RR was confirmed in randomised trials. In one study, docetaxel 100 mg/m$^2$ over 1 hour was compared to mitomycin C plus vinblastine in patients with anthracycline-resistant metastatic breast cancer. Patients treated with docetaxel had significantly better RR (30% versus 11.6%), time to progression (19 versus 11 weeks), and overall survival (11.4 versus 8.7 months) (Nabholtz *et al.* 1999). Another study compared docetaxel (100 mg/m$^2$ over 1 hour) with sequential methotrexate (200 mg/m$^2$ day 1) and 5-FU (600 mg/m$^2$ days 1, 8) administered to patients with advanced anthracycline-resistant breast cancer (Sjostrom *et al.* 1999). The results from this phase III trial indicate that docetaxel appears to be more active than the sequential combination of methotrexate and 5-FU. RR (42% versus 19%) and median time to progression (6 months versus 3 months) were significantly better in the docetaxel arm, again demonstrating that docetaxel is effective therapy against anthracyline-resistant breast cancer.

A randomised trial compared docetaxel (100 mg/m$^2$ over 1 hour) with doxorubicin (75 mg/m$^2$ bolus) in patients with metastatic breast cancer who had failed an alkylating agent-containing regimen (Chan *et al.* 1999). Docetaxel demonstrated significantly better RR compared to doxorubicin in these patients (47% versus 32%). Of the 326 evaluable patients, 49% were classified with resistant disease, having progressed on prior chemotherapy, 70% of patients received docetaxel or doxorubicin as second-line therapy for metastatic breast cancer, and 30% received this regimen as first-line therapy for metastatic disease after having relapsed >12 months after adjuvant therapy. These results suggest that docetaxel may be a more active agent against breast cancer than doxorubicin. Docetaxel also appears to have activity in breast cancer patients that exhibit resistance to paclitaxel (Valero *et al.* 1998).

## Weekly taxanes

The taxanes can be safely administered on weekly schedules with preserved efficacy. However, administration of taxanes on a weekly schedule significantly changes their toxicity profile. Both agents cause mild myelosuppression and less hypersensitivity reactions compared to 3-weekly schedules, even if they are administered without interruption. The dose-limiting toxicity for weekly paclitaxel is peripheral neuropathy.

The optimal starting dose is 80 mg/m$^2$/week. Seidman et al. reported a RR of 53% in patients treated with weekly paclitaxel. A multi-centre study reported a lower RR of 21.5% (95% confidence interval, 15.4% to 27.5%) (Perez *et al.* 1999). For weekly docetaxel, the optimal dose is 35–40 mg/m$^2$/week, and the most common limiting toxicities are neutropenia and fatigue (Fumoleau *et al.* 1995). In a phase II study of weekly docetaxel, the RR was 41% (95% confidence interval, 24% to 61%), all occurring within the first two cycles (Burstein *et al.* 2000). A recently published Japanese phase II study confirms the efficacy and tolerability of weekly docetaxel (objective response rate of 38%; 95% confidence interval (CI) 22% to 53%) (Aihara *et al.* 2002). A series of non-randomised studies of weekly paclitaxel at the Memorial Hospital have raised interest in this schedule. Toxicity was low and response rates possibly superior to the standard three-weekly schedule. A trial is underway in the UK comparing weekly versus three-weekly paclitaxel in advanced breast cancer.

In summary, both taxanes are excellent choices for the first- and second-line treatment of patients with metastatic breast cancer. In patients with anthracycline-resistant breast cancer, docetaxel activity is impressively and consistently high in all trials reported in the literature. Compared to paclitaxel, docetaxel appears to produce superior results in this subset of patients. However, comparisons are indirect and potentially biased due to the lack of direct comparative data.

## Capecitabine

Capecitabine is the first oral fluoropyrimidine approved by the Food and Drug Administration (FDA) for the treatment of patients with metastatic breast cancer who failed prior doxorubicin and paclitaxel chemotherapy. Capecitabine is a prodrug that is activated at the tumour site by a series of enzymatic reactions. Clinically, its activity mimics continuous infusional 5-FU. Capecitabine is well-absorbed and not altered by the small bowel intestinal mucosa. It then undergoes a three-step conversion process to the active form, 5-FU. The first step of this process occurs in the liver, where it is converted to 5'-deoxy-5-fluorocytidine by carboxylesterase. It is then converted to 5'-deoxy-5-fluorouridine (5'-DFUR) by cytidine deaminase in liver and also tumour tissues. Further metabolism of 5'-DFUR occurs selectively within tumours by thymidine synthetase to 5-FU. This causes less direct 5-FU release into the bowel, and reduces the potential for diarrhoea.

The first phase II study of capecitabine in breast cancer involved 162 women previously treated with paclitaxel for metastatic disease (Blum *et al.* 1999). Of these, 37 (23%) were classified as paclitaxel failures, and 124 (77%) as paclitaxel-resistant. Of the 147 patients who had also received previous anthracycline treatment, 42 were designated as having failed therapy, and 67 as being anthracycline-resistant. Capecitabine was administered as 2,510 mg/m$^2$/day in two divided doses for 14 days, followed by 1 week of rest at 3-weekly cycles. Using this regimen, 27 (20%) of the 135 women with measurable disease demonstrated complete ($n = 3$) or partial ($n = 24$)

responses. All women who responded to therapy were resistant to or had failed paclitaxel, and all had received an anthracycline. The median duration of response for these women was 8.1 months, and median survival time was 12.8 months. Furthermore, of 51 patients with considerable tumour-related pain at baseline, capecitabine treatment reduced the pain intensity on a visual analogue scale by more than half in 47%. Two additional phase II studies confirmed this response to treatment in women with previously treated breast cancer (O'Shaughnessy *et al.* 1998 and O'Reilly *et al.* 1998). O'Shaughnessey and colleagues randomized older women (>55 years) to CMF (cyclophosphamide 600 mg/m$^2$, methotrexate 40 mg/m$^2$, 5-FU 600 mg/m$^2$) or capecitabine as front-line chemotherapy for metastatic breast cancer. The overall RR was 30% for capecitabine and 16% for CMF. Five CRs were observed in the capecitabine group. There was no difference in the median time to progression. Similar levels of vomiting, stomatitis, and fatigue were observed for both groups, whereas more cases of diarrhoea (8%) and hand-foot syndrome (16%) were seen in patients treated with capecitabine. Alopecia and myelosuppression were more common for patients receiving CMF. These studies demonstrated that capecitabine is an active agent in the treatment of metastatic breast cancer, and that significant responses can be achieved in women already treated with anthracyclines and taxanes. Retrospective studies suggest that a slightly lower starting dose (2,000 mg/m$^2$/day) is better tolerated with preserved efficacy (O'Shaughnessy *et al.* 2000, Michaud *et al.* 2000).

## Vinorelbine

Vinorelbine is a novel vinca alkaloid that has shown significant activity against breast cancer. Vinorelbine is a cell cycle-specific microtubule inhibitor. In contrast to the taxanes, vinorelbine destabilises the microtubules. In vitro studies showed a selective effect on non-neuronal microtubules, which may explain the decreased neurotoxicity of vinorelbine compared with other vinca alkaloids (Johnson *et al.* 1996). As a single agent, vinorelbine produced RR of 20–40% when delivered i.v. at 25–35 mg/m$^2$ on days 1 and 8 of a 3-week cycle. Objective RR have been reported in patients who had progressed after anthracyclines and taxanes (Canobbio *et al.* 1989, Degardin *et al.* 1994, Romero *et al.* 1994, Marty *et al.* 1992). This agent is particularly well-tolerated in elderly patients (Vogel *et al.* 1999). Long infusions and dose-intense regimens administered with the addition of hematopoietic growth factors to support blood counts are feasible (Ibrahim *et al.* 1996, Livingston *et al.* 1997). However, it is not clear that these approaches would be superior to the standard weekly administration of vinorelbine.

The low incidence of alopecia and other non-haematological toxicities makes vinorelbine particularly attractive as a safe agent for the palliative treatment of metastatic breast cancer. Granulocytopenia, the dose-limiting toxicity of this agent, is transient and, at current recommended dose levels, rarely results in life-threatening consequences. Perhaps one of the main applications of vinorelbine will be in combination with novel biologic agents, as shown with trastuzumab monoclonal antibody therapy (Burstein *et al.* 2000).

## Gemcitabine

Gemcitabine is a nucleotide analogue that inhibits DNA synthesis. Gemcitabine is an effective cytotoxic against a variety of solid tumour cell lines in vitro and in vivo (von Hoff 1996). Carmichael *et al.* evaluated the safety and efficacy of gemcitabine as a single agent (800 mg/m$^2$/week for 3 weeks of a 4-week cycle), in patients with metastatic breast cancer. The RR quoted was 25% with a median survival of 11.5 months. The main toxicity was haematological, although only 1 of 44 patients developed neutropenic sepsis. Other phase II studies suggest that single-agent gemcitabine is safe and effective and should be an option as salvage chemotherapy for patients who failed anthracycline-, taxane-, and fluorocytidine-based therapy.

## Combination versus sequential chemotherapy

The role of single-agent chemotherapy versus combination chemotherapy has been a controversial area for more than 30 years. When evaluating older regimens such as FAC, FEC, or CMF, polychemotherapy regimens produce higher rates than single agents. Anthracycline-containing regimens are superior to non-anthracycline-containing regimens. However, it is not clear that polychemotherapy regimens result in improved survival when compared to the same agents administered sequentially. Chlebowski *et al.* randomised 222 women with metastatic breast cancer to CMFP ± V versus sequential single-agent therapy. In this study there was no difference in overall survival among both groups; RR was higher in the combination arm, particularly for patients with liver metastases, and combination chemotherapy was associated with greater toxicity. Another study compared an FEC-MV (MV = methotrexate and vinblastine) combination to single-agent epirubicin followed by MV. The RR was higher for FEC-MV, but survival was the same for both groups (Joensuu *et al.* 1998).

With the emergence of the taxanes as one of the most effective classes of treatments for breast cancer, clinical trials were launched to determine the efficacy and safety of anthracycline/taxane combinations.

## Paclitaxel in combination with anthracycline

Many studies have reported the feasibility of combining the taxanes with doxorubicin or epirubicin. Of these, the doxorubicin/paclitaxel (AT) combinations have been studied in detail and extensive data are available regarding their clinical activity. Early trials incorporated prolonged infusions of both drugs, but were associated with pharmacokinetic interactions between the agents which resulted in severe neutropenia and gastrointestinal toxicity (Holmes *et al.* 1996, Holmes 1995, O'Shaughnessy *et al.* 1994). The increased gastrointestinal toxicity was found to be sequence-dependent and mostly seen when paclitaxel preceded doxorubicin, secondary to delayed doxorubicin clearance (Holmes *et al.* 1996). Steps taken to reduce toxicity and maintain efficacy were accomplished in two ways: A) giving both agents as short infusions or bolus, or B) separating the agents to avoid pharmacokinetic interactions that lead to increased acute toxicity. Gianni and colleagues reported a very high RR of 94% in one early trial utilising bolus administration of doxorubicin (60 mg/m$^2$) and a 3-hour infusion of paclitaxel (200 mg/m$^2$). In this study, 20% of the patients developed CHF. In the ECOG study that compared A versus T, versus AT the incidence of severe cardiac toxicity was no different between the doxorubicin-alone arm and the combination arm (9% versus 9%), perhaps due to the delay between the administration of doxorubicin and paclitaxel (Sledge *et al.* 1997). This trial did not confirm the high RR seen in earlier trials; however, it did demonstrate a superior RR and median-time-to-treatment failure for the combination compared to either single agent. Overall survival was similar for all three arms of the study. Methods to reduce the cardiac toxicity associated with this regimen include substituting epirubicin for doxorubicin, and limiting the cumulative amount of doxorubicin administered. In the bolus combination regimens, if the cumulative dose of doxorubicin is limited to 300–360 mg/m$^2$ and the paclitaxel continued until progression, the RR is maintained and the incidence of CHF drops to about 1–5% (Gianni *et al.* 1995). In another randomised trial the AT combination (50 mg/m$^2$ day 1,220 mg/m$^2$ day 2, respectively) was shown to be superior to FAC (500 mg/m$^2$, 50 mg/m$^2$, 500 mg/m$^2$, respectively) as first-line therapy of patients with metastatic breast cancer. In this study, RR (68% versus 55%), time-to-progression (8.3 months versus 6.2 months), and overall survival (22.7 months versus 18.3 months) were significantly higher in the AT arms (Pluzanska *et al.* 1999).

The safety and efficacy of paclitaxel in combination with epirubicin has been evaluated in several phase I and II studies (Carmichael *et al.* 1997, Catimel *et al.* 1996, Luck *et al.* 1997). Conte and colleagues (Conte *et al.* 1995, Conte *et al.* 1996) escalated the dose of paclitaxel up to 225 mg/m$^2$ given over 3 hours in combination with epirubicin, given at 90 mg/m$^2$ as a bolus. The RR was 80%, and the regimen was well-tolerated. The most frequent dose-related toxicity was grade 4 neutropenia, which occurred in 59% of courses. The cardiac toxicity was low. Only 2 of 29 patients experienced a decrease of left ventricular ejection fraction below 50% after six courses, and no signs of anthracycline-induced CHF were noted. A phase II study conducted by the EORTC compared epirubicin plus paclitaxel (EP) with epirubicin plus cyclophosphamide (EC) as front-line therapy for patients with metastatic breast cancer. Preliminary data from this study showed that EP is as active as EC, although there was no difference in time to progression between the two groups (Luck *et al.* 2000).

## Docetaxel in combination with anthracycline

The combination of doxorubicin with docetaxel (AD) has been shown to be a highly active regimen for the treatment of metastatic breast cancer. Docetaxel is administered over 1 hour and doxorubicin is given as either short infusions or bolus injections. High RR of 81% were reported in phase I trials of AD at doses ranging from 40–60 mg/m$^2$ for doxorubicin and 50–85 mg/m$^2$ for docetaxel (Bozec *et al.* 1997). The dose-limiting toxicity with this regimen was neutropenic sepsis. The recommended phase II doses were doxorubicin 50 mg/m$^2$ bolus plus docetaxel 75 mg/m$^2$ over 1 hour or doxorubin 60 mg/m$^2$ bolus plus docetaxel 60 mg/m$^2$ over 1 hour. In a phase II study conducted by the National Surgical Adjuvant Breast and Bowel Project (NSABP B-57), AD produced a RR of 53% (PR = 47%; CR = 6%) with manageable toxicity (Lembersky *et al.* 2000). Interestingly, an excess of cardiac toxicity was not seen with this combination, one advantage over some of the paclitaxel-doxorubicin combinations. Ongoing phase III trials comparing the AD combination to standard regimens for metastatic and primary breast cancer will assist in determining the optimal combination chemotherapy regimen for breast cancer. Preliminary data indicated that AD produced a superior RR (60% versus 47%) and longer time to progression (37.1 weeks versus 31.9 weeks), at the expense of higher haematological toxicity (Nabholtz 1999). Overall survival data from this study have yet to be reported.

Pagani *et al.* reported a phase I-II study of docetaxel in combination with epirubicin as first-line chemotherapy in 70 patients with metastatic breast cancer. The dose-limiting toxicity was neutropenia and G-CSF was required in 44% of patients. Otherwise the regimen was well-tolerated. Only one patient developed symptomatic CHF, and six additional patients had decreases in left ventricular ejection fraction with no symptoms. The RR was reported as 66%.

## Other chemotherapy combinations

There is great interest in developing non-anthracycline combination regimens. The taxanes have been studied in combination with a variety of agents. Perez and colleagues (Perez *et al.* 2000) conducted a phase II study of paclitaxel (200 mg/m$^2$ over 3 hours) in combination with carboplatin (area under the curve AUC6 mg/ml per minute) administered as first-line therapy for patients with metastatic breast cancer. The main toxicity was haematological and 16% of patients developed peripheral neuropathy. The RR was 62%. Sawada and colleagues (Sawada *et al.* 1998) showed that both taxanes enhance the efficacy of capecitabine and 5'-dFUrd in vivo, probably by modulating dThdPase activity in tumor tissues. In a human xenograft model, these authors showed a synergistic interaction between docetaxel and capecitabine. O'Shaughnessy and collaborators have completed a phase III study of docetaxel in combination with capecitabine versus single-agent docetaxel for patients with metastatic breast cancer previously exposed to anthracyclines. Data from this large randomised study indicate that the docetaxel/capecitabine combination is superior to docetaxel monotherapy. The combination resulted in significantly superior efficacy in time to disease progression (TTP) (hazard ratio, 0.652; 95% confidence interval [CI], 0.545 to 0.780; $p$ = .0001; median, 6.1 v 4.2 months), overall survival (hazard ratio, 0.775; 95% CI, 0.634 to 0.947; $p$ =.0126; median, 14.5 v 11.5 months), and objective tumour response rate (42% v 30%, $p$ = .006) compared with docetaxel (O'Shaughnessy 2002).

Vinorelbine has been studied in combination with other agents commonly administered for the treatment of metastatic breast cancer. Early phase II clinical trials showed high RR for a vinorelbine/doxorubicin combination (Spielmann *et al.* 1994). However, the superiority of this combination could not be reproduced in a large randomized phase III trial conducted by the National Cancer Institute of Canada (Norris *et al.* 2000). In this study, vinca alkaloid- and anthracycline-naive patients with metastatic breast cancer were randomised to receive vinorelbine plus doxorubicin or doxorubicin alone. The RR, quality of life, and time to progression were not significantly different between the arms, suggesting that the vinorelbine/doxorubicin combination is not superior to doxorubicin as a single agent for metastatic breast cancer. Vinorelbine has been studied in combination with other chemotherapy drugs including paclitaxel, docetaxel, and 5-FU (Dieras *et al.* 1996).

Gemcitabine is also being evaluated in combination with anthracyclines, taxanes, and vinorelbine. In general, these combinations are active but toxicities are usually cumulative. In the absence of randomised trial data, the role of these combinations remains uncertain.

In summary, chemotherapy combinations produce higher RR compared with sequential single-agent therapy. The taxane/anthracycline combinations are the most effective regimens and are rapidly becoming the first-line therapy of choice for patients with metastatic breast cancer. However, the impact of polychemotherapy regimens in overall survival is modest. Except for the commonly used two/three-drug regimens (i.e., FAC, FEC, CMF, ATx), there is little rationale to support the use of more sophisticated chemotherapy combinations.

## High dose chemotherapy

A retrospective study conducted by Hryniuk and colleagues suggested that patients with metastatic breast cancer who had received the planned full dose of chemotherapy had a better response compared with patients who had received a less intense regimen (Hryniuk *et al.* 1984). Phase I studies showed that the dose of "standard" chemotherapy regimens could be increased by 30% to 50% using haematopoietic growth factors (e.g., G-CSF). Higher doses could be achieved using haematopoietic stem cells isolated from the bone marrow or peripheral blood. One of the major limitations of this approach has been the extra-medullary toxicity of many of the agents used for the treatment of metastatic breast cancer. Because of this limitation, most of the drugs employed for high dose-intensity regimens are restricted to alkylating agent therapy.

With high-dose combination alkylating agents, overall RR between 70% to 100% can be obtained in patients with previously untreated metastatic breast cancer. More importantly, CR rates with these regimens range between 40% and 60%. However, median duration of response and survival have not been modified by high dose-intensity regimens, and, while 15–25% of patients so treated remain progression-free at two and three years after the initiation of therapy, it is unclear whether this represents patient selection or improved therapeutic efficacy (Rahman *et al.* 1997). With the exception of the PEGASE 03 and 04 trials, multi-centre, randomised studies have failed to confirm the efficacy of high-dose chemotherapy regimens over standard-dose chemotherapy (Stadtmauer *et al.* 2000). Until these issues are resolved, the use of high-dose chemotherapy with haematopoietic stem cell support should be considered experimental.

## Monoclonal antibody therapy

The field of mAb therapy for breast cancer is moving forward both in the experimental and clinical settings (Esteva *et al.* 1998). Trastuzumab (Herceptin) is a humanized recombinant mAb directed against the anti-Her-2/neu protein. This is being used as a single-agent therapy or in combination with chemotherapy. The evidence supporting its use is reviewed by Miles in the chapter which follows.

## New agents

The development of novel anticancer agents continues on several fronts. One approach is to develop analogues of older drugs with improved efficacy and/or safety profiles. Examples include novel anthracyclines (e.g., annamycin), novel formulations (e.g., liposomal doxorubicin), water-soluble taxanes, and new oral fluoropyrimidines. A second approach is to study agents that belong to classes of compounds that historically have had little activity against breast cancer cells. These include gemcitabine and topoisomerase I inhibitors. A third strategy is to interfere with mechanisms of drug resistance using inhibitors of the multi-drug resistance pump.

In addition to cytotoxic chemotherapy, there is great interest in developing novel molecular-based therapeutics targeted at inhibition of tumour cell proliferation pathways. Promising targets include growth factor receptors and their ligands, intracellular signal transduction molecules, cell-cycle regulatory proteins, and transcription factors. These agents are not likely to produce CRs in patients with metastatic solid tumours and it may be necessary to combine or sequence them with chemotherapy in order to affect maximal tumour reduction (Pusztai *et al.* 1999).

## Conclusion

The role of chemotherapy is well-established for patients with oestrogen receptor-negative and hormone-refractory breast cancer. Although poly-chemotherapy regimens produce higher RR compared with single-agent therapy, the survival impact is modest.

Anthracycline plus taxane regimens are the most effective therapy, at the price of higher toxicity, and should be considered for patients with rapidly growing visceral metastases, lymphangitic spread, or locally advanced breast cancer. For the majority of patients, the available data support the sequential use of single-agent chemotherapy or the usual two- to three-drug combination regimens (e.g., FAC, FEC, CMF). It must be remembered that there is still a law of diminishing returns with successive lines of chemotherapy as a paper by Tannock's group demonstrates (McLachlan *et al.* 1999). Particularly as more complex adjuvant chemotherapy combination regimens are being used routinely, it is likely that well-tolerated novel agents or combinations will replace anthracycline-based regimens in the palliation and management of relapsed disease. Marked progress has been made to make chemotherapy more tolerable using more effective anti-emetics, antibiotics, and haematopoietic growth factors. Development of novel therapeutic agents continues, based on expanded biological understanding of tumour development and progression. Anti-angiogenic therapy and signal transduction inhibitors are the biologic agents most likely to be combined or sequenced with chemotherapy in the near term.


## *References*

Abrams, J. S., Vena, D. A., Baltz, J. *et al.* (1995). Paclitaxel activity in heavily pretreated breast cancer: a National Cancer Institute Treatment Referral Center trial. *Journal of Clinical Oncology* **13**, 2056–2065.

A'Hern, R. P., Smith, I. E., Ebbs, S. R. (1993). Chemotherapy and survival in advanced breast cancer: the inclusion of doxorubicin in Cooper type regimens. *British Journal of Cancer* **67**, 801–805.

Aihara, T., Kim, Y., Takatsuka, Y. (2002). Phase II study of weekly docetaxel in patients with metastatic breast cancer. *Annals of Oncology* **13**(2), 286–92.

Aisner, J., Weinberg, V., Perloff, M. *et al.* (1987). Chemotherapy versus chemoimmunotherapy (CAF v CAFVP v CMF each +/- MER) for metastatic carcinoma of the breast: a CALGB study. Cancer and Leukemia Group *British Journal of Clinical Oncology* **5**, 1523–1533.

Bishop, J. F., Dewar, J., Toner, G. C. *et al.* (1999). Initial paclitaxel improves outcome compared with CMFP combination chemotherapy as front-line therapy in untreated metastatic breast cancer. *Journal of Clinical Oncology* **17**, 2355–2364.

Blum, J. L., Jones, S. E., Buzdar, A. U. *et al.* (1999). Multicenter phase II study of capecitabine in paclitaxel-refractory metastatic breast cancer. *Journal of Clinical Oncology* **17**, 485–493.

Bozec, I., Nabholtz, J-M., Dieras, V. *et al.* (1997). Docetaxel (D) in combination with doxorubicin (Dx) (AT) and with cyclophosphamide (CTX) (TAC) as first-line chemotherapy (CT) in metastatic breast cancer (MBC): high activity and absence of cardiotoxicity. *Proceedings of the American Society of Clinical Oncology* **16**, A566.

Bull, J. M., Tormey, D. C., Li, S. H. *et al.* (1978). A randomized comparative trial of adriamycin versus methotrexate in combination drug therapy. *Cancer* **41**, 1649–1657.

Burstein, H. J., Manola, J., Younger, J. *et al.* (2000). Docetaxel administered on a weekly basis for metastatic breast cancer. *Journal of Clinical Oncology* **18**, 1212–1219.

Burstein, H. J., Kuter, I., Richardson, P. G. *et al.* (2000). Herceptin and vinorelbine for Her2-positive metastatic breast cancer: a phase II study. *Proceedings of the American Society of Clinical Oncology* **19**, 392.

Camaggi, C. M., Strocchi, E., Carisi, P. *et al.* (1993). Epirubicin metabolism and pharmacokinetics after conventional- and high-dose intravenous administration: a cross-over study. *Cancer Chemotherapy and Pharmacology* **32**, 301–309.

Canobbio, L., Boccardo, F., Pastorino, G. *et al.* (1989). Phase II study of Navelbine in advanced breast cancer. *Seminars in Oncology* **16**(suppl 4), 33–36.

Carmichael, J., Possinger, K., Phillip, P. *et al.* (1995). Advanced breast cancer: a phase II trial with gemcitabine. *Journal of Clinical Oncology* **13**, 2731–2736.

Carmichael, J., Jones, A., Hutchinson, T. (1997). A phase II trial of epirubicin plus paclitaxel in metastatic breast cancer. United Kingdom Coordinating Committee for Cancer Research Breast Cancer Sub-Committee. *Seminars in Oncology* **24**(suppl 17), S44–S47.

Catimel, G., Spielmann, M., Dieras, V. *et al.* (1996). Phase I study of paclitaxel and epirubicin in patients with metastatic breast cancer: a preliminary report on safety. *Seminars in Oncology* **23**, 24–27.

Chan, S., Friedrichs, K., Noel, D. *et al.* (1999). Prospective randomized trial of docetaxel versus doxorubicin in patients with metastatic breast cancer. The 303 Study Group. *Journal of Clinical Oncology* **17**, 2341–2354.

Chlebowski, R. T., Smalley, R. V., Weiner, J. M. *et al.* (1989). Combination versus sequential single agent chemotherapy in advanced breast cancer: associations with metastatic sites and long-term survival. The Western Cancer Study Group and The Southeastern Cancer Study Group. *British Journal of Cancer* **59**, 227–230.

Coates, A., Gebski, V., Bishop, J. F. *et al.* (1987). Improving the quality of life during chemotherapy for advanced breast cancer. A comparison of intermittent and continuous treatment strategies. *New England Journal of Medicine* **317**(24), 1490–1495.

Conte, P. F., Michelotti, A., Baldini, E. *et al.* (1995). The Italian Experience: Activity and Safety of Paclitaxel Plus Epirubicin in the Treatment of Advanced Breast Cancer. Abstracts of Paclitaxel (Taxol)-Current Practices and Future Directions in Breast Cancer Management-London, September 16, 11–12.

Conte, P. F., Michelotti, A., Baldini, E. *et al.* (1996). A dose-finding study of epirubicin in combination with paclitaxel in the treatment of advanced breast cancer. *Seminars in Oncology* **23**, 28–31.

Cortes, J. E., Pazdur, R. (1995). Docetaxel. *Journal of Clinical Oncology* **13**, 2643–2655.

Degardin, M., Bonneterre, J., Hecquet, B. *et al.* (1994). Vinorelbine (navelbine) as a salvage treatment for advanced breast cancer. *Annals of Oncology* **5**, 423–426.

Dieras, V., Extra, J. M., Bellissant, E. *et al.* (1996). Efficacy and tolerance of vinorelbine and fluorouracil combination as first-line chemotherapy of advanced breast cancer: results of a phase II study using a sequential group method. *Journal of Clinical Oncology* **14**, 3097–3104.

Ellis, M. J., Hayes, D. F., Lippman, M. E. (2000). Treatment of metastatic breast cancer. In: Harris, J. R., Lippman, M. E., Morrow, M. *et al.*, eds. Diseases of the Breast. Philadelphia: Lippincott Williams & Wilkins pg749.

Esteva, F. J., Hortobagyi, G. N. (1999). Adjuvant systemic therapy for primary breast cancer. *Surgical Clinics of North America* **79**, 1075–1090.

Esteva, F. J., Hayes, D. F. (1998). Monoclonal antibody-based therapy of breast cancer. In: Grossbard ML, ed. Monoclonal Antibody-Based Therapy of Cancer. New York: Marcel Decker, pp309–338.

French Epirubicin Study Group (1988). A prospective randomized phase III trial comparing combination chemotherapy with cyclophosphamide, fluorouracil and either doxorubicin or epirubicin. *Journal of Clinical Oncology* **6**, 679–688.

French Epirubicin Study Group (1991). A prospective randomized trial comparing epirubicin monochemotherapy to two fluorouracil, cyclophosphamide, and epirubicin regimens differing in epirubicin dose in advanced breast cancer patients. *Journal of Clinical Oncology* **9**, 305–312.

French Epirubicin Study Group (2000). Epirubicin-based chemotherapy in metastatic breast cancer patients: role of dose-intensity and duration of treatment. *Journal of Clinical Oncology* **18**, 3115–3124.

Fumoleau, P., Chevallier, B., Kerbrat, P. *et al.* (1995). Current status of Taxotere (docetaxel) as a new treatment in breast cancer. *Breast Cancer Research and Treatment* **33**, 39–46.

Gianni, L., Munzone, E., Capri, G. *et al.* (1995). Paclitaxel by 3-hour infusion in combination with bolus doxorubicin in women with untreated metastatic breast cancer: high antitumor efficacy and cardiac effects in a dose-finding and sequence-finding study. *Journal of Clinical Oncology* **13**, 2688–2699.

Greenberg, P. A., Hortobagyi, G. N., Smith, T. L. *et al.* (1996). Long-term follow-up of patients with complete remission following combination chemotherapy for metastatic breast cancer. *Journal of Clinical Oncology* **14**, 2197–2205.

Greenspan, E. M. (1965). Combination cytotoxic chemotherapy in advanced disseminated breast carcinoma. *Journal of Mount Sinai Hospital NY* **32**, 1–27.

Gregory, W. M., Smith, P., Richards, M. A. *et al.* (1993). Chemotherapy of advanced breast cancer: outcome and prognostic factors. *British Journal of Cancer* **68**(5), 988–95.

Haldar, S., Jena, N., Croce, C. M. (1995). Inactivation of Bcl-2 by phosphorylation. *Proceedings of the National Academy of Sciences USA* **92**, 4507–4511.

Haldar, S., Basu, A., Croce, C. M. (1997). Bcl2 is the guardian of microtubule integrity. *Cancer Research* **57**, 229–233.

Henderson, I. C. (1991). Chemotherapy for metastatic disease. In: Harris, J. R., Hellman, S., Henderson, I. C. *et al.*, eds. Breast Diseases. Philadelphia: J.B. Lippincott Company, 604–665.

Holmes, F. A., Walters, R. S., Theriault, R. L. *et al.* (1991). Phase II trial of taxol, an active drug in the treatment of metastatic breast cancer. *Journal of the National Cancer Institute* **83**, 1797–1805.

Holmes, F. A., Valero, V., Walters, R. S. *et al.* (1993). The M. D. Anderson Cancer Center experience with Taxol in metastatic breast cancer. *Journal of the National Cancer Institute Monographs* **15**, 161–169.

Holmes, F. A., Madden, T., Newman, R. A. *et al.* (1996). Sequence-dependent alteration of doxorubicin pharmacokinetics by paclitaxel in a phase I study of paclitaxel and doxorubicin in patients with metastatic breast cancer. *Journal of Clinical Oncology* **14**, 2713–2721.

Holmes, F. A. (1995). Update: the M.D. Anderson Cancer Center experience with paclitaxel in the management of breast carcinoma. *Seminars in Oncology* **22**, 9–15.

Hortobagyi, G. N. (1998). Treatment of breast cancer. *New England Journal of Medicine* **339**, 974–984.

Hortobagyi, G. N., Gutterman, J. U., Blumenschein, G. R. *et al.* (1979). Combination chemoimmunotherapy of metastatic breast cancer with 5-fluorouracil, adriamycin, cyclophosphamide, and BCG. *Cancer* **43**, 1225–1233.

Hryniuk, W. M., Bush, H. (1984). The importance of dose intensity in chemotherapy of metastatic breast cancer. *Journal of Clinical Oncology* **2**, 1281–1288.

Ibrahim, N.K., Hortobagyi, G. N., Valero, V. *et al.* (1996). Phase I study of Navelbine (vinorelbine) administered by 96-hour infusion in metastatic breast cancer patients. *Breast Cancer Research and Treatment* **41**, 511a.

Joensuu, H., Holli, K., Heikkinen, M. *et al.* (1998). Combination chemotherapy versus single-agent therapy as first- and second-line treatment in metastatic breast cancer: a prospective randomized trial. *Journal of Clinical Oncology* **16**, 3720–3730.

Johnson, S. A., Harper, P., Hortobagyi, G. N. *et al.* (1996). Vinorelbine: an overview. *Cancer Treatment Reviews* **22**, 127–142.

Lembersky, B. C., Anderson, S., Smith, R. *et al.* (2000). Phase II trial of doxorubicin and docetaxel for locally advanced and metastatic breast cancer: preliminary results from NSABP BP-57. *Proceedings of the American Society of Clinical Oncology* **19**, 403.

Livingston, R. B., Ellis, G. K., Gralow, J. R. *et al.* (1997). Dose-intensive vinorelbine with concurrent granulocyte colony-stimulating factor support in paclitaxel-refractory metastatic breast cancer. *Journal of Clinical Oncology* **15**, 1395–1400.

Luck, H. J., Thomssen, C., du, B. A. *et al.* (1997). Phase II study of paclitaxel and epirubicin as first-line therapy in patients with metastatic breast cancer. *Seminars in Oncology* **24**(suppl 17), S35–S39.

Luck, H. J., Thomssen, C., Untch, M. *et al.* (2000). Multicentric phase III study in first line treatment of advanced metastatic breast cancer (ABC). Epirubicin/paclitaxel (ET) vs epirubicin/cyclophosphamide (EC). A study of the Ago Breast Cancer Group. *Proceedings of the American Society for Clinical Oncology* **19**, 280.

Marty, M., Extra, J. M., Dieras, V. *et al.* (1992). A review of the antitumour activity of vinorelbine in breast cancer. *Drugs* **44**(suppl 4), 29–35.

McLachlsn, S. A., Pintilie, M. & Tannock, I. F. (1999). Third line chemotherapy in patients with matastatic breast cancer: an evaluation of quality of life and cost. *Breast Cancer Research and Treatment* **54**(3), 213–23.

Michaud, L. B., Gauthier, M. A., Wojdylo, J. R. *et al.* (2000). Improved therapeutic index with lower dose capecitabine in metastatic breast cancer patients. *Proceedings of the American Society for Clinical Oncology* **19**, 402.

Muss, H. B., White, D. R., Richards, F. *et al.* (1978). Adriamycin versus methotrexate in five-drug combination chemotherapy for advanced breast cancer. *Cancer* **42**, 2142–2148.

Nabholtz, J. M., Gelmon, K., Bontenbal, M. *et al.* (1996). Multicenter, randomized comparative study of two doses of paclitaxel in patients with metastatic breast cancer. *Journal of Clinical Oncology* **14**, 1858–1867.

Nabholtz, J. M., Senn, H. J., Bezwoda, W. R. *et al.* (1999). Prospective randomized trial of docetaxel versus mitomycin plus vinblastine in patients with metastatic breast cancer progressing despite previous anthracycline-containing chemotherapy. 304 Study Group. *Journal of Clinical Oncology* **17**, 1413–1424.

Nabholtz, J. M. (1999). Docetaxel (Taxotere) plus doxorubicin-based combinations: the evidence of activity in breast cancer. *Seminars in Oncology* **26**, 7–13.

Nabholtz, J-M., Falkson, C., Campos, D. *et al.* (1999). Doxorubicin and docetaxel (AT) is superior to standard doxorubicin and cyclophosphamide (AC) as first line CT for MBC: randomized phase III trial. *Breast Cancer Research and Treatment* **57**, 330a.

Norris, B., Pritchard, K. I., James, K. *et al.* (2000). Phase III comparative study of vinorelbine combined with doxorubicin versus doxorubicin alone in disseminated metastatic/recurrent breast cancer: National Cancer Institute of Canada Clinical Trials Group Study MA8. *Journal of Clinical Oncology* **18**, 2385–2394.

O'Reilly, S. M., Moiseyenko, V. M., Talbot, D. C. *et al.* (1998). A randomized phase II study of Xeloda (capecitabine) vs paclitaxel in breast cancer patients failing previous anthracycline therapy. *Proceedings of the American Society for Clinical Oncology* **17**, 627a.

O'Shaughnessy, J., Moiseyenko, V. M., Bell, D. *et al.* (1998). A randomized phase II study of Xeloda (capecitabine) vs CMF as first line chemotherapy of breast cancer in women aged 55 years. *Proceedings of the American Society for Clinical Oncology* **17**, 398a.

O'Shaughnessy, J., Blum, J. (2000). A retrospective evaluation of the impact of dose reduction in patients treated with Xeloda (capecitabine). *Proceedings of the American Society for Clinical Oncology* **19**, 400.

O'Shaughnessy, J. A., Fisherman, J. S., Cowan, K. H. (1994). Combination paclitaxel (Taxol) and doxorubicin therapy for metastatic breast cancer. *Seminars in Oncology* **21**(suppl 8),19–23.

O'Shaughnessy, J., Miles, D., Vukelja, S. *et al.* (2002). Superior survival with capecitabine plus docetaxel combination therapy in anthracycline-pretreated patients with advanced breast cancer: phase III trial results. *Journal of Clinical Oncology* **20**(12), 2812–23.

Pagani, O., Sessa, C., Nole, F. *et al.* (2000). Epidoxorubicin and docetaxel as first-line chemotherapy in patients with advanced breast cancer: a multicentric phase I-II study. *Annals of Oncology* **11**, 985–991.

Paridaens, R., Biganzoli, L., Bruning, P. *et al.* (2000). Paclitaxel versus doxorubicin as first-line single-agent chemotherapy for metastatic breast cancer: a European Organization for Research and Treatment of Cancer randomized study with cross-over. *Journal of Clinical Oncology* **18**, 724–733.

Perez, E. A., Vogel, C. L., Irwin, D. H. *et al.* (2001). Multicenter phase II trial of weekly paclitaxel in women with metastatic breast cancer. *Journal of Clinical Oncology* **19**(22), 4216–23.

Perez, E. A., Hillman, D. W., Stella, P. J. *et al.* (2000). A phase II study of paclitaxel plus carboplatin as first-line chemotherapy for women with metastatic breast carcinoma. *Cancer* **88**, 124–131.

Pluzanska, A., Pienkowski, T., Jelic, S. *et al.* (1999). Phase III multicenter trial comparing Taxol/doxorubicin (AT) vs 5-fluorouracil/doxorubicin and cyclophosphamide (FAC) as a first line treatment for patients with metastatic breast cancer. *Breast Cancer Research and Treatment* **57**, 21a.

Pouillart, P., Fumoleau, P., Romieu, G. *et al.* (1999). Final results of a phase II randomized, parallel study of doxorubicin/cyclophosphamide (AC) and Doxorubicin/Taxol (paclitaxel) (AT) as neoadjuvant treatment of local-regional breast cancer. *Proceedings of the American Society for Clinical Oncology* **19**, 275a.

Pusztai, L., Esteva, F. J., Cristofanilli, M. *et al.* (1999). Chemo-signal therapy, an emerging new approach to modify drug resistance in breast cancer. *Cancer Treatment and Reviews* **25**, 271–277.

Rahman, Z. U., Frye, D. K., Buzdar, A. U. *et al.* (1997). Impact of selection process on response rate and long-term survival of potential high-dose chemotherapy candidates treated with standard-dose doxorubicin-containing chemotherapy in patients with metastatic breast cancer. *Journal of Clinical Oncology* **15**, 3171–3177.

Ravdin, P. M., Burris, H. A., Cook, G. *et al.* (1995). Phase II trial of docetaxel in advanced anthracycline-resistant or anthracenedione-resistant breast cancer. *Journal of Clinical Oncology* **13**, 2879–2885.

Romero, A., Rabinovich, M. G., Vallejo, C. T. *et al.* (1994). Vinorelbine as first-line chemotherapy for metastatic breast carcinoma. *Journal of Clinical Oncology* **12**, 336–341.

Sawada, N., Ishikawa, T., Fukase, Y. *et al.* (1998). Induction of thymidine phosphorylase activity and enhancement of capecitabine efficacy by taxol/taxotere in human cancer xenografts. *Clinical Cancer Research* **4**, 1013–1019.

Schiff, P. B., Fant, J., Horwitz, S. B. (1979). Promotion of microtubule assembly in vitro by Taxol. *Nature* **277**, 665–667.

Seidman, A. D., Reichman, B. S., Crown, J. P. *et al.* (1995). Paclitaxel as second and subsequent therapy for metastatic breast cancer: activity independent of prior anthracycline response. *Journal of Clinical Oncology* **13**, 1152–1159.

Seidman, A. D. (1999) Single-agent paclitaxel in the treatment of breast cancer: phase I and II development. *Seminars in Oncology* **26**, 14–20.

Sjostrom, J., Blomqvist, C., Mouridsen, H. *et al.* (1999). Docetaxel compared with sequential methotrexate and 5-fluorouracil in patients with advanced breast cancer after anthracycline failure: a randomised phase III study with crossover on progression by the Scandinavian Breast Group. *European Journal of Cancer* **35**, 1194–1201.

Sledge, G. W. Jr., Neuberg, D., Ingle, J. N. *et al.* (1997). Phase III trial of doxorubicin (A) vs. paclitaxel (T) vs. doxorubicin + paclitaxel (A + T) as first-line therapy for metastatic breast cancer: an Intergroup trial. *Proceedings of the American Society for Clinical Oncology* **16**, 2a.

Smalley, R. V., Carpenter, J., Bartolucci, A. *et al.* (1977). A comparison of cyclophosphamide, adriamycin, 5-fluorouracil (CAF) and cyclophosphamide, methotrexate, 5-fluorouracil, vincristine, prednisone (CMFVP) in patients with metastatic breast cancer: a Southeastern Cancer Study Group Project. *Cancer* **40**, 625–632.

Smith, R. E., Brown, A. M., Mamounas, E. P. *et al.* (1999). Randomized trial of 3-hour versus 24-hour infusion of high-dose paclitaxel in patients with metastatic or locally advanced breast cancer: National Surgical Adjuvant Breast and Bowel Project Protocol B-26. *Journal of Clinical Oncology* **17**, 3403–3411.

Spielmann, M., Dorval, T., Turpin, F. *et al.* (1994). Phase II trial of vinorelbine/doxorubicin as first-line therapy of advanced breast cancer. *Journal of Clinical Oncology* **12**, 1764–1770.

Stadtmauer, E. A., Goldstein, L. J., Glick, J. H. (2000). High-dose chemotherapy plus hematopoietic stem-cell rescue for metastatic breast cancer-reply. *New England Journal of Medicine* **343**, 440–441.

Sutherland, H. J., Lockwood, G. A., Boyd, N. F. (1990). Ratings of the importance of quality of life variables: therapeutic implications for patients with metastatic breast cancer. *Journal of Clinical Epidemiology* **43**(7), 661–666.

Tannock, I. F., Boyd, N. F., DeBoer, G. *et al.* (1998). A randomised trial of two dose levels of cyclophosphamide, methotrexate and fluorouracil chemotherapy for patients with metastatic breast cancer. *Journal of Clinical Oncology* **6**(9), 1377–1387.

Tormey, D. C., Weinberg, V. E., Leone, L. A. *et al.* (1984). A comparison of intermittent vs. continuous use of adriamycin vs. methotrexate 5-drug chemotherapy for advanced breast cancer: a Cancer and Leukemia Group B Study. *American Journal of Clinical Oncology* (CCT) **7**, 231–239.

Valero, V. (1997). Docetaxel as single-agent therapy in metastatic breast cancer: clinical efficacy. *Seminars in Oncology* **24**, S13-1–S13-18.

Valero, V., Holmes, F. A., Walters, R. S. *et al.* (1995). Phase II trial of docetaxel: a new, highly effective antineoplastic agent in the management of patients with anthracycline-resistant metastatic breast cancer. *Journal of Clinical Oncology* **13**, 2886–2894.

Valero, V., Jones, S. E., von Hoff, D. D. *et al.* (1998). A phase II study of docetaxel in patients with paclitaxel-resistant metastatic breast cancer. *Journal of Clinical Oncology* **16**, 3362–3368.

Verweij, J., Clavel, M., Chevallier, B. (1994). Paclitaxel (Taxol) and Docetaxel (Taxotere): not simply two of a kind. *Annals of Oncology* **5**, 495–505.

Vogel, C., O'Rourke, M., Winer, E. *et al.* (1999). Vinorelbine as first-line chemotherapy for advanced breast cancer in women 60 years of age or older. *Annals of Oncology* **10**, 397–402.

von Hoff, D. D. (1996). Activity of gemcitabine in a human tumor cloning assay as a basis for clinical trials with gemcitabine. San Antonio Drug Development Team. *Investigational New Drugs* **14**, 265–270.

Wani, M. C., Taylor, H. L., Wall, M. E. *et al.* (1971). Plant antitumor agents. VI. The isolation and structure of taxol, a novel antileukemic and antitumor agent from Taxus brevifolia. *Journal of the American Chemical Society* **93**, 2325–2327.

Winer, E., Berry, D., Duggan, D. *et al.* (1998). Failure of higher dose paclitaxel to improve outcome in patients with metastatic breast cancer-results from CALGB 9342. *Proceedings of the American Society for Clinical Oncology* **17**, 101a.

# Chapter 17

# Update on trastuzumab (Herceptin) in the clinical setting

*David W. Miles*

## Introduction

Targeted therapies are not a new concept in the field of breast cancer. Strategies aimed at targeting the oestrogen receptor having been with us for several decades. The identification and exploitation of other targets has taken longer than had been hoped. It is over 30 years since growth receptors were identified, but only in the past couple of years has a treatment targeting these receptors been available.

Women whose tumours express HER2 at high levels have a relatively poor prognosis with a median survival of 3 years, compared with 6–7 years for HER2-negative cases (Slamon *et al.* 1987). Many studies published subsequently, have demonstrated that HER2 overexpression is associated with other features of a poor prognosis, namely high tumour grade/S-phase fraction, oestrogen and progesterone receptor negativity, etc. (Ross & Fletcher 1999). In many series, however, HER2 status remains an independent poor prognostic feature. Whether HER2 status is a predictor of response to other treatment modalities in breast cancer, namely hormonal and cytotoxic therapy, remains contentious. Conflicting data are presented in the literature regarding the ability of HER2 positivity to predict relative resistance to hormonal therapy and chemotherapy. The major difficulties in interpreting these studies are that they are retrospective analyses and in many instances, there is no satisfactory 'control' arm against which to test attributable benefit of a treatment intervention in different HER2 subgroups. Although debate on this area is bound to continue, it seems unlikely that prospective studies of adjuvant hormonal and/or chemotherapy will be stratified according to HER2 status. Such is the conflicting nature of the literature about HER2 as a predictive factor that a rational view would be that no active therapeutic option should be disregarded based solely on the HER2 status of a patient's tumour (Yamauchi *et al.* 2001).

## Herceptin: pivotal trials

The two studies that led to the licensing of trastuzumab (referred to throughout this chapter by its trade name Herceptin) as treatment for metastatic breast cancer have now been published (Cobleigh *et al.* 1999; Slamon *et al.* 2001a). A re-analysis of data from both these studies supports the pre-clinical observation of a relation between

HER2 expression and growth inhibition of tumour cell lines by antibodies to the receptor (Mass *et al.* 2001; Genentech, unpublished data).

In the pivotal phase II study, heavily pre-treated patients whose tumour overexpressed HER2 at the 2 and 3+ level by immunohistochemistry were treated with Herceptin as a single agent. After re-analysis by a 'response evaluation committee', the overall response rate in this group was 15%, with a median survival of 9.1 months (Cobleigh *et al.* 1999). Although this response rate appears modest, it is noteworthy that most of these patients had already received anthracyclines and taxoids, and about one-quarter of patients had received a high-dose regimen of chemotherapy. In addition, those patients who did respond to Herceptin had a longer duration of response after treatment, compared with their previous regimen of chemotherapy (9.1 versus 5.2 months). Retrospective analysis of response rate and median survival restricted to the patients whose tumours who overexpress HER2 at the highest levels (immunohistochemical (IHC) score 3+) had a response rate of 18% and a median survival of 16.4 months.

In the pivotal phase III study (Slamon *et al.* 2001a), patients were randomised to receive chemotherapy with or without Herceptin. Patients were stratified according to whether or not adjuvant chemotherapy contained an anthracycline such that most patients who did not have adjuvant chemotherapy or whose adjuvant therapy did not contain an anthracycline were randomised to doxorubicin and cyclophosphamide (AC) with or without Herceptin (H). In the subgroup of patients who had received an anthracycline in the adjuvant setting, patients were randomised to paclitaxel (P) with or without Herceptin (H). The principal endpoint of this study was median time to progression, which for groups as a whole was significantly longer in those patients receiving chemotherapy with Herceptin, compared with chemotherapy alone (7.4 versus 4.6 months, $p < 0.05$). Time to progression was significantly longer in each of the chemotherapy subgroups (AC versus H+AC, 6.1 versus 7.8 months, P versus H+P 2.7 versus 6.9 months). When both chemotherapy subsets were considered a survival benefit attributable to Herceptin plus chemotherapy versus chemotherapy alone was noted (median survival 25 versus 20 months). This observed survival difference was despite the fact that nearly three-quarters of patients treated initially with chemotherapy alone crossed over to Herceptin as commonly as a single agent and often in the context of the pivotal phase II trial previously mentioned. It is likely therefore that any observed survival difference attributable to Herceptin has been somewhat underestimated. Interestingly, when the benefits of Herceptin were analysed retrospectively in those patients expressing HER2 at the highest level (immunohistochemical score 3+) it became apparent that the difference in most parameters (time to progression, response rate and survival) were greater in those patients whose tumours expressed HER2 at the 3+ level, compared with the group as a whole. For example, survival in the 3+ subgroup was 29 months for those patients receiving chemotherapy with Herceptin, compared with 20 months for those receiving chemotherapy alone (Mass *et al.* 2001).

The current limitation of Herceptin use in combination chemotherapy remains the cardiac dysfunction observed as part of the pivotal phase III study when Herceptin was combined with anthracycline. Some level of cardiac dysfunction was observed in 27% of patients treated with doxorubicin, cyclophosphamide with Herceptin compared with only 7% treated with AC alone. Cardiac dysfunction reached grade III and IV levels of the New York Heart Association rating in 16% of patients at some point during therapy, reducing to 6% of patients once treatment had been completed. The aetiology of the cardiac dysfunction remains unclear, and combinations of Herceptin with other anthracyclines including epirubicin and liposomal doxorubicin remain the subject of clinical trials. The licence for Herceptin in combination with chemotherapy is therefore restricted to its use with paclitaxel where the addition of Herceptin increased median survival from 18 to 25 months.

In summary, Herceptin is currently licensed for use as a single agent after anthracycline and taxoid or in those patients for whom such therapies are unsuitable and also in combination with paclitaxel. In both incidences, the current licence restricts its use to those patients who tumours overexpress HER2 at the highest level (3+) as assessed by immunohistochemistry.

As well as conventional endpoints, health-related quality of life using the European Organisation for Research and Treatment of Cancer Quality of Life questionnaire QLQ-C30 was administered at baseline, week 8 and every three months thereafter. The five primary prospectively defined quality of life domains examined included global quality of life, physical, social and role functioning as well as fatigue. The use of Herceptin with chemotherapy was associated with improvements in all these domains when compared with chemotherapy alone (Osoba & Burchmore 1999).

## Testing of Samples for HER2 Status

Debate continues about the best way of testing tissue samples for the presence of high levels of HER2 receptor. Most studies examining the use of HER2 overexpression as a prognostic and predictive factor have been done using immunohistochemistry. This is obviously a well-established and easy to use technique that is widely available. Part of the problem encountered in interpreting the prognostic and predictive data from HER2 is also an issue for testing the suitability of patients for Herceptin; immunohistochemical analysis may be subject to the vagaries of differences in tissue fixation. In addition, the use of different antibodies, other methodologies and scoring systems may render this technique less than completely objective. Fluorescent *in situ* hybridisation (FISH) detects HER2 at the DNA level and is specific and very sensitive. As a technique, however, it has limited availability, is more expensive than immunohistochemistry and requires specialised equipment. Comparisons between immunohistochemical analysis and analysis by FISH of many of the samples from the phase II and phases III pivotal studies show a good concordance between the two techniques. Nevertheless, from the data presented by Mass *et al.* (2001), it is clear that

11% of cases that were 3+ by immunohistochemistry are actually FISH negative and conversely, a significant proportion (24%) of cases which are 2+ by immunohistochemistry are FISH positive. Given the inherent variability of testing by immunohistochemistry, it is a concern that cases that are FISH positive, but only 2+ by immunohistochemistry might indeed benefit from Herceptin though this has not been evaluated prospectively. Nevertheless, it is worthy of note that for the monotherapy study, objective response rate in the FISH positive group is 21% compared with 18% in the patients whose tumours were 3+ by immunohistochemistry. Time to progression in these two groups (IHC 3+ and FISH positive) was identical at 3.2 months. Similarly, in the pivotal phase III study, response rates, time to progression and survival were similar in those patients who were FISH positive compared with the group whose tumours were IHC 3+. On these grounds it has been suggested that although patients whose tumours express HER2 at the 3+ level are those most likely to benefit from Herceptin, patients whose tumours express HER2 at the 2+ level, but who are FISH positive should also be considered for treatment with Herceptin. It is expected that a licence variation will be applied for to account for this group of patients.

## Future development of Herceptin

### First-line monotherapy

Herceptin has been tested in the first line treatment of metastatic breast cancer in patients who were unsuitable for or who declined chemotherapy. Vogel *et al.* (2001) performed a randomised phase II study comparing two different dose schedules of Herceptin. One hundred and fourteen HER2-positive patients were randomised to receive Herceptin at standard doses (4 mg/kg loading dose followed by 2 mg/kg weekly) or high dose (8 mg/kg loading dose followed by 4 mg/kg weekly). Response rates in the two groups were similar. When combined, the overall response rate (complete plus partial responses) for the group as a whole was 26% (95% confidence interval (CI), 18–34%). In those patients who overexpressed HER2 at the 3+ level by immunohistochemistry, the response rate was 35% (95% CI, 24–44%). If disease stabilisation for more than six months was added to the complete and partial responders to define a clinical benefit rate, then in the patients whose tumours expressed HER2 at the IHC 3+ level, the clinical benefit rate was 48%. It is noteworthy that no complete or partial responses were noted in patients whose tumours expressed HER2 at the IHC 2+ level. If only patients whose tumours expressed HER2 by FISH were considered, then the overall response rate (CR and PR) was 41% (95% CI, 26–56%). The 95% confidence intervals on these response rate estimates, taking all comers, IHC 3+ or FISH positive patients, all overlap. There is, however, a trend towards higher response rate in those patients who are perhaps better defined by FISH. Cross trial comparisons between Dr Vogel's study and the pivotal phase III study suggest that the use of Herceptin as monotherapy in FISH positive patients rather than in combination may not ultimately compromise outcome. The median survival in 41 patients who were FISH positive receiving Herceptin as first line monotherapy was 23 months, compared with a median survival of 26.8 months in a 125 patients from the pivotal study who had Herceptin in combination with chemotherapy. Although logistically difficult, a sequential versus combination study would be informative in this respect.

## Herceptin in combination with other agents

The combination of Herceptin and navelbine has been tested in the phase II setting Burstein *et al.* 2001). The overall response rate to the combination in patients with metastatic disease was 75% in considering patients whose tumours overexpressed HER2 at the IHC 3+ level, overall response rate was 80%. The combination was well tolerated and clearly warrants further investigation. Given the weekly schedule of Herceptin and the observations that weekly paclitaxel has relatively high activity, the combination of Herceptin and weekly paclitaxel was a logical one to pursue. Seidman *et al.* (2001) examined the use of Herceptin and paclitaxel in patients with metastatic disease irrespective of HER2 status. The original intention of the study was to compare roughly equal numbers of HER2-positive and HER2-negative patients and make comparisons of response rate according to different assay techniques. Overall, the combination was associated with response rates of 80% in patients who were HER2 positive and only 43% in patients who were HER2 negative. Responses were probably better defined by the use of the monoclonal antibody, TAB 250, rather than the now more widely HercepTest kit. Given the other data on the relative lack of effect of Herceptin in HER2-negative patients, it seems unlikely that this will be the subject of much further study. However, whether the weekly schedule of paclitaxel in combination with Herceptin is superior to three weekly in those patients whose tumours overexpress HER2 will clearly need to be tested in a randomised study.

Given the observed cardiotoxicity in the pivotal phase III trial, current combinations of Herceptin and anthracyclines are in the minority. Some groups are, however, investigating the possible use of the slightly less cardiotoxic epirubicin as well as liposomal doxorubicin. A current randomised phase II study is examining the contribution of Herceptin to docetaxel as first line therapy for metastatic disease. Pre-clinical data suggest that one of the more potent 'synergistic' combinations of Herceptin would be with a platinum and a taxoid. Studies by Slamon *et al.* (2001b) have examined this combination.

## **Herceptin dose scheduling**

Increasing the dose interval of Herceptin would obviously be more convenient, increase patient compliance and render more feasible studies of Herceptin in the adjuvant setting. Pharmacokinetic modelling suggest that a three weekly administration may be feasible. This is largely on the basis that Herceptin demonstrates dose-dependent nonlinear pharmacokinetics, with faster clearance and shorter half-life at doses of less than 100 mg. More recent data from Gelman *et al.* (2001) assess the toxicity and safety of three weekly Herceptin and paclitaxel. Herceptin was given at a loading dose of 8 mg/kg with subsequent doses of 6 mg/kg every three weeks. Overall, the half-life of Herceptin in this study was of the order of 21 days. Biological relevant trough levels were attained in a similar time period to the schedule of weekly administration. A similar profile of toxicity in reduction in left ventricular ejection fraction was noted as for weekly administration. Herceptin given every three weeks is clearly a feasible schedule. It is noteworthy, however, that with a half-life of 21 days, total clearance of Herceptin could take up to 18 weeks, which might have implications for anthracycline regimens after discontinuation of Herceptin.

## Herceptin in the adjuvant setting

HER2 amplification and overexpression is clearly an early event in the pathogenesis of breast cancer. Indeed, overexpression in ductal carcinoma in situ is significantly higher than in invasive disease (reviewed by Ross & Fletcher 1999). With the observation of the activity of Herceptin as single-agent therapy and considering its capacity to improve survival in metastatic disease when used in combination with chemotherapy, the development of adjuvant studies was clearly logical.

The NSABP B31 study compares paclitaxel with paclitaxel and concurrent Herceptin after four cycles of AC. Eligible patients are those whose tumours overexpress HER2 at the 3+ level by immunohistochemistry or those who are FISH positive. Two thousand seven hundred patients are expected to accrue to this study. The inter-group trial N9831 is similar to an NSABP B31, but as a three arm study which compared paclitaxel alone with paclitaxel and concurrent Herceptin versus paclitaxel followed by Herceptin. Again, eligible patients are those who express HER2 at the highest levels by immunohistochemistry or FISH. A thousand patients per arm will be accrued over four and a half years. In both these studies, cardiac safety is being monitored carefully with safety analyses after predetermined levels of accrual. The BCIRG trial of Herceptin in the adjuvant setting is also a three arm study which tests the use of docetaxel following four courses of AC with docetaxel and Herceptin given on a weekly schedule for a year. A third arm of this study aims to compare these 'standard' anthracycline style regimens with docetaxel and cisplatin or carboplatin times 6 with weekly Herceptin for one year. The Herceptin adjuvant trial (HERA trial) is a slightly more pragmatic study in which eligible patients (tumour HER2 3+ or FISH positive) complete primary management with chemotherapy and possibly radiotherapy, and are stratified by type of chemotherapy to one of three arms: namely observation, Herceptin given on a three weekly schedule for 12 months, and Herceptin given on a three weekly schedule for 24 months. This is the only current randomised adjuvant trial proposed that uses the three-weekly schedule and is also testing two durations of Herceptin. Again, cardiac function is being monitored closely.

## Conclusions

HER2 testing should be considered in patients with breast cancer, less perhaps because of its usefulness as a prognostic or predictive factor, but more to define whether the humanised monoclonal antibody to this growth factor receptor may be of use in patient management. The use of Herceptin with chemotherapy has been demonstrated to prolong survival in women with metastatic breast cancer. Sadly, very few agents have shown such a benefit in this setting and certainly the additional toxicity associated with this benefit seems small. New combinations and schedules using Herceptin seem very promising, but will need to be tested further. The role of this agent and the adjuvant treatment of breast cancer will be tested in the adjuvant studies that are currently ongoing.


*References*

Burstein, H. J., Juter. I., Campos, S. M., Gelman, R. S., Tribou, L., Parker, L. M., Manola, J., Younger, J., Matulouis, U., Bunnell, C. A. *et al.* (2001). Clinical activity of trastuzumab and vinorelbine in women with HER2-overexpressing metastatic breast cancer. *Journal of Clinical Oncology* **19**, 2722–2730.

Cobleigh, M. A., Vogel, C. L., Tripathy, D., Robert, N. J., Scholl, S., Fehrenbacher, L., Wolter, J. M., Paton, V., Shak, S., Lieberman, G. & Slamon, D. J. (1999). Multinational sutdy of the efficacy and saftey of humanised anti-HER2 monoclonal antibody in women who have HER2-overexpressing metastatic breast cancer that has progressed after chemotherapy for metastatic disease. *Journal of Clinical Oncology* **17**, 2639–2648.

Gelmon, K., Arnold, A., Verma, S., Ayoub, J., Hemmings, F. & Leyland-Jones, B. (2001). Pharmacokinetics (PK) and safety of trastuzumab (Herceptin) when administered every three weeks to women with metastatic breast cancer. *Proceedings of the American Society of Clinical Oncology* **20**, 69a (abstract 271).

Mass, R. D., Sanders, C., Charlene, K., Johnson, L., Everett, T. & Anderson, S. (2001). The concordance between the clinical trials assay (CTA) and fluorescence in situ hybridisation (FISH) in the Herceptin pivotal trials. *Proceedings of the American Society of Clinical Oncology* **20**, 75a (abstract 291).

Osoba, D. & Burchmore, M. (1999). Health-related quality of life in women with metastatic breast cancer treated with trastuzumab (Herceptin). *Seminars in Oncology* **4** (Suppl. 12), 84–88.

Ross, J. S. & Fletcher, J. A. (1999). HER-2/neu (c-erb-B2) gene and protein in breast cancer. *American Journal of Clinical Pathology* **112** (Suppl. 1), S53–S67.

Seidman, A. D., Fornier, M. N., Esteva, F. J., Tan, L., Kaptain, S., Bach, A., Panageas, K. S., Arroyo, C., Valero, V., Currie, V. *et al.* (2001). Weekly trastuzumab and paclitaxel therapy for metastatic breast cancer with analysis of efficacy by HER2 immunophenotype and gene amplification. *Journal of Clinical Oncology* **19**, 2587–2595.

Slamon, D. J., Clark, G. M., Wong, S. G., Levin, W. J., Ullrich, A. & McGuire, W. L. (1987). Human breast cancer: correlation of relapse and survival with amplification of the HER-2/neu oncogene. *Science* **235**, 177–182.

Slamon, D. J., Leyland-Jones, B., Shak, S., Fuchs, H., Paton, V., Bejamonde, A., Fleming, T., Eiermann, W., Wolter, J., Pegram, M., Beselga, J. & Norton, L. (2001a). Use of chemotherapy plus a monoclonal antibody against HER2 for metastatic breast cancer that overexpress HER2. *New England Journal of Medicine* **44**, 783–792.

Slamon, D.J., Pate,l R., Northfelt, R., Pegram, M., Rubin, J., Sebastian, G., Tannenbaum, S., Sanchez, J., Quan, E., Toppmeyer, D., Overmoyer, B. & Nabholtz, J. (2001b). Phase II pilot study of Herceptin combined with taxotere and carboplatin (TCH) in metastatic breast cancer (MBC) patients overexpressing the HER2-neu proto-oncogene: a pilot study of the UCLA network. *Proceedings of the American Society of Clinical Oncology* **20**, 49a (abstract 193).

Vogel, C., Cobleigh, M., Tripathy, D., Harris, L., Fehrenbacher, L., Slamon, D., Ash, M., Novotny, W., Stewart, S. & Shak, S. (2001). First-line, non-hormonal, treatment of women with HER2 overexpressing metastatic breast cancer with Herceptin (trastuzumab, humanised anti-HER2 antibody). *Proceedings of the American Society of Clinical Oncology* **20**, 71a (abstract 275).

Yamauchi, H., Stearns, V. & Hayes, D. F. (2001). When is a tumour marker ready for prime time? A case study of c-erbB-2 as a predictive factor in breast cancer. *Journal of Clinical Oncology* **19**, 2334–2356.

# Chapter 18

# New generation aromatase inhibitors in the preoperative, adjuvant and metastatic settings

*Stephen R. D. Johnston*

A significant proportion of breast cancers are oestrogen dependent and therefore amenable to endocrine therapy. Since the original description of the therapeutic response to ovarian ablation over 100 years ago (Beatson 1896), several advances have been made within the last decade in developing effective new hormone treatments and expanding their role from the management of advanced disease into adjuvant therapy. Although tamoxifen, a competitive non-steroidal anti-oestrogen, has been the mainstay of treatment for over 20 years, new agents such as the third-generation aromatase inhibitors have entered the clinic as a result of their superior activity and improved safety profile.

## Role of tamoxifen in advanced breast cancer

In women with advanced breast cancer who have received no prior endocrine therapy and are unselected for oestrogen receptor (ER) status, a review of the literature shows that the overall objective response rate to tamoxifen is 34%, with disease stabilisation in a further 20% and a median duration of response of 12–18 months (Arafah and Pearson 1986; Jackson *et al.* 1991). The likelihood of responding to tamoxifen was highest (60–70%) in postmenopausal women with ER-positive disease (McGuire 1978; Kuss *et al.* 1997). Tamoxifen is well tolerated in women with advanced breast cancer: less than 3% of women discontinue tamoxifen as a result of toxicity, and reported adverse effects include minor gastrointestinal upset (8%), hot flushes (27%), and menstrual disturbance in premenopausal women (13%) (Litherland and Jackson, 1988). For those with bone metastases, tumour flare may occur in less than 5% and can result in increased pain or symptomatic hypercalcaemia. A key problem in advanced breast cancer is that most women (> 90%) who initially respond to tamoxifen eventually relapse and develop acquired resistance to tamoxifen, although it is clear that they may still respond to further hormonal interventions (Johnston 1997). The most recent questions have been what is the most effective second-line treatment when tamoxifen has failed, and is there a more effective therapy than tamoxifen which may delay the time to progression.

## Previous second-line endocrine therapy

Although previously progestins (megestrol acetate or medroxyprogesterone acetate) were the standard treatment of choice after tamoxifen failure, considerable progress has been made with the development of potent oral aromatase inhibitors, which provide maximal oestrogen deprivation in postmenopausal women. The first generation non-steroidal aromatase inhibitor was aminoglutethimide, but its major problem was the lack of specificity for the aromatase enzyme and the fact that it inhibited the adrenal synthesis of both glucocorticoids and mineralocorticoids (which required concomitant use of hydrocortisone). Although aminoglutethimide suppressed plasma oestrogens and induced clinical responses, the drug also had several side effects including lethargy and skin rash (Harris *et al.* 1986). Second-generation inhibitors included the non-steroidal compound fadrozole (Afema) and the steroidal agent formestane (Lentaron) (Figure 18.1), both of which were more potent than aminoglutethimide (Coombes *et al.* 1984; Dowsett *et al.* 1990). However, clinical trials with both agents failed to show superiority over second-line progestin therapy (Buzdar *et al.* 1996; Thurlimann *et al.* 1997), and further clinical development was limited by specific problems including lack of selectivity caused by inhibition of aldosterone production (fadrozole) or inconvenient intramuscular route of administration (formestane).

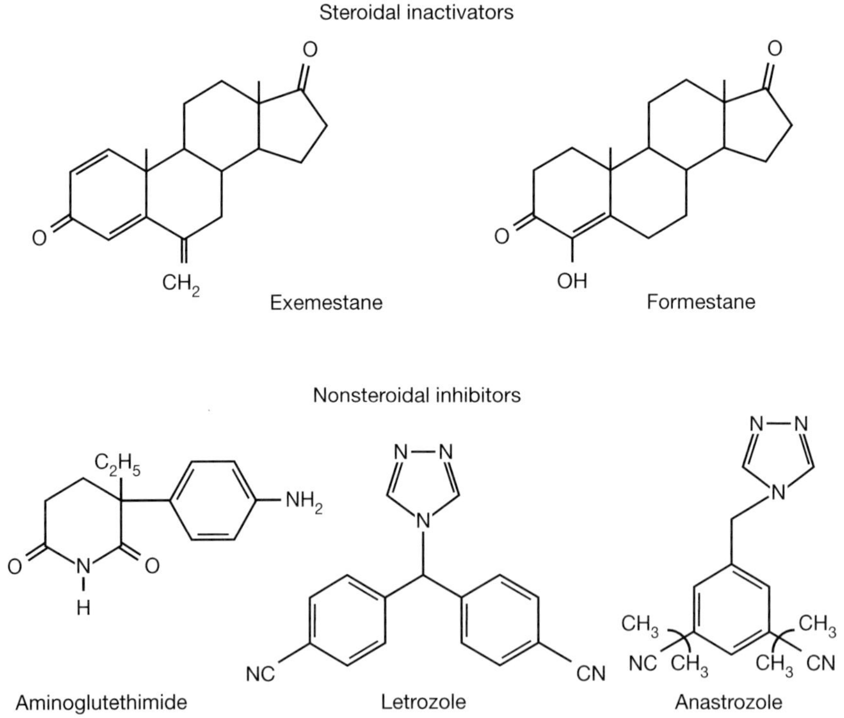

**Figure 18.1** Structures of non-steroidal and steroidal aromatase inhibitors.

## Potent and selective third-generation aromatase inhibitors

Considerable clinical progress has been made with the development of third-generation potent oral aromatase inhibitors, including the non-steroidal inhibitors anastrozole (Arimidex) and letrozole (Femara), together with the steroidal inhibitor exemestane (Aromasin) (see Figure 18.1). These novel agents are two to three orders of magnitude more potent than aminoglutethimide and are very effective in reducing serum oestrogen levels in postmenopausal women (Evans *et al.* 1992; Iveson *et al.* 1993; Plourde *et al.* 1994). In addition they are highly selective for the aromatase enzyme without affecting mineralocorticoid or glucocorticoid synthesis.

In the metastatic setting, phase III trials have been conducted in over 2000 postmenopausal women comparing each of the third-generation aromatase inhibitors with megestrol acetate as second-line therapy after failure on tamoxifen, and each trial has demonstrated clinical superiority for the aromatase inhibitors (Buzdar *et al.* 1998; Dombernowsky *et al.* 1998; Kaufmann *et al.* 2000). For anastrozole 1 mg daily, this was manifest as a significant improvement in overall survival (Buzdar *et al.* 1998), although there was no difference in response rate or time to progression. In contrast two large (> 550 patients each) randomised phase III trials compared letrozole 0.5 mg or 2.5 mg with standard second-line hormonal treatments, either megestrol acetate (Dombernowsky *et al.* 1998) or the non-selective and less potent aromatase inhibitor aminoglutethimide (Gershanovich *et al.* 1998). Both trials were in postmenopausal women with metastatic breast cancer unresponsive to tamoxifen (median age 64–65, 55% ER positive, 45% ER status unknown). Letrozole was significantly more effective than either of the standard drugs: compared with megestrol acetate; letrozole 2.5 mg was associated with a significantly higher response rate (hazard ratio [HR] 1.82, 95% confidence interval [95%CI] 1.02–3.25, $p$ = 0.04), longer duration of response (HR 0.42, 95%CI 0.2–0.86, $p$ = 0.02), and longer time to treatment failure (HR 0.77, 95%CI 0.61–0.99, $p$ = 0.04). Compared with the aminoglutethimide, letrozole achieved better overall survival (HR 0.64, 95%CI 0.49–0.85, $p$ = 0.002) and time to progression (HR 0.72, 95%CI 0.57–0.92, $p$ = 0.008) (Gershanovich *et al.* 1998). Likewise, in the recently reported trial with exemestane, time to disease progression, time to treatment failure and overall survival were all significantly better than megestrol acetate (Kaufmann *et al.* 2000).

These improvements in clinical endpoints, together with the superior tolerability profile shown for the new third-generation oral aromatase inhibitors over megestrol acetate, have defined the role for these drugs as the standard endocrine treatment after tamoxifen failure. What is particularly impressive from some of these trials are the substantial improvements seen in response duration for those who benefited, e.g. in the letrozole study the median response duration was > 33 months compared with 18 months for megestrol acetate (Dombernowsky *et al.* 1998). However, not all patients derived such clinical benefit (< 50% in each of the three trials), and as discussed below it remains important to see whether predictive factors (prior response to tamoxifen, ER expression post-tamoxifen) can be used to identify subgroups of patients with advanced breast cancer for whom this treatment is likely to be of greatest significance.

## First-line therapy – a challenge to tamoxifen?

As clinical trials showed substantial improvements in clinical efficacy for the novel aromatase inhibitors when given as second-line therapy, it became obvious to design trials that asked whether these drugs should challenge tamoxifen as the first-line agent of choice. The great potential of these studies was to see whether complete oestrogen blockade provided greater control of hormone-sensitive breast cancer than tamoxifen, thus circumventing the problem of acquired tamoxifen resistance whereby a proportion of ER-positive tumours re-grow following an initial response to tamoxifen (Johnston 1997). However, previous randomised clinical trials versus tamoxifen of the early generation aromatase inhibitors, such as aminoglutethimide (Smith *et al.* 1982), fadrozole (Falkson and Falkson 1996; Thurlimann *et al.* 1996) and formestane (Perrez-Carrion *et al.* 1994), had all failed to show improved time to treatment failure/ disease progression or prolonged response duration.

Data have emerged from trials that have evaluated the third-generation aromatase inhibitors as potential first-line therapy in advanced postmenopausal breast cancer challenging tamoxifen as the agent of choice. In a US trial of 353 postmenopausal women, anastrozole was associated with a significant improvement in time to disease progression from 5.6 to 11.1 months compared with tamoxifen ($p = 0.005$) (Nabholtz *et al.* 2000), although in a second larger European study of 668 patients the two drugs were equivalent, but anastrozole had significantly fewer thromboembolic and vaginal side effects (Bonneterre *et al.* 2000). One explanation for the differences in results between these two trials was the higher incidence of ER-positive confirmed patients in the American rather than the European study (89% vs 48%). A retrospective combined analysis of ER-positive patients from both studies confirmed that a third-generation aromatase inhibitor such as anastrozole was associated with a significant improvement in time to disease progression (Buzdar *et al.* 2000).

More recently, results were published from a single large prospective trial of letrozole versus tamoxifen as first-line endocrine therapy in 973 postmenopausal women with advanced breast cancer. There was a highly significant improvement in both response rate (30% vs 20%, $p = 0.0001$) and time to disease progression (9.2 vs 6.3 months, $p = 0.00001$) for patients treated with letrozole compared with tamoxifen (Mouridsen *et al.* 2001). The improved likelihood of benefit was seen in all subgroups and the tolerability profile for letrozole was excellent, with a reduced number of drug-related adverse events compared with tamoxifen. Recent data have suggested that these improvements for letrozole as first-line therapy may translate into an early gain in survival over tamoxifen (Mouridsen *et al.* 2003).

## Who benefits most from aromatase inhibitors?

Clinical predictors of response to endocrine therapy in advanced disease have traditionally included factors such as soft tissue versus visceral sites of disease, long disease-free interval and prior response to tamoxifen. The enhanced efficacy of the more potent aromatase inhibitors, including evidence for activity in groups of patients previously deemed to have a low chance of endocrine response, means that some of these traditional clinical factors may be less of a discriminator. Subset analyses of the recent second-line phase III trials with third-generation aromatase inhibitors (Buzdar *et al.* 1998; Dombernowsky *et al.* 1998; Gershanovich *et al.* 1998; Kaufmann *et al.* 2000) have demonstrated significant efficacy in sites of visceral disease for aromatase inhibitors compared with progestins, e.g. in the first-line trial of letrozole versus tamoxifen, superior response rates were seen both in those with soft-tissue or visceral sites of disease (Mouridsen *et al.* 2001). As a consequence, the presence of asymptomatic visceral metastases as the dominant site of disease in those with hormone-sensitive breast cancer should no longer be the sole reason to favour chemotherapy over and above effective endocrine therapy.

Prior sensitivity to tamoxifen in advanced disease has been a clinical factor often cited as a predictor for the likelihood of response to a further endocrine agent in the second-line setting (Johnston 1997). Patients who have received tamoxifen for advanced disease may be categorised as responders if they show an objective response (complete regression [CR] or partial regression [PR]), or have stabilisation of disease for at least 6 months (SD). It is well recognised that patients who were previously sensitive to tamoxifen and then developed acquired resistance are more likely to respond to further endocrine therapy. We previously reported, from our own historical series of studies with various aromatase inhibitors, that 70% of tamoxifen responders had an objective response (CR/PR) or SD to second-line aromatase inhibitors, compared with less than 15% who had shown *de novo* resistance to tamoxifen (Dowsett *et al.* 1995). However, in the recent randomised trials of letrozole, significant response rates have also been seen in so-called tamoxifen non-responders (Dombernowsky *et al.* 1998) and in those who had received tamoxifen previously in the adjuvant setting (Mouridsen *et al.* 2001). The enhanced efficacy of these agents may mean that a benefit can be seen in patients deemed to have shown no initial sensitivity to tamoxifen, or who have been exposed to tamoxifen in the past at some stage.

## Preoperative endocrine therapy – biological predictors of response

Recently, supportive data from a randomised trial of preoperative endocrine therapy have demonstrated an improvement in clinical efficacy for letrozole over tamoxifen in 453 postmenopausal women with primary ER-positive breast cancer (Ellis *et al.* 2001). The results confirmed a higher response rate in terms of tumour shrinkage whether defined clinically, by ultrasonography or mammography. This resulted in a higher rate of breast-conserving surgery after 4 months of planned preoperative endocrine therapy. Although the ultimate role and clinical benefit for preoperative (neoadjuvant) endocrine therapy remain to be defined, these data can be seen as confirmatory evidence for the enhanced efficacy of letrozole over tamoxifen. For women with large ER-positive primary breast cancers for whom surgery is not indicated and in whom tamoxifen has been the previous standard of care (i.e. locally advanced disease or the more elderly patient), it is clear that an aromatase inhibitor is now a more effective treatment option.

The presence of a functional oestrogen receptor in breast cancer implies a hormone-sensitive tumour which is dependent on oestrogen to grow. Thus, ER-positive tumours should be highly sensitive to oestrogen deprivation therapy in comparison with tumours that are completely ER negative. In the setting where tamoxifen has been used as initial therapy in elderly patients, ER expression has proved the best predictor of response (Gaskell *et al.* 1992; Low *et al.* 1992). In the Edinburgh series of primary neoadjuvant tamoxifen in ER-positive operable breast cancer, the quantitative value of ER became a significant discriminator for response in such patients as determined by ultrasonography after 3 months of tamoxifen (Millet *et al.* 1991). In particular, all tumours with an ER > 200 fmol/mg protein responded, whereas tumours with ER values below this were equally likely to respond or not. In terms of similar data for predicting response to aromatase inhibitors, the response rates and median reduction in tumour volume by ultrasonography of primary ER-positive cancers appeared much higher with either anastrozole or letrozole than tamoxifen in sequential non-randomised groups of patients in the Edinburgh series (Miller *et al.* 1991; Dixon *et al.* 1999). In the recent randomised preoperative study of letrozole versus tamoxifen, although quantitative ER score was predictive of response to both endocrine treatments, tumours with intermediate ER scores were more likely to respond to letrozole than tamoxifen. In addition tumours that co-expressed HER-2 and ER had a very low likelihood of response to tamoxifen, consistent with previous data that this phenotype predicts for endocrine resistance. In contrast there was a significantly greater chance of responding to letrozole in ER-positive HER-2-positive tumours (Ellis *et al.* 2001), although the biological basis for this result remains unclear.

When patients develop recurrent disease, it has been of concern as to whether hormone sensitivity resulting from the presence of ER in the original primary tumour is lost over time. This could account for lower response rates seen with tamoxifen in advanced metastatic breast cancer compared with studies when given as primary preoperative therapy. However, several studies have confirmed that a significant number of patients retain ER expression when they develop recurrent metastatic disease (Encarnacion *et al.* 1993; Johnston *et al.* 1995; Kuukasjarvi *et al.* 1996). Knowledge of change in ER status may be more helpful in predicting response to endocrine therapy in the metastatic setting than relying on the ER status of the previous primary tumour. We examined the role of intervening tamoxifen given in the adjuvant or first-line setting on preservation of ER status from the primary tumour to the relapsed sample in 95 patients who developed tamoxifen resistance. Overall, we confirmed that ER expression was often retained, and that preservation of ER at relapse on tamoxifen may prove the best predictor of response to second-line endocrine therapy, especially to aromatase inhibitors (Johnston *et al.* 2001).

## Future role of aromatase inhibitors – adjuvant therapy

In view of the recent data which have demonstrated a significant improvement in clinical efficacy for aromatase inhibitors over tamoxifen as first-line therapy in postmenopausal women with advanced ER-positive breast cancer, much interest awaits the results of large randomised trials in the adjuvant setting. Tamoxifen taken for 5 years is established as the endocrine treatment of choice for ER-positive breast cancer in view of the world overview data, which demonstrated a 50% improvement in 10-year relapse free survival and a 25% improvement in 10-year overall survival for those with ER-positive tumours (Early Breast Cancer Trialists' Group [EBCTG] 1998). The possibility exists that, if efficacy for aromatase inhibitors is much greater than for tamoxifen, significant further improvements in relapse-free and overall survival could be seen in the current trials in comparison with tamoxifen. The design of these trials has varied, and addresses several questions in relation to optimal use of these drugs (Figure 18.2). Many of these trials are still ongoing and are scheduled to recruit over 40,000 women. Only one trial, the so-called Adjuvant Tamoxifen, Anastrozole or the Combination trial (ATAC) has reported early results (ATAC Trialist's Group. 2002). A total of 9366 postmenopausal patients with early breast cancer were randomized to the 3 treatment arms. After a median of 33 months follow-up there was a significant improvement in 3-year disease-free survival for anastrozole compared with tamoxifen. There was also a significantly reduced incidence of contra-lateral invasive breast cancers, suggesting an even greater effect for an aromatase inhibitor than tamoxifen in the possible chemo-prevention of breast cancer. Further follow up of this trial is needed to see if overall survival is improved. The Femara versus Tamoxifen Adjuvant Study (FEMTA) has directly compared 5 years of letrozole versus tamoxifen, but in addition has examined sequential therapy of tamoxifen for 2 years followed by letrozole for 3 years, or the reverse sequence. This trial will therefore determine whether resistance to tamoxifen manifest by relapse during years 3–5 can be overcome or prevented by switching to an aromatase inhibitor. A preliminary report of this trial was presented at the St. Gallen meeting in January of this year (2005). Essentially, the results replicate those of the ATAC trial in respect of the main end-points, confirming superiority of aromatase inhibitors versus tamoxifen over the first 3 years. Further supporting data for sequential therapy of tamoxifen followed by a steroidal aromatase inhibitor (exemestane), indicate that

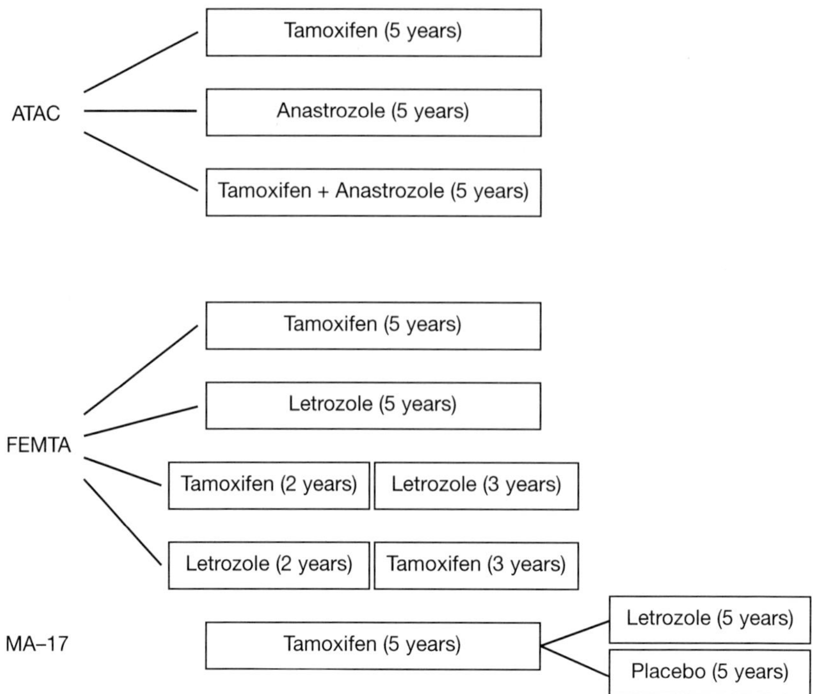



**Figure 18.2** Design of current adjuvant therapy trials of non-steroidal aromatase inhibitors in early breast cancer. ATAC, Adjuvant Tamoxifen, Anastrozole or the Combination trial; FEMTA, Femara versus Tamoxifen Adjuvant Study; MA-17, Canadian study.

5 years of tamoxifen monotherapy after surgery may be suboptimal for post-menopausal patients with ER-positive breast cancer (Coombes *et al.* 2004). The authors recommend that clinicians should consider switching patients to exemestane between 2 and 3 years after the start of tamoxifen therapy. Finally, while the optimal duration of adjuvant tamoxifen remains unclear, MA-17 is examining an alternative strategy of changing to 5 years of letrozole. All of these trials are large (5000–9000 patients), and will require several years of follow-up before we know the results. At the same time, there is concern about the potential effects of long-term oestrogen deprivation in those postmenopausal women with a potent third-generation aromatase inhibitor, and sub-protocols are examining bone mineral density in these women.

## Conclusions

The development of third-generation aromatase inhibitors has resulted in a significant advance in endocrine therapy of breast cancer. Their role has been clearly established as second-line therapy after tamoxifen failure, with the consistent finding being that they significantly enhance tumour response duration, time to progression and overall survival compared with progestins. Likewise, recent trials in first-line therapy have demonstrated, for the first time, significant improvement in both response rate and time to disease progression for aromatase inhibitors compared with tamoxifen. These new data have generated significant optimism that in the adjuvant setting an aromatase inhibitor could yield further substantial gains in outcome over tamoxifen for postmenopausal women with endocrine-sensitive breast cancer.

## *References*

Arafah, B. M., Pearson, O. H. (1986). Endocrine treatment of advanced breast cancer. In: Jordan, V. C. (ed.), *Estrogen/Antiestrogen Action and Breast Cancer Therapy*. Madison, C. T.: University of Wisconsin Press, pp. 417–429.

ATAC Trialists Group. (2002). Anastrozole alone or in combination with tamoxifen versus tamoxifen alone for adjuvant treatment of postmenopausal women with early breast cancer; first results of the ATAC randomised trial. *Lancet* **359**, 2131–2139.

Beatson, G. T. (1896). On the treatment of inoperable cases of carcinoma of the mamma: suggestions for a new method of treatment with illustrative cases. *The Lancet* **ii**, 104–107.

Bonneterre, J., Thurlimann, B., Robertson, J. F. R. *et al.* (2000). Anastrozole versus tamoxifen as first-line therapy for advanced breast cancer in 668 postmenopausal women: results of the tamoxifen or arimidex randomised group efficacy and tolerability study. *Journal of Clinical Oncology* **18**, 3748–3757.

Buzdar, A. U., Smith, R., Vogel, C. *et al.* (1996). Fadrozole HCL (CGS-16949A) versus megestrol acetate in treatment of postmenopausal patients with metastatic breast cancer. *Cancer* **77**, 2503–2513.

Buzdar, A., Jonat, W., Howell, A. *et al.* (1998). Anastrozole versus megestrol acetate in the treatment of postmenopausal women with advanced breast carcinoma: results of a survival update based on a combined analysis of data from two mature phase III trials. *Cancer* **83**, 1142–1152.

Buzdar, A. W., Nabholtz, J. M., Robertson, J. F. R *et al.* (2000). Anastrozole (Arimidex) versus tamoxifen as first-line therapy for advanced breast cancer in postmenopausal women; combined analysis from two identically designed multicenter trials. *Proceedings of the American Society of Clinical Oncology* **19**, 154 (A609).

Coombes, R. C., Goss, P., Dowsett, M., Gazet, J. C., Brodie, A. (1984). 4-Hydroxyandrostenedione in treatment of postmenopausal women with advanced breast cancer. *The Lancet* **ii**, 1237–1239.

Coombes, R. C., Hall, E., Cubson, L. J. *et al.* (2004). A randomised trial of exemestane after 2 to 3 years of tamoxifen therapy in post-menopausal women with primary breast cancer. *New England Journal of Medicine* **350**, 1081–1092.

Dixon, J. M., Love, C. D. B., Renshaw, L. *et al.* (1999). Lessons from the use of aromatase inhibitors in the neoadjuvant setting. *Endocrine-Related Cancer* **6**, 227–230.

Dombernowsky, P., Smith, I. E., Falkson, G. *et al.* (1998). Letrozole, a new oral aromatase inhibitor for advanced breast cancer: double-blind randomised trial showing a dose-effect and improved efficacy and tolerability compared with megestrol acetate. *Journal of Clinical Oncology* **16**, 453–461.

Dowsett, M., Stein, R. C., Mehta, A., Coombes, R. C. (1990). Potency and selectivity of the non-steroidal aromatase inhibitor CGS 16949A in postmenopausal breast cancer patients. *Clinical Endocrinology* **32**, 623–624.

Dowsett, M., Johnston, S. R. D., Iveson, T. J., Smith, I. E. (1995). Response to pure anti-estrogen (ICI 182,780) in tamoxifen-resistant breast cancer. *The Lancet* **345**, 525.

Early Breast Cancer Trialists' Group (1998) Tamoxifen for early breast cancer; an overview of the randomised trials. *The Lancet* **351**, 1451–1467.

Ellis, M., Singh, B., Miller, W. R. *et al.* (2001). Letrozole (Femara) is a more effective inhibitor of estrogen activity than tamoxifen: evidence from a randomised phase III trial of 4 months preoperative endocrine therapy for postmenopausal women with primary invasive breast cancer. *Proceedings of the American Society of Clinical Oncology* **20**, 416A (A1661).

Encarnacion, C. A., Ciocca, D. R., McGuire, W. L., Clark, G. M., Fuqua, S. A. W., Osborne, C. K. (1993). Measurement of steroid hormone receptors in breast cancer patients on tamoxifen. *Breast Cancer Research Treatment* **26**, 237–246.

Evans, T. R. J., Di Salle, E., Ornati, G. *et al.* (1992). Phase I endocrine study of exemestane (FCE 24304), a new aromatase inhibitor, in postmenopausal women. *Cancer Research* **52**, 5933–5939.

Falkson, C. I,. Falkson, H. C. (1996). A randomized study of GCS 16949A (fadrozole) versus tamoxifen in previously untreated postmenopausal patients with metastatic breast cancer. *Annals of Oncology* **7**, 465–469.

Gaskell, D. J., Hawkins, R. A., Sangster, K., Chetty, U., Forrest, A. P. M. (1992). Relation between immunocytochemical estimation of estrogen receptor in elderly patients with primary breast cancer and response to tamoxifen. *The Lancet* **i**, 1044–1046.

Gershanovich, M., Chaudri, H. A., Campos, D. *et al.* (1998). Letrozole, a new oral aromatase inhibitor: randomised trial comparing 2.5 mg daily, 0.5 mg daily and aminoglutethimide in postmenopausal women with advanced breast cancer. *Annals of Oncology* **9**, 639–645.

Harris, A. L., Dowsett, M., Cantwell, B. M. *et al.* (1986). Endocrine effects of low-dose aminoglutethimide with hydrocortisone – an optimal hormonal suppressive regimen. *Breast Cancer Research and Treatment* **7**, 69–72.

Iveson, T. J., Smith, I. E., Ahern, J., Smithers, D. A., Trunet, P. F., Dowsett, M. (1993). Phase I study of the oral nonsteroidal aromatase inhibitor CGS 20267 (letrozole) in postmenopausal patients with advanced breast cancer. *Cancer Research* **53**, 266–270.

Jackson, I. M., Litherland, S., Wakeling, A. E. (1991). Tamoxifen and other antioestrogens. In: Powles, T. J., Smith, I. E. (eds), *Medical Management of Breast Cancer*. London: Martin Dunitz, pp. 51–59.

Johnston, S. R. D. (1997). Acquired tamoxifen resistance in human breast cancer – potential mechanisms and clinical implications. *Anti-Cancer Drugs* **8**, 911–930.

Johnston, S. R. D., Saccani-Jotti, G., Smith, I. E. *et al.* (1995). Changes in estrogen receptor, progesterone receptor and pS2 expression in tamoxifen-resistant human breast cancer. *Cancer Research* **55**, 3331–3338.

Johnston, S. R. D., Smith, I. E., Dowsett, M. (2001). Place of aromatase inhibitors in the endocrine therapy of breast cancer. In: Miller, W. R., Santen, R. J. (eds), *Aromatase Inhibition and Breast Cancer*. New York: Marcel Dekker Inc., pp. 29–49.

Kaufmann, M., Bajetta, E., Dirix, L. Y. *et al.* (2000). Exemestane is superior to megestrol acetate after tamoxifen failure in postmenopausal women with advanced breast cancer; results of a phase III randomised double-blind study. *Journal of Clinical Oncology* **18**, 1399–1411.

Kuss, J. T., Muss, H. B., Hoen, H., Case, L. D. (1997). Tamoxifen as initial endocrine therapy for metastatic breast cancer: long term follow-up of two Piedmont Oncology Association (POA) trials. *Breast Cancer Research and Treatment* **42**, 265–274.

Kuukasjarvi, T., Kononen, J., Helin, H., Holli, K., Isola, J. (1996). Loss of estrogen receptor in recurrent breast cancer is associated with poor response to endocrine therapy *Journal of Clinical Oncology* **14**, 2584–2589.

Litherland, S., Jackson, I. M. (1988). Antioestrogens in the management of hormone-dependent cancer. *Cancer Treatment Reports* **15**, 183–194.

Low, S. C., Dixon, A. R., Bell, J. (1992). Tumour oestrogen receptor content allows selection of elderly patients with breast cancer for conservative tamoxifen treatment. *British Journal of Surgery* **79**, 1314–1316.

McGuire, W. L. (1978). Hormone receptors; their role in predicting prognosis and response to endocrine therapy. *Seminars in Oncology* **5**, 428–443

Miller, W. R., Anderson, T. J., Hawkins, R. A., Keen, J., Dixon, J. M. (1991). Neoadjuvant endocrine treatment; the Edinburgh experience. In: Howell, A., Dowsett, M. (eds), *European School of Oncology Update*, Vol 4 – *Primary Medical Therapy for Breast Cancer*. Amsterdam: Elsevier Science B.V., pp. 89–99.

Mouridsen, H,. Gershanovich, M., Sun, Y. *et al.* (2001). Superior efficacy of Letrozole (Femara) versus tamoxifen as first-line therapy for postmenopausal women with advanced breast cancer: results of a phase III study of the International Letrozole Breast Cancer Group. *Journal of Clinical Oncology* **19**, 2596–2606.

Mouridsen, H., Gershanovich, M., Sun, Y. & *et al.* (2003). Phase III study of letrozole versus tamoxifen as first-line therapy of advanced breast cancer in post-menopausal women: analysis of survival and update of efficacy from International Letrozole Breast Cancer Group. *Journal of Clinical Oncology* **21**, 2101–2109.

Nabholtz, J. M., Buzdar, A., Pollak, M. *et al.* (2000). Anastrozole is superior to tamoxifen as first-line therapy for advanced breast cancer in postmenopausal women: results of a North American multicentre randomised trial. *Journal of Clinical Oncology* **18**, 3758–3767.

Perrez-Carrion, R., Alberola Candel, V., Calabresi, F. (1994). Comparison of the selective aromatase inhibitor formestane with tamoxifen as first-line hormonal therapy in postmenopausal women with advanced breast cancer. *Annals of Oncology* **5** (suppl 7), 19–24.

Plourde, P. V., Dyroff, M., Dukes, M. (1994). Arimidex: a potent and selective fourth generation aromatase inhibitor. *Breast Cancer Research and Treatment* **30**, 103–111.

Smith, I. E., Harris, A. L., Morgan, M. (1982). Tamoxifen versus aminoglutethimide versus combined tamoxifen and aminoglutethimide in the treatment of advanced breast carcinoma. *Cancer Research* **42**, 3430–3433.

Thurlimann, B., Beretta, K., Bacchi, M. *et al.* (1996). First-line fadrozole HCL (CGS 16949A) versus tamoxifen in postmenopausal women with advanced breast cancer. *Annals of Oncology* **7**, 471–479.

Thurlimann, B., Castiglione, M., Hsu-Schmitz, S. F. *et al.* (1997). Formestane versus megestrol acetate in postmenopausal breast cancer patients after failure of tamoxifen; a phase III prospective randomized cross-over trial of second-line hormonal treatment (SAKK 20/90). *European Journal of Cancer* **33**, 1017–1024.

# Chapter 19

# The future treatment of breast cancer: scientific advances and clinical innovations

*Stephen R. D. Johnston*

## Introduction

The late 1990s saw the introduction into routine clinical practice of several new drugs for the management of breast cancer. These included aromatase inhibitors, taxanes, bisphosphonates, and the monoclonal antibody trastuzumab targeted against the growth factor receptor HER-2. Much enthusiasm exists around the next generation of potential 'breakthrough drugs'. The rapid expansion in knowledge of the molecular pathogenesis of breast cancer has created several opportunities for novel strategies in anti-cancer drug design, including better and more effective endocrine therapies such as selective oestrogen receptor modulators (SERMs) that may have fewer side-effects than tamoxifen, and novel signal transduction inhibitors (STIs) targeted against various abnormal growth and cell survival pathways. In addition it is accepted that we require better selection of patients for individual therapies, and molecular profiling of primary carcinomas is set to re-define how we classify breast cancer both for prognosis, and for prediction of response to individual therapies. This chapter specifically reviews recent advances in the development of SERMs and STIs for breast cancer.

## Selective oestrogen receptor modulators: an improvement on tamoxifen?

Ever since evidence emerged that human breast carcinomas may be associated with oestrogen, attempts have been made to block or inhibit oestrogen's biological effects as a therapeutic strategy for women with breast cancer. Tamoxifen is one of the most effective treatments for breast cancer though its ability to antagonise oestrogen-dependent growth by binding oestrogen receptors (ERs) and inhibiting breast epithelial cell proliferation. However, tamoxifen has oestrogenic agonist effects on other tissues such as bone and endometrium because of liganded ER-activating target genes in these different cell types. Several new anti-oestrogens are termed SERMs, which have an altered agonist profile on breast and gynaecological tissues. These SERMs were developed with the expectation that they may offer enhanced efficacy and reduced toxicity compared with tamoxifen (Johnston 2001).

For breast cancer therapy, a meta-analysis has shown that five years of tamoxifen in women with in early stage ER-positive breast cancer significantly reduced the risk of recurrence (47% reduction in annual odds) and death (26% reduction in annual odds) (Early Breast Cancer Trialists' Group 2001). This benefit was greatest in women with ER-rich tumours and occurred across all age groups, irrespective of nodal involvement. In addition, tamoxifen's anti-oestrogenic effects on normal breast epithelial cells resulted in a 50% reduction in new contra-lateral breast cancers, evidence that provided much of the impetus to develop tamoxifen in chemoprevention. At the same time, the oestrogenic effects of tamoxifen therapy on bone and cholesterol are of clinical benefit for these women in terms of reducing risk from osteoporosis and cardiovascular disease (Love *et al.* 1991, 1992). In the adjuvant setting, tamoxifen's increased risk of endometrial cancer has been perceived as small in relation to the substantial benefit from reduction in breast cancer related-events (Fisher *et al.* 1994). However, both in adjuvant and metastatic therapy with tamoxifen, breast epithelial cells and established tumours adapt to chronic anti-oestrogen exposure and develop resistance to tamoxifen, which may relate to the partial agonist effect of tamoxifen in stimulating tumour growth (Johnston 1997). Experimental models have shown that novel anti-oestrogens (SERMs) devoid of agonist effects can antagonise tamoxifen-stimulated growth, and as treatment of hormone-sensitive tumours may delay the emergence of resistance (Osborne *et al.* 1995; Johnston *et al.* 1997). This generated hope that better SERMs with an improved anti-oestrogen/oestrogen profile may overcome this form of resistance and improve further on the efficacy of tamoxifen in treating breast cancer.

## Pre-clinical profile of selective oestrogen receptor modulators

Non-steroidal SERMs fall into two broad categories: those that are structurally similar to the triphenylethylene structure of tamoxifen (Figure 19.1), and those that are structurally different and more related to the benzothiophene structure of raloxifene (Figure 19.2). A third class of anti-oestrogen includes the steroidal anti-oestrogen ICI-182,780 (fulvestrant) which is a structural derivative of estradiol with a long hydrophobic side-chain at the 7 alpha position (Figure 19.2). Pharmacologically, these last compounds are pure anti-oestrogens that not only impair ER dimerisation but also induce ER degradation (Dauvois *et al.* 1993), and thus act as potent anti-oestrogens in all tissues including the breast, uterus and probably bone. Although some may argue that fulvestrant is not a true SERM because it lacks selective agonist/antagonist effects in different tissues and possesses a fundamentally different mechanism of action, others have suggested that it represents one extreme end (i.e. a pure anti-oestrogen) of the SERM spectrum, with oestrogen as a pure agonist at the other end, and that all other SERMs fall somewhere in between.

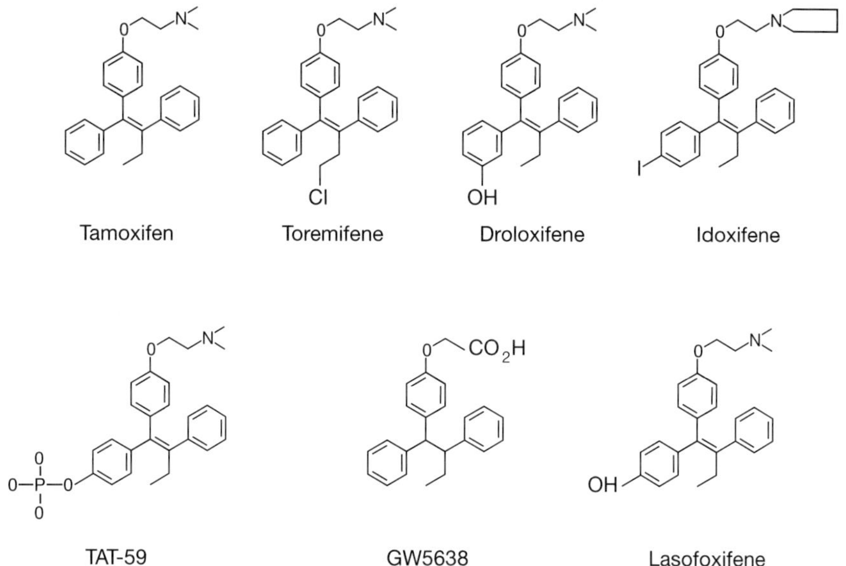



**Figure 19.1** Tamoxifen-like selective oestrogen receptor modulators that have been developed for breast cancer.

Each of the SERMs demonstrated pharmacological or pharmacodynamic benefit over tamoxifen in various pre-clinical studies, and as a consequence had a profile that supported clinical development in women with advanced breast cancer, in the hope of producing a more effective and beneficial anti-oestrogen. The potential pre-clinical advantage for these SERMs included either greater potency due to enhanced affinity for ER, greater efficacy compared with tamoxifen against breast cancer *in vitro* or *in vivo*, and reduced risk of toxicity compared with tamoxifen on end organs such as the liver and endometrium (reviewed in Johnston (2001)). If resistance to tamoxifen occurs in part because of the agonist effects of the drug stimulating tumour re-growth, then SERMs would be expected to either be active against tamoxifen-resistant tumours, or delay the emergence of resistance. In the clinic, this profile might be expected to produce either superior response rates, or delay the emergence of resistance during long-term therapy.

## Clinical efficacy of selective oestrogen receptor modulators

As second-line therapy after failure of tamoxifen in advanced breast cancer, overall little significant activity has been observed with the first-generation tamoxifen-like SERMs (toremifene, droloxifene and idoxifene), with a median response rate from all studies of only 5% (range 0–15%) (Johnston 2001). The reduced agonist profile seen with droloxifene and idoxifene in pre-clinical studies may have been tissue or cell

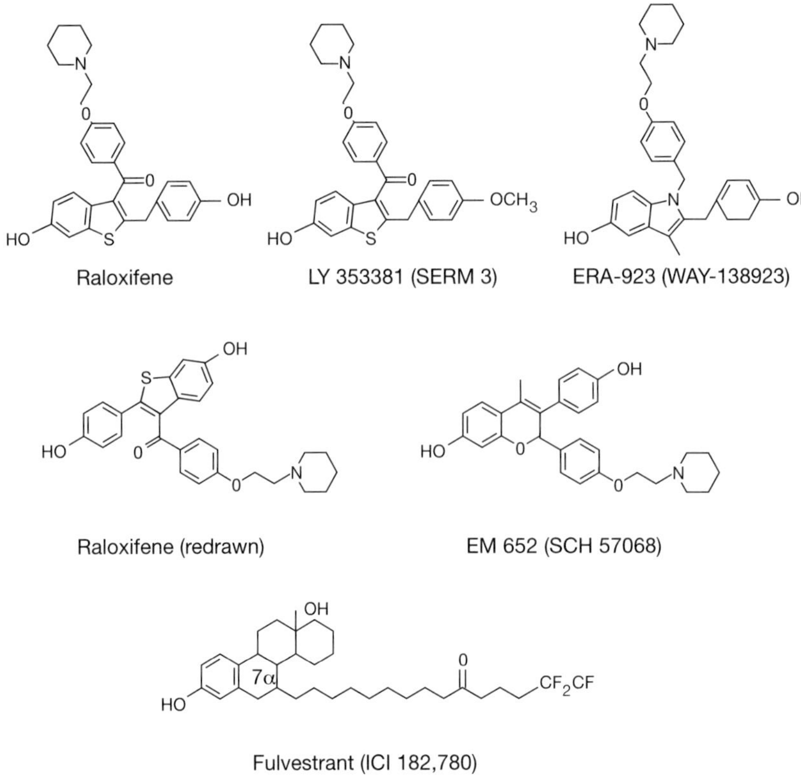

**Figure 19.2** Second- and third-generation selective oestrogen receptor modulators, based primarily on the benzothiophene structure of raloxifene. Fulvestrant is a steroidal anti-oestrogen devoid of agonist effects.

specific, and did not appear to manifest itself as any improved efficacy in treating or preventing tamoxifen resistance in patients with breast cancer. In contrast, fulvestrant acts by down-regulating ER expression (Dauvois *et al.* 1993), and this may explain why the drug appears to have much better activity in tamoxifen-resistant breast cancer than the tamoxifen-like SERMs (Howell *et al.* 1995), with efficacy similar to the non-steroidal anti-oestrogen anastrozole (Osborne *et al.* 2002; Howell *et al.* 2002).

As first-line therapy, the combined phase II/III clinical trial data for tamoxifen-like SERMs (toremiphene, droloxifene, idoxifene) suggest a median response rate of 31% (range 20–68%), with a median time to disease progression of 6.9 months (Table 19.1). In the randomised first-line trials in hormone-sensitive advanced breast cancer, both toremifene and idoxifene were shown to be very similar to tamoxifen in terms of both clinical efficacy and toxicity, whereas droloxifene appeared to be inferior (reviewed in Johnston 2001). The toxicity profile was the same, including gynaecological effects seen with idoxifene. On the basis of these current data, therefore, it is unlikely that the first-generation triphenylethylene SERMs will replace tamoxifen for advanced breast cancer as they have failed to show superiority or any significant clinical advantage in terms of tolerability and toxicity.

**Table 19.1** Efficacy of tamoxifen-like SERMs in advanced breast cancer

|  | *Tam resistant ORR (SD)* | *1st line Phase III (*II) ORR (median TTP)* |
| --- | --- | --- |
| Toremifene | 0–14% (16–30%) | 21–38% (4.9–11.9 mo) |
| Droloxifene | 15% (19%) | *30–51% (5.6–8.3 mo) |
| Idoxifene | 9% (9%) | 20% (6.5 mo) |
| Median | 5% (18%) | 31% (6.9 mo) |

Greater optimism has surrounded the profile of 'fixed ring' SERMs (Figure 19.2), in particular that this may translate into an improved clinical benefit for breast cancer patients. Much of the initial enthusiasm related to the fact that these drugs appeared devoid of any agonist activity in the endometrium, while appearing to be potent anti-oestrogens in the breast, which retained agonist activity in bone. The development of the lead benzothiophene compound raloxifene has been in osteoporosis, with the potential for this drug to prevent breast cancer (Cummings *et al.* 1999). These new compounds in pre-clinical models appear to offer a greater increase in potency and tumour growth inhibition, together with an improved SERM profile on other tissues, in comparison with the tamoxifen-like SERMs. However, there are too few clinical data to know whether these potential advantages will translate into beneficial effects for breast cancer patients. However, in tamoxifen-resistant patients, the level of activity reported for raloxifene (Gradishar *et al.* 1997), arzoxifene (Buzdar *et al.* 2003), and EM-800 (Labri *et al.* 1997) are all low, with a median response rate of 6.5%, which is very similar to that observed with the tamoxifen-like SERMs (Table 19.2). It is probable that activity in first-line will be similar to tamoxifen, and the only phase II data with raloxifene and arzoxifene give a median response rate of 30% with a median time to progression of 9.4 months (Table 19.2). Large-scale randomised trials versus tamoxifen with arzoxifene were abandonded when the drug proved no better.

**Table 19.2** Efficacy of 2nd/3rd generation SERMs in advanced breast cancer

|  | *Tam resistant ORR (SD)* | *1st line Phase III ORR (median TTP)* |
| --- | --- | --- |
| Raloxifene | 0% (–) | 19% |
| Arzoxifene | 3–10% (3–7%) | 30–36% (8.3–10.4 mo) |
| EM-800 | 14% (23%) | – |
| Median | 6.5% (7%) | 30% (9.4 mo) |

## Future role for selective oestrogen receptor modulators

It is unclear where or whether any further progress with SERMs will be made in the treatment of breast cancer. The failure of the pre-clinical promise to be translated into substantial differentiation from tamoxifen in the clinical trials reported above has been disappointing. At the same time, tamoxifen's pre-eminent position in the first-line management of breast cancer has been surpassed by the enhanced efficacy seen with the new third-generation aromatase inhibitors. Whether SERMs would have any efficacy in breast cancer after failure of aromatase inhibitors is unclear. Concerns have been raised that in cells resistant to long-term oestrogen deprivation, ER expression is enhanced and super-sensitised such that the agonist effects of SERMs (however minimal) may become enhanced resulting in SERM-stimulated breast cancer growth. To that end, greater emphasis has been put on developing the selective oestrogen receptor downregulator (SERD) fulvestrant, and preliminary clinical data have shown encouraging activity in the post-aromatase inhibitor setting (Perey *et al.* 2002; Steger *et al.* 2003). The other clinical arena in which SERMs could be developed is the adjuvant or prevention setting, where the protective effects on bone may be beneficial compared with long-term aromatase inhibitor therapy. However, the lack of convincing improvement over tamoxifen so far would make drug development in this area with the existing SERMs both risky and challenging.

## Signal transduction inhibitors: targeted therapies for the future

Whereas there is little clinical evidence to suggest that in advanced breast cancer substantial improvements in efficacy will be made over tamoxifen with any novel anti-oestrogens or SERMs, the major clinical issue that remains is the emergence of endocrine resistance. Our understanding of the mechanisms involved has revealed that various growth factor pathways and oncogenes in the signal transduction cascades become activated and used by cells to bypass normal endocrine responsiveness. As such, these represent attractive targets for pharmacological intervention with drugs which may inhibit the function of an aberrantly or excessively expressed oncogene products. Figure 19.3 illustrates the several different signal transduction pathways from the external growth factor receptors (discussed above) that operate through to the cell nucleus and ultimately may influence both the cell cycle and transcription of genes involved in cell proliferation. In breast cancers that become resistant to endocrine therapy, oestrogen receptor signalling still plays a crucial role in many tumours. However, evidence has started to emerge that the various signalling pathways 'cross-talk' at several levels with the ER pathway, and that this interaction becomes the dominant pathway when tumours become resistant to endocrine therapy (Nicholson & Gee 2000). At present, the emphasis in drug development has focused on antibodies to growth factor receptors, tyrosine kinase inhbitors, farnesyl transferase inhibitors, and drugs that target the cell cycle.

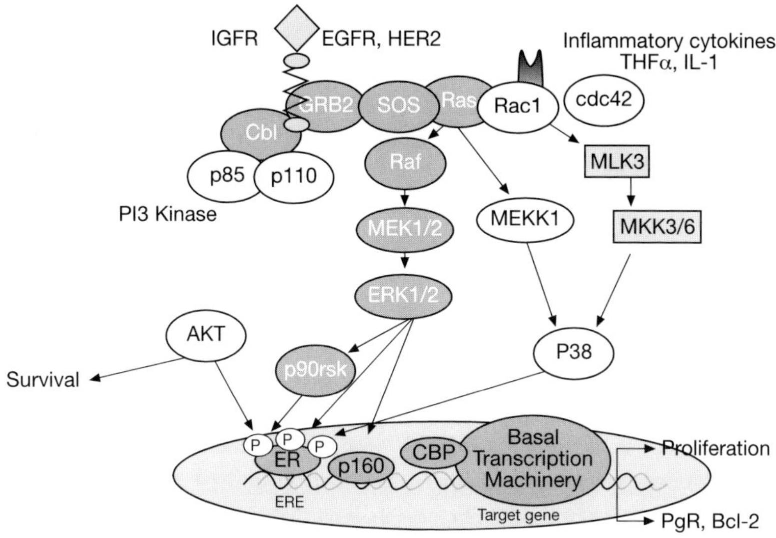


**Figure 19.3** A current understanding of the important signal transduction pathways that operate in breast cancer cells and how these cross-talk with the oestrogen receptor pathway.

## Antibodies to growth factor receptors

Among the first oncogenes to be identified in human breast cancer were the transmembrane growth factor receptors, which include epidermal growth factor receptor (EGFR) and c-erbB2 (or HER2). HER2 gene amplification occurs in 25–30% of tumours and contributes to malignant transformation and breast cancer growth (Slamon *et al.* 1987). Recently, there has been considerable interest about the role of trastuzumab (Herceptin), a humanised monoclonal antibody directed against HER2 (see Chapter 17). Tumours that are HER2 positive are thought to be resistant to both endocrine and conventional chemotherapies, and Herceptin given either alone or in conjunction with conventional therapy offers an opportunity to modulate aberrant growth factor activity in patients with resistant disease. In patients with HER2-positive tumours, Herceptin administered as a weekly intravenous infusion produced response rates of up to 35% as first-line therapy for metastatic breast cancer (Vogel *et al.* 2002). In a randomised phase III trial in 469 women with HER-2-positive metastatic breast cancer (Slamon *et al.* 2001), the addition of Herceptin to taxane or anthracycline-based chemotherapy significantly enhanced both response rates (50% versus 32%, $p < 0.001$) and time to disease progression (median 7.4 versus 4.6 months, $p < 0.001$), which in turn significantly improved overall survival (median 25 versus 20 months, $p < 0.046$). As such, this represents this first example of a targeted biological therapy for advanced breast cancer successfully entering the clinic.

Several large-scale adjuvant trials in women with HER2-positive breast cancer are now underway to establish whether Herceptin can further improve survival after early breast cancer.

Likewise, over-expression of EGFR is common in several epithelial tumours and occurs in 15–20% of breast cancers. Mouse-human chimeric monoclonal antibodies such as C225 (cetuximab) inhibit EGFR activity and may also enhance the sensitivity to other treatment modalities such as radiotherapy and chemotherapy (Baselga *et al.* 2000). So far, however, clinical development of cetuximab has predominantly been in squamous cell carcinomas of lung or head and neck.

## Tyrosine kinase inhibitors

When growth factor receptors are bound by their natural ligand they undergo dimerisation, which activates their tyrosine kinase activity located on the cytosolic side, which in turn phosphorylates the next set of proteins involved in the signal transduction cascade. Small molecules such as imatinib (Glivec) which target internal tyrosine kinase activity, in particular that associated with the *bcr–abl* oncogene, have been approved for chronic myeloid leukaemia and gastrointestinal stromal tumours based on clear evidence of enhanced clinical activity, with the added advantage of an oral based therapy with minimal toxicity (Druker *et al.* 2001).

Several inhibitors of EGFR tyrosine kinase are in development (Table 19.3), including gefitinib (Iressa), an orally active low molecular mass synthetic anilinoquinazoline, which is a potent and selective inhibitor of EGFR-TK. In experimental models, including human breast cancer cells, Iressa given as a single agent induced a dose-dependent anti-proliferative effect which delayed tumour growth (Ciardiello *et al.* 2000). The effect appears to be cytostatic, as after drug withdrawal tumour growth continued. Additional pre-clinical studies suggested that when given in combination of several different cytotoxic drugs including taxanes and anthracyclines, Iressa enhanced their antitumour activity (Sirotnak *et al.* 2000). This interaction did not always appear to be dependent on over-expression of EGFR, and the mechanism of any enhanced cytotoxic effect with chemotherapy remains unclear. In models of human non-invasive breast cancer (DCIS) implanted in athymic mice, many tumours that are ER negative have been shown to be dependent on EGFR over-expression for their growth, and in this model Iressa was found to be an effective inhibitor of cell proliferation (Bundred *et al.* 2001). Recent evidence also suggested that peptide growth factor receptors such as EGFR or HER2 become up-regulated or activated in endocrine-resistant breast cancer (Jang *et al.* 2000; McClelland *et al.* 2001), and experiments demonstrated that an EGFR-TK inhibitor such as Iressa may treat, or perhaps even prevent, endocrine resistance in breast cancer cells (Knowlden *et al.* 2003).

Based on the scientific rationale outlined above, several phase II clinical trials were undertaken in breast cancer with EGFR tyrosine kinase inhibitors (Albain *et al.*

**Table 19.3** EGFR/HER2 tyrosine kinase inhibitors

| Compound | Source | EGFR $IC_{50}$ (µM) | HER2 $IC_{50}$ (µM) | Clin. Devt. Br Cancer |
|---|---|---|---|---|
| *EGFR TK Inhibitor* | | | | |
| ZD-1839 | AstraZeneca | 0.023 | 3.7 | Phs II |
| OSI-774 | Roche | 0.02 | 0.4 | Phs II |
| EKB-569 | Wyeth | 0.039 | 1.3 | Phs I |
| | | | | |
| *Dual Inhibitor* | | | | |
| PKI-166 | Novartis | 0.025 | 0.1 | Phs I |
| GW-572016 | GSK | 0.01 | 0.009 | Phs II |
| | | | | |
| *Pan-erbB Inhibitor* | | | | |
| CI-1033 | Pfizer | 0.001 | 0.009 | Phs II |

2002; Winer *et al.* 2002; Baslega *et al.* 2003; Robertson *et al.* 2003;). The results so far from the four separate trials are summarised in Table 19.4. There was no selection on the basis of EGFR or HER2 expression in these trials, and in several studies patients had been heavily pre-treated with other therapies. Overall, the data are relatively disappointing, with low clinical response rates. The only trial to report a significant number of response included patients with ER-positive tamoxifen-resistant breast cancer, the scenario in which pre-clinical models had shown evidence of activity for gefitinib (Knowlden *et al.* 2003). More work needs to be done to establish tumour phenotypes in responding versus non-responding patients. For example, recent evidence suggests that over-expression of the PI-3 kinase/Akt pathway may play an important role in resistance to tyrosine-kinase inhibitor therapy (Jin *et al.* 2003). Ultimately combinations of different signal transduction inhibitors may prove a more effective strategy.

**Table 19.4** Clinical trials of EGFR TKIs in breast cancer

| Phase II studies | No pts | ORR | CBR | TTP |
|---|---|---|---|---|
| Robertson (ASCO 2003) | 33 | 7% | 30% | ? |
| Baselga (ASCO 2003) | 32 | 0% | 6% | 8 wk |
| Albain (San Antonio 2002) | 63 | 2% | 5% | 8 wk |
| Winer (ASCO 2002) | 69 | 3% | 6% | 6 wk |

Challenges for Clinical Development:
- selection & predictors of response (EGFR expression; pAKT)
- use earlier in natural history of disease
- hormone-resistant (modest Rx) vs. sensitive disease (minimal Rx)
- better rationale for combination Rx

## Farnesyl transferase inhibitors

A key component of the signal transduction pathway is the ras protein, which becomes attached to the inner plasma membrane, thus providing a link between activated transmembrane growth factors and downstream intra-cellular kinases which ultimately trigger cell growth (Figure 19.3). The rate-limiting processing event of the ras protein involves attachment to the inner membrane by addition of a 15-carbon isoprenoid (lipid) moiety called farnesyl. Thus ras functions as a relay switch whose activity is dependent upon the enzyme farnesyl transferase. Specific inhibitors of farnseyl transferase (FTIs) were initially developed to prevent the post-translational processing of ras, thereby inhibiting cell growth.

Breast carcinomas are known to contain a very low frequency of *Ras* mutations (less than 2%), although aberrant function of the *Ras* signal transduction pathway is thought to be common in human breast cancer because of permanent upstream growth factor activation (Clark & Der 1995). Hormone-sensitive ER-positive MCF-7 breast cancer xenografts established in athymic mice are growth inhibited with increasing oral doses of the farnesyl transferase inhibitor R115777, with inhibition of cell proliferation, induction of apoptosis and enhanced expression of the cyclin-dependent kinase inhibitor p21 (Kelland *et al.* 2001). A phase II clinical study of R115777 in 76 women with advanced breast cancer demonstrated clinical activity for an FTI, including partial responses and prolonged stable disease seen in sites of visceral and soft tissue disease in 25% of patients (Johnston *et al.* 2003). The drug was well tolerated, although dose-related myelosuppression was the most frequent drug-related toxicity. Because of pre-clinical data suggesting synergy with endocrine therapy (Johnston *et al.* 2002), studies are now examining how FTIs can be combined with aromatase inhibitors in breast cancer patients previously treated with tamoxifen.

## Cell cycle inhibitors

Cyclins are downstream proteins expressed at different points in the cell cycle which regulate the progression of cells through various checkpoints. Cyclin activity is regulated by cyclin-dependent kinases (CDKs), which form various protein–protein complexes; these in turn are regulated by small proteins known as cyclin-dependent kinase inhibitors (CDKIs). Many of the latter have been considered tumour suppressor genes which if lost may contribute to uncontrolled progression through the cell cycle (i.e. loss of p16 in melanoma). Equally, therapeutic strategies have been conceived to abrogate cell cycle checkpoints, in particular by developing pharmacological inhibitors of CDKs. Two compounds (flavopiridol and 7-hydroxys-taurosporine, or UCN-01) derived from microbial and plant sources have CDKI activity, and have shown anti-tumour activity in various pre-clinical models including breast cancer and entered early clinical development (Sampath & Plunkett 2001; Senderowicz & Sausville 2000).

Other signalling pathways important in breast cancer include the insulin-like growth factor pathway, which activates phosphatidylinositol 3×-kinase (PI3K), a family of lipid kinases that phosphorylate second messenger phosphoinositides and contribute to cell survival through suppression of apoptosis (Figure 19.3). In addition, activation of PI3K by Akt activates mTOR (the mammalian target of rapamycin), which in turn facilitates progression through the cell cycle by enhancing synthesis and stabilising several cell-cycle proteins including cyclin D1 and c-myc. The rapamycin ester CCI-779 targets mTOR function and has been found to inhibit proliferation of a panel of breast cancer cell lines, including those that were either oestrogen dependent or over-expressed HER-2 (Yu *et al.* 2001). There was good correlation between activation of the Akt pathway, including loss of the regulatory PTEN tumour suppressor gene, and sensitivity to CCI-779 in breast cancer models, and a phase II clinical trial in advanced breast cancer with CCI-779 has shown evidence of clinical activity (Chan *et al.* 2003).

## Conclusions: integration of novel therapies into clinical practice

Over the past 5 years the development of future systemic treatments for breast cancer has focused on improving current endocrine therapies, and exploiting novel information about biological pathways involved in breast cancer cell growth. To a large extent the various SERMs have been eclipsed by the success of the aromatase inhibitors that have now become the standard of care in post-menopausal breast cancer, and may indeed replace tamoxifen in the adjuvant setting. There may remain a niche for a potent selective anti-oestrogen that retains a protective effect on bone and lacks any agonist effect on endometrium, but its development in an adjuvant or preventive setting will be extremely difficult in the absence of clear superiority over tamoxifen. Much greater hope lies with the SERD fulvestrant, but once again it may have to re-define its role in the setting following prior aromatase inhibitors.

Unlike conventional cytotoxic chemotherapy used in routine clinical practice, many of the new STI therapies represent non-cytotoxic modulators that target specific identified molecular abnormalities associated with malignancy. As one of the major limitations of conventional endocrine and chemotherapy in metastatic disease is the emergence of drug resistance, these therapies offer a novel approach that in some situations may circumvent resistance to conventional therapies. Another opportunity for these STIs may be in the setting of minimal residual disease, where some trials are examining maintenance therapy after chemotherapy-induced remission so as to prolong time to disease progression. As each of these STIs evolves towards the clinic, the challenge to oncologists will be whether their potential to selectively target molecular abnormalities in breast cancer cells can be matched by further substantial improvements in clinical outcome. In particular, the design of clinical trials will need to assess pharmaco-dynamic endpoints to establish the optimal dose and schedule, remembering that the biologically effective dose may be substantially less than the maximally tolerated dose. There is a need to be aware that clinical activity as monotherapy in early phase II studies may be relatively modest, but that effective combinations with existing therapies and also between different signal transduction inhibitors may be a more effective strategy. Ultimately, if these novel approaches are effective, their use in the adjuvant setting could offer further incremental improvements in survival from breast cancer.

## References


Albain, K., Elledge, R., Gradishar, W. *et al.* (2002). Open-label phase II multicenter trial of ZD1839 (Iressa) in patients with advanced breast cancer. *Breast Cancer Research and Treatment* **76**, A20.

Baselga, J., Pfister, D., Cooper, M. R. *et al.* (2000). Phase I studies of anti-epidermal growth factor receptor chimeric antibody C225 alone and in combination with cisplatin. *Journal of Clinical Oncology* **18**, 904–914.

Baslega, J., Albanelli, J., Ruiz, A. *et al.* (2003). Phase II and tumor pharmacodynamic study of gefitinib in patients with advanced breast cancer. *Proceedings of the American Society of Clinical Oncology* **22**, A24.

Bundred, N. J., Chan, K. & Anderson, N. G. (2001). Studies of epidermal growth factor inhibition in breast cancer. *Endocrine-Related Cancer* **8**, 183–189.

Buzdar, A., O'Shaughnessy, J. & Booser, D. J. (2003). Phase II randomised double-blind study of two dose levels of arzoxifene in patients with locally advanced or metastatic breast cancer. *Journal of Clinical Oncology* **21**, 1007–1014.

Chan, S., Scheulen, M. E., Johnston, S. R. D. *et al.* (2003). A phase II study of two dose levels of CCI-779 in locally advanced or metastatic breast cancer failing prior anthracyclines and/or taxanes regimens. *Proceedings of the American Society of Clinical Oncology* **22**, A774.

Ciardiello, F., Caputo, R., Bianco, R. *et al.* (2000). Antitumor effect and potentiation of cytotoxic drugs activity in human cancer cells by ZD1839 (Iressa), an epidermal growth factor receptor-selective tyrosine kinase inhibitor. *Clinical Cancer Research* **6**, 2053–2063.

Clark, G. J. & Der, C. J. (1995). Aberrant function of the Ras signal transduction pathway in human breast cancer. *Breast Cancer Research and Treatment* **35**, 133–144.

Cummings, S. R., Eckert, S. *et al.* (1999). The effect of raloxifene on risk of breast cancer in postmenopausal women: results from the Multiple Outcomes of Raloxifene Evaluation (MORE) randomised trial. *Journal of the American Medical Association* **281**, 2189–2197.

Dauvois, S., White, R. & Parker, M. G. (1993). The anti-estrogen ICI 182780 disrupts estrogen receptor nucleocytoplasmic shuttling. *Journal of Cell Science* **106**, 1377–1388.

Druker, B. J., Talpaz, M., Resta, D. *et al.* (2001). Efficacy and safety of a specific inhibitor of the BCR-abl tyrosine kinase in chronic myeloid leukaemia. *New England Journal of Medicine* **344**, 1031–1037.

Early Breast Cancer Trialists Collaborative Group (1998). Tamoxifen for early breast cancer; an overview of the randomised trials. *The Lancet* **351**, 1451–1467.

Fisher, B., Costantino, J. P., Redmond, C. K., Fisher, E. R., Wickerham, D. L., Cronin, W. M. *et al.* (1994). Endometrial cancer in tamoxifen-treated breast cancer patients: findings from the NSABP B-14. *Journal of the National Cancer Institute* **86**, 527–537.

Gradishar, W. J., Glusman, J. E., Vogel, C. L. *et al.* (1997). Raloxifene HCL, a new endocrine agent, is active in estrogen receptor positive (ER+) metastatic breast cancer. *Breast Cancer Research and Treatment* **46**, 53 (A209).

Howell, A., DeFriend, D. *et al.* (1995). Response to a specific antiestrogen (ICI182,780) in tamoxifen-resistant breast cancer. *The Lancet* **345**, 29–30.

Howell, A., Robertson, J. R. F., Albano, J. Q. *et al.* (2002). Fulvestrant, formerly ICI 182,780, is as effective as anastrozole in postmenopausal women with advanced breast cancer progressing after prior endocrine treatment. *Journal of Clinical Oncology* **20**, 3396–3403.

Jeng, M.-H., Yue, W., Eischied, A. *et al.* (2000). Role of MAP kinase in the enhanced cell proliferation of long-term estrogen deprived human breast cancer cells. *Breast Cancer Research and Treatment* **62**, 167–175.

Jin, W., Wu, L., Liang, K., Liu, B., Lu, Y. & Fan, Z. (2003). Roles of the PI-3K and MEK pathways in Ras-mediated chemoresistance in breast cancer cells. *British Journal of Cancer* **89**, 185–191.

Johnston, S. R. D. (1997). Acquired tamoxifen resistance in human breast cancer; potential mechanisms and clinical implications. *Anticancer Drugs* **8**, 911–930.

Johnston, S. R. D., Riddler, S., Haynes, B. P. *et al.* (1997). The novel antioestrogen idoxifene inhibits the growth of human MCF-7 breast cancer xenografts and reduces the frequency of acquired antiestrogen resistance. *British Journal of Cancer* **75**, 804–809.

Johnston, S. R. D. (2001) Endocrine manipulation in advanced breast cancer; recent advances with SERM therapies. *Clinical Cancer Research* **7**, 4376–4387.

Johnston, S. R. D., Head, J., Valenti, M., Detre, S. & Dowsett, M. (2002). Endocrine therapy combined with the farnesyltransferase inhibitor R115777 produces enhanced tumour growth inhibition in hormone-sensitive MCF-7 human breast cancer xenografts in-vivo. *Breast Cancer Research and Treatment* **76**, A245.

Johnston, S. R. D., Hickish, T., Ellis, P. A. *et al.* (2003). Phase II study of the efficacy and tolerability of two dosing regimens of the farnesyltransferase inhibitor R115777 (Zarnestra) in patients with advanced breast cancer. *Journal of Clinical Oncology* **21**, 2492–2499.

Kelland, L. R., Smith, V., Valenti, M. *et al.* (2001) Preclinical antitumor activity and pharmacodynamic studies with the farnesyl protein transferase inhbitor R115777 in human breast cancer. *Clinical Cancer Research* **7**, 3554–3550.

Knowlden, J. M., Hutcheson, I. R., Jones, H. E. *et al.* (2003). Elevated levels of epidermal growth factor receptor cerbB2 heterodimers mediate an autocrine growth regulatory pathways in tamoxifen-resistant MCF-7 cells. *Endocrinology* **144**, 1032–1044.

Labrie, F., Champagne, P., Labrie, C., Belanger, A., Roy, J., Laverdiere, J. *et al.* (1997). Response to the orally active specific antiestrogen EM-800 (SCH-57070) in tamoxifen-resistant breast cancer. *Breast Cancer Research and Treatment* **46**, 53 (A211).

Love, R. R., Mazess, R. B., Barden, H. S., Epstein, S., Newcomb, P. A., Jordan, V. C., Carbone, P. P. & DeMets, D. L. (1992). Effects of tamoxifen on bone mineral density in postmenopausal women with breast cancer. *New England Journal of Medicine* **326**, 852–856.

Love, R. R., Wiebe, D. A., Newcomb, P. A., Cameron, L., Leventhal, H., Jordan, V. C., Feyzi, J. & DeMets, D. L. (1991). Effects of tamoxifen on cardiovascular risk factors in postmenopausal women. *Annals of Internal Medicine* **115**, 860–864.

McClelland, R. A., Barrow, D., Madden, T. A. *et al.* (2001). Enhanced epidermal growth factor receptor signaling in MCF7 breast cancer cells after long-term culture in the presence of the pure antiestrogen ICI 182,780 (Faslodex). *Endocrinology* **142**, 2776–2788.

Nicholson, R. I. & Gee, J. M. (2000). Oestrogen and growth factor cross-talk and endocrine insensitivity and acquired resistance in breast cancer. *British Journal of Cancer* **82**, 501–513.

Osborne, C. K., Coronado–Heinsohn, E. B., Hilsenbeck, S. G. *et al.* (1995). Comparison of the effects of a pure steroidal antioestrogen with those of tamoxifen in a model of human breast cancer. *Journal of the National Cancer Institute* **87**, 746–750.

Osborne, C. K., Pippen, J., Jones, S. E. *et al.* (2002). Double-blind, randomised trial comparing the efficacy and tolerability of fulvestrant versus anastrozole in postmenopausal women with advanced breast cancer progressing on prior endocrine therapy: results of a North American trial. *Journal of Clinical Oncology* **20**, 3386–3395.

Perey, L., Thurlimann, B., Hawle, H. *et al* (2002). Fulvestrant (Faslodex) as hormonal treatment in postmenopausal patients with advanced breast cancer progressing after treatment with tamoxifen and aromatase inhibitors: an ongoing phase II SAAK trial. *European Journal of Cancer* **38**, S98 223.

Robertson, J. F. R., Gutteridge, L., Cheung, K. L. *et al.* (2003). Gefitinib (ZD1839) is active in acquired tamoxifen-resistant oestrogen receptor positive and ER-negative breast cancer: results from a phase II study. *Proceedings of the American Society of Clinical Oncology* **22**, A23.

Sampath, D. & Plunkett, W. (2001). Design of new anticancer therapies targeting cell cycle checkpoint pathways. *Current Opinion in Oncology* **13**, 484–490.

Senderowicz, A. M. & Sausville, E. A. (2000). Preclinical and clinical development of cyclin-dependent kinase modulators. *Journal of the National Cancer Institute* **92**, 376–387.

Sirotnak, F. M., Zakowski, M. F., Miller, V. A. *et al.* (2000). Efficacy of cytotoxic agents against human tumor xenografts is markedly enhanced by co-administration of ZD1839 (Iressa), an inhibitor of EGFR tyrosine kinase. *Clinical Cancer Research* **6**, 4885–4892.

Slamon, D. J., Clark, G. M., Wong, S. G. *et al.* (1987). Human breast cancer: correlation of relapse and survival with amplification of the HER-2/neu oncogene. *Science* **235**, 177–182.

Slamon, D., Leyland-Jones, B., Shak, S. *et al.* (2001). Use of chemotherapy plus a monoclonal antibody against HER-2 for metastatic breast cancer that overexpresses HER2. *New England Journal of Medicine* **344**, 783–792.

Smith, I. E. (2001). Future directions in the adjuvant treatment of breast cancer: the role of trastuzumab. *Annals of Oncology* **12**, S75–S79.

Steger, G. C., Bartsch, R., Wenzel, C. *et al.* (2003). Fulvestrant beyond the second hormonal treatment in metastatic breast cancer. *Proceedings of the American Society of Clinical Oncology* **22**, 20 (A78).

Vogel, C., Cobleigh, M. A., Tripathy, D. *et al.* (2002). Efficay and safety of trastuzumab as a single agent in first-line treatment of HER2-overexpressing metastatic breast cancer. *Journal of Clinical Oncology* **20**, 719–726.

Winer, E., Cobleigh M., Dickler, M. *et al.* (2002). Phase II multicenter study to evaluate the efficacy and safety of Tarceva (erlotinib, OSI-774) in women with previously treated locally advanced or metastatic breast cancer. *Breast Cancer Research and Treatment* **76**, A445.

Yu, K., Toral-Barza, L., Discafani, C. *et al.* (2001). mTOR, a novel target in breast cancer: the effect of CCI-779, an mTOR inhibitor, in preclinical models of breast cancer. *Endocrine-Related Cancer* **8**, 249–258.

# Chapter 20

# Bisphosphonate treatment for the prevention and management of bone metastases

*Robert Coleman*

## Introduction

Advanced cancers frequently metastasise to the bone, and the resulting bone destruction is associated with a variety of skeletal complications, including pathologic fractures, bone pain, impaired mobility, spinal cord compression, and hypercalcaemia. It is estimated that more than 1.5 million cancer patients worldwide have bone metastases. Current treatment options for patients with bone metastases include radiation therapy, surgery, bisphosphonates and analgesics, in addition to standard anti-cancer therapy. The primary goal of therapy is to minimise bone pain and morbidity and improve mobility and quality of life.

Bone is not an inert organ. Throughout adult life, normal bone undergoes a continuous remodelling process of resorption and formation. This is normally a tightly coordinated process in which initial osteoclast resorption takes place in discrete 'packets', known as bone remodelling units, over a period of about 8 days. This is followed by a more prolonged phase of bone formation over about 3 months and mediated by osteoblasts to repair the defect. There is normally a fine balance between bone formation and bone resorption, so that the total amount of bone tends to remain fairly constant.

There are many factors involved in the regulation of bone resorption, including signalling molecules that enhance or inhibit proliferation of osteoclast progenitors. Of these, osteoprotogerin (OPG) (Kong *et al.* 1999) is a natural inhibitor of osteoclast production and activity and is a member of the tumour necrosis factor superfamily. Recent studies on OPG and its binding to RANK (osteoclast differentiation factor) ligand have led to the possibility of new therapeutic agents, based on OPG, which are able to inhibit cancer-induced bone destruction (Body *et al.* 2003). Hormonal effects also play a role, and in women oestrogen is of key importance, a fact that is highlighted by the accelerated rate of bone loss around the menopause, that corresponds to the decrease in oestrogen levels.

Recent research has increased our understanding of the development of bone metastases as well as the continual interaction between cancer cells and active bone (Roodman 2003). Tumour cells in the bone marrow cavity secrete a variety of paracrine factors that stimulate bone cell activity, including parathyroid hormone related protein, interleukin-6 and endothelin-1. Stimulation of osteoclast function is of key importance resulting in osteolysis. Overall, there is a disruption of the normal coupling signals between osteoblast and osteoclast function.

## Treatment of bone metastases

In recent years, the opportunities for improving the management of metastatic bone disease have increased steadily. These include improvements in reconstructive orthopaedic surgery, the development of bone-seeking radiopharmaceuticals, new endocrine and cytotoxic treatments, and in particular the development of bisphosphonates to prevent and treat skeletal complications.

All bisphosphonates are characterised by a P–C–P containing central structure, which promotes their binding to the mineralised bone matrix, and a variable side chain which determines the relative potency and side effects. After administration, bisphosphonates bind avidly to exposed bone mineral around resorbing osteoclasts leading to very high local concentrations of bisphosphonate in the resorption lacunae (up to 1000 μM). On release from the bone surface, bisphosphonates are internalised by the osteoclast, where they cause disruption of the biochemical processes involved in bone resorption (Rogers *et al.* 1997).

Bisphosphonates also cause osteoclast apoptosis, with the appearance of distinctive changes in cell and nuclear morphology (Hughes *et al.* 1995). Although the molecular targets responsible for promoting this apoptosis are unknown, the bisphosphonates have recently been shown to inhibit enzymes of the mevalonate pathway (Luckman *et al.* 1998) which are ultimately responsible for events that lead to the post-translational modification of GTP-binding proteins such as Ras and Rho. Recent studies also suggest that bisphosphonates may have direct apoptotic effects on tumour cells (Neville-Webbe *et al.* 2002).

### Bisphosphonates for hypercalcaemia of malignancy

Hypercalcaemia is the most common metabolic complication of malignancy producing many unpleasant gastrointestinal and neurological symptoms. Focal osteolysis by tumour cells, generalised osteolysis by humoral factors secreted by the tumour, increased renal tubular reabsorption of calcium and impaired renal glomerular function may all contribute to the pathophysiology. Intravenous bisphosphonates, in conjunction with rehydration, are now established as the treatment of choice for hypercalcaemia. Seventy to ninety per cent of patients will achieve normocalcaemia resulting in relief of symptoms and improved quality of life (Coleman 1998). Zoledronic acid is the most effective bisphosphonate for the acute treatment of this metabolic emergency (Major *et al.* 2001).

### Bisphosphonates for bone pain

Radiotherapy remains the treatment of choice for localised bone pain but many patients have widespread poorly localised, non-mechanical bone pain, while others will experience recurrence of pain in previously irradiated skeletal sites. The bisphosphonates provide an alternative treatment approach to the management of these patients with clinically meaningful pain improvement in around 50% of patients. To obtain optimal effects, the intravenous route is necessary, at least until more potent and well tolerated oral bisphosphonates have been developed, as it has not been convincingly demonstrated that any of the currently available oral bisphosphonates, in the absence of systemic anti-cancer treatment, can significantly reduce metastatic bone pain.

The effect of bisphosphonates on pain seems to be independent of the nature of the underlying tumour or radiographic appearance of the metastases, with sclerotic lesions responding similarly to lytic metastases. Additionally, there appears to be an important link between metastatic bone pain and the rate of bone resorption, with subjective response correlating with biochemical response (Vinholes *et al.* 1996, 1997).

## Bisphosphonates to prevent skeletal related events

In 1983, a small study from Elomaa and colleagues reported that oral clodronate could inhibit ostoclastic activity, and that this resulted in symptomatic improvement in patients with metastatic breast cancer ((Elomaa *et al.* 1983). This study stimulated other investigators, particularly in Europe, to evaluate either regular intravenous infusions of pamidronate, enteric coated oral pamidronate, or either oral or parenteral clodronate in advanced breast cancer (Body *et al.* 1998). In addition to the effects on bone pain, sclerosis of lytic lesions was seen in phase II studies of intravenous pamidronate in the absence of specific anti-cancer treatments while a reduction in skeletal morbidity was reported in the randomised studies of oral bisphosphonates (van Holten-Verzantvoort *et al.* 1987; Paterson *et al.* 1993).

Subsequently other randomised trials were performed (Table 20.1) (Theriault *et al.* 1999; Hortobagyi *et al.* 1996; Conte *et al.* 1996; Hultborn *et al.* 1996; Body *et al.* 2003), including in advanced breast cancer a study comparing chemotherapy plus intravenous pamidronate 45 mg every three weeks with chemotherapy alone (Conte *et al.* 1996). This study reported a 48% improvement in time to progression in bone (249 versus 168 days) in favour of combination therapy. Subsequently, large placebo-controlled studies were perfomed of endocrine therapy (Theriault *et al.* 1999) or chemotherapy (Hortobagyi *et al.* 1996) with and without pamidronate for metastatic bone disease in advanced breast cancer. In both studies pamidronate was given monthly at a dose of 90 mg by intravenous infusion. These trials showed that pamidronate significantly reduced skeletal morbidity in advanced breast cancer. Differences began to show after three months of treatment and were maintained for two years. In addition, in the pamidronate treated patients, quality of life was maintained and a reduction in pain and analgesic use observed in comparison to the placebo group. No significant overall effects on survival have yet been seen, although

**Table 20.1** Effects of bisphosphonates on skeletal morbidity: results of randomised trials

| Agent and Route | n | Results (Bisphosphonate versus placebo/control) | Reference |
|---|---|---|---|
| Pamidronate 600 mg (300 mg) p.o. versus placebo | 161 | Reduced SMR: 94 versus 52 events per 100 woman–years ($p < 0.01$); 600 mg poorly tolerated. No benefit with reduced dose (300 mg). | Van Holten *et al.* (1987) |
| Clodronate 1600 mg p.o. versus placebo | 173 | Reduced SMR: 305 versus 219 events per 100 woman–years ($p < 0.001$). | Paterson *et al.* (1993) |
| Pamidronate 45 mg i.v. versus control | 295 | Increased time to bone progression: 168 versus 249 days ($p = 0.02$). | Conte *et al.* (1996) |
| Pamidronate 90 mg i.v. versus placebo | 382 | Reduced proportion experiencing SRE: 65% versus 46% ($p < 0.001$) Delay in first SRE 7.0 months versus 13.1 ($p = 0.0005$). | Hortobagyi *et al.* (1996) |
| Pamidronate 60 mg i.v. versus control | 401 | Median time to skeletal progression: 9 versus 14 months ($p < 0.01$). | Hultborn *et al.* (1996) |
| Pamidronate 90 mg i.v. versus placebo | 374 | Reduced proportion experiencing SRE: 67% versus 56% ($p = 0.027$). Delay in first SRE 6.9 months versus 10.4 ($p = 0.049$). | Theriault *et al.* (1999) |
| Ibandronate 2/6 mg i.v.. versus placebo | 467 | Reduced SMR with 6 mg dose. 2 mg ineffective: SMR 2.18 versus 1.61 ($p = 0.03$). | Body *et al.* (1999) |

p.o., per oral; i.v., intravenous; SRE, skeletal-related event; SMR, skeletal morbidity rate.

unconfirmed and exploratory subgroup analyses have suggested that young patients (younger than 50 years) appear to gain a small survival advantage.

Zoledronic acid is the most potent bisphosphonate in clinical development and in in vitro systems has around 100–1000 times the potency of pamidronate. A phase I study in thirty patients with hypercalcaemia indicated dose levels as low as 0.02 mg/kg (1–2 mg total dose) were effective in achieving normocalcaemia (Body *et al.* 1999). In normocalcaemic patients receiving zoledronic acid, a dose dependent reduction in deoxypyridinoline, a specific marker of bone resorption was identified (Berenson *et al.* 2001a). These biochemical responses were at least as large as those previously reported after infusions of pamidronate 90 mg. Subsequently, a randomised double-blind, dose finding, phase II study of zoledronic acid tested doses of 0.5, 2 and 4 mg zoledronic acid given on a 4 weekly schedule. This study showed that 4 mg zoledronic acid was of similar efficacy to pamidronate (Berenson *et al.* 2001b).

More recently, a large international, multicentre, stratified, randomised double-blind, phase III trial of zoledronic acid compared with pamidronate in the treatment of malignant bone disease in patients with breast cancer has been completed (Rosen *et al.* 2001). The trial was designed as a non-inferiority trial in which the primary efficacy variable was the proportion of patients experiencing at least one skeletal-related event (SRE). Secondary efficacy variables included the time to first SRE, skeletal morbidity rate (SMR), and an Andersen-Gill multiple events analysis. The proportion of patients experiencing individual SREs, time to progression, response, performance status, analgesic and pain scores, and markers of bone resorption and formation were also assessed.

A total of 1,130 patients with advanced breast cancer, and at least one metastatic bone lesion, were randomised to receive either 4mg zoledronic acid or 8 mg zoledronic acid via a short intravenous infusion, or 90 mg pamidronate through a 2 hour infusion. Treatments were administered every three to four weeks. Initially zoledronic acid was administered as a 5 minute infusion in 50 ml of 0.9% saline or 5% dextrose. This was amended to 15 minute infusion in 100 ml of saline or dextrose due to concerns over renal toxicity. Similarly, the 8 mg dose of zoledronic acid was reduced to 4mg due to continuing concerns over renal safety. Due to this protocol change, statistical comparisons between the 8/4 mg zoledronic acid group and 4 mg zoledronic acid group or pamidronate group were dropped from the primary endpoint analyses.

An initial analysis of the first 13-months on study has been published (Rosen *et al.* 2001). Forty-four to forty-six per cent of patients experienced at least one SRE. This was similar across all three treatment groups. Differences that were seen included a reduction in radiotherapy requirements between the zoledronic acid 4mg and pamidronate groups (15% versus 20%; $p = 0.031$). This difference was most marked in the breast cancer patients receiving hormonal therapy (16% versus 25%; $p = 0.022$). More recently, the final 25 month data have become available (Rosen *et al.* 2003). These show superiority for zoledronic acid. Using the pre-planned Andersen-Gill multiple event analysis, a reduction of 20% in the risk of developing an SRE was observed (hazard ratio 0.799; $p = 0.025$; see Figure 20.1).

There were no significant differences between the groups in pain scores, analgesic use or performance status. Pain was reduced in all groups, and analgesic use was decreased or stabilised. There were no appreciable differences in the response of bone lesions to therapy or the time to progression between the study groups. All markers of bone resorption or formation decreased from baseline to the end-of-study. At all time points the urinary marker of bone resorption NTX was significantly less in the zoledronic acid 4 mg group compared to the pamidronate group (e.g. 64% versus 57% below baseline at the end of one year; $p = 0.015$). Median overall survival was similar at approximately 2 years in the study groups.

The most common adverse events were bone pain, nausea, fever and fatigue, and as with the other adverse effects, they occurred generally with a similar frequency in each group. The incidence of renal dysfunction with 4 mg zoledronic acid (given on the 15 minute schedule) was indistinguishable from pamidronate.

Ibandronate is another highly potent amino-bisphosphonate which is licensed in Europe for the treatment of hypercalcaemia of malignancy and the treatment of metastatic bone disease, and in development for the prevention and treatment of osteoporosis. A phase III placebo-controlled trial of monthly infusions in breast cancer has shown a significant reduction in skeletal related morbidity with ibandronate 4 mg (Body *et al.* 2003). Additionally, a film-coated tablet has been developed which has been shown to produce a dose dependent reduction, at doses which are generally well tolerated, in both urinary calcium and collagen crosslink

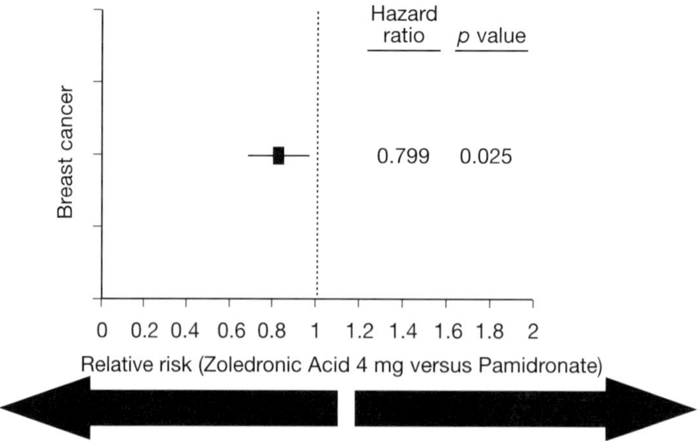


**Figure 20.1** Risk reduction for skeletal related events as determined by Andersen–Gill multiple event analysis (Andersen & Gill 1982). Point estimate (hazard ratio) and 95% confidence intervals displayed.

excretion (Coleman *et al.* 1999). Recent reports of phase III placebo-controlled trials of the oral formulation indicate that the oral ibandronate is active with a broadly similar impact on skeletal morbidity to that observed in earlier placebo controlled trials with other bisphosphonates (Body *et al.* 2004). The oral formulation has obvious attractions to both patients and health care providers but the place of ibandronate cannot be defined until comparative data with zoledronic acid are available.

## Monitoring skeletal health and assessment of response

Because of the increasing range of treatment options for metastatic bone disease, there is an increased requirement for practical and accurate methods for assessment of the response to therapy in bone. An ideal approach would be simple and non-invasive to perform, would report changes using a quantitative measure, and would be sufficiently sensitive so that an early assessment of response to treatment could be obtained. Although several methods for assessment are available, no single method in current use approaches this ideal.

For metastases in visceral and soft tissues, assessment of treatment response by measurement of tumour dimensions using imaging methods is relatively straightforward. However, in the case of bone metastases, this is much more difficult and controversial because of the length of time before response is detectable by imaging methods, as well as the difficulties in distinguishing between metastatic progression and bone healing in response to treatment. Although imaging methods are likely to remain central to the management of bone metastases, there is intensive current research into the possible role of bone markers in this context (Coleman 2002).

Recently, highly specific biochemical markers of bone metabolism have been developed and are increasingly used to predict outcome and monitor therapies for benign bone disease such as osteoporosis. These assays, based on the measurement of bone breakdown and formation products, are now relatively straightforward and convenient to perform. Data are emerging that suggest that bone markers may be useful in oncology and could be used to augment the imaging techniques currently used for diagnosis and assessment of response. For example, they could be used to identify patients at risk of developing skeletal complications, to aid in diagnosis of skeletal abnormalities, for assessment of response to systemic therapy, and to help define patients who may or may not benefit from bisphosphonate therapy (Coleman 2002).

Objective assessment of response in bone metastases from breast cancer takes up to 6 months using radiological techniques, and bone markers have been studied with the aim of providing an earlier indication of response. These markers include several unique breakdown products of type I collagen, including the pyridinium crosslinks pyridinoline (PYD) and deoxypyridinoline (DPD), and the peptide-bound crosslinks

N-telopeptide (NTX) and C-telopeptide (CTX). Both PYD and DPD crosslinks are specific to bone, and can be quantified in the urine using reverse-phase high-performance liquid chromatography (HPLC) and/or an enzyme-linked immunosorbent assay (ELISA). Their excretion relative to creatinine is only minimally affected by renal function, but does vary substantially throughout the day with a circadian rhythm, and from day to day. Therefore, samples must be taken at the same time each day, and collection of two samples on consecutive days is ideal to establish a reliable baseline value. The peptide-bound crosslinks NTX and CTX constitute the major fraction of crosslinks from collagen degradation in both the serum and the urine. Therefore, changes in bone metabolism result in greater changes in serum and urine concentrations of NTX and CTX compared with PYD and DPD. This is reflected in the greater decreases in NTX and CTX compared with PYD and DPD observed in response to bisphosphonate therapy (Brown & Coleman 2002).

Walls *et al.* (1999) studied the collagen crosslinks PYD and DPD as markers in 36 breast cancer patients with bone metastases. In 19 women who developed progressive disease over a median follow-up time of 4 months, both markers increased with significant changes becoming apparent by 8 weeks. This evidence preceded radiological evidence by a median of 2 months. By contrast, in 17 women who responded to hormone therapy the markers did not change significantly over a median time of 6 months.

In a study designed to evaluate bone resorption and tumour markers as possible alternatives to plain radiographs for the assessment of response to bisphosphonate therapy, Vinholes *et al.* (1999) studied 37 patients with newly diagnosed bone metastases from breast cancer. NTX levels were significantly lower compared to baseline values ($p \leq 0.05$) at 1 and 4 months in responding patients as opposed to patients with progressive disease. Similarly, NTX levels at 4 months in patients were significantly lower in patients with a time to progression of more than 7 months compared with patients who progressed in not more than 7 months. Furthermore, an increase in NTX excretion of more than 50% correctly predicted disease progression in 78% of patients. Compared with urinary calcium, hydroxyproline and the tumour markers CA15-3 and cancer associated serum antigen (CASA), Ntx was reported to be the most sensitive marker for assessing response to therapy or progression.

In a larger more recent study, 97 evaluable patients with metastatic bone disease from a variety of primary sites were followed during systemic therapy in order to correlate marker changes with response to treatment (Costa *et al.* 2002). Good correlations between urinary NTX, ICTP and bone alkaline phosphatase changes and response were observed with a rise in NTX of not less than 52% having the highest positive predictive value (71%) for identifying progression.

Although it is now well accepted that bone-targeted systemic therapy, particularly the use of the bisphosphonates, can substantially reduce morbidity of skeletal metastases of breast cancer, the optimisation and timing of these therapies remains to be established. Bone markers potentially offer a powerful and relatively simple tool to assist the clinician in developing the most appropriate treatment strategies. Moreover, there is the prospect that it may be possible to use bone markers to tailor treatment to the individual patient. Both NTX and CTX are typically increased 2- to 7-fold in 70–80% of patients with bone metastases compared with healthy controls, and typically decrease by 60–80% in response to bisphosphonate therapy (Brown & Coleman 2002). Similar dramatic reductions in urinary PYD, DPD, CTX and NTX levels have been reported in patients with postmenopausal osteoporosis treated with 20 to 30 mg/day risedronate (Zegels *et al.* 2001).

Several comparative trials have examined bone resorption markers in patients with bone metastases who were treated with bisphosphonates (Brown & Coleman 2002). Firstly, in a study of 19 breast cancer patients with extensive bone metastases, mean baseline levels of urinary calcium, hydroxyproline, CTX, and collagen crosslinks (PYD and DPD) were elevated in 47%, 74%, 83% and 100% of patients, respectively (Body *et al.* 1997). All of these markers decreased following pamidronate therapy, with the largest decrease observed in CTX. In a second study of 29 breast cancer patients with progressing bone metastases, the mean baseline values of NTX, CTX, and DPD were elevated approximately 2-fold compared with age-matched controls (Vinholes *et al.* 1997), and after pamidronate therapy, levels of NTX and CTX again decreased significantly ($p = 0.001$). Thirdly, in a double-blind study of 32 patients with hypercalcaemia of malignancy, mean baseline levels of NTX were 7-fold above normal, and mean DPD and CTX levels were each 5-fold higher than normal (Vinholes *et al.* 1997). Again, NTX and CTX showed the greatest decrease following pamidronate therapy, reaching 15% and 2% of the baseline values, respectively ($p < 0.01$).

As well as these changes observed in the mean values of resorption marker values following bisphosphonate treatment, there is also evidence that the individual pre-treatment values of a bone marker, particularly NTX, is correlated with response to treatment. In a study of patients with metastatic bone pain treated with 120 mg pamidronate, the baseline values of NTX in non-responding patients were significantly higher ($p < 0.02$) than those of the clinical responders. None of the patients with an initial NTX value above twice the upper limit of normal responded, compared with over 50% of those whose initial marker values were normal or below twice the upper level of normal. This study showed also that normalisation of bone resorption markers correlated with response to treatment. Clinical benefit, as indicated by an improvement in a pain score, was only seen in those patients (17/32 (60%)) achieving a normal bone resorption rate after pamidronate. No response was seen in the 11 patients (35%) with persistently elevated levels ($p \leq 0.01$). This suggested that the aim of bisphosphonate therapy ought to be to produce a fall in marker levels, preferably into the normal range.

A subsequent study (Jagdev *et al.* 2001) has shown that this principle may be extended to the use of bone markers to distinguish between the benefits of different bisphosphonates. Fifty-one patients, including 24 with metastatic breast cancer, were randomly allocated to treatment with either oral clodronate, intravenous clodronate or intravenous pamidronate. Symptomatic response was more frequent in the pamidronate group than in patients receiving clodronate and this was reflected in a correspondingly greater decrease in the bone resorption markers CTX and NTX. Additionally, biochemical changes correlated with the evolution of a composite pain score after bisphosphonate treatment ($p = 0.01$).

The reduction in skeletal events associated with bisphosphonate therapy also appears to be correlated with a reduction in bone resorption markers. Lipton *et al.* (1998) investigated the fracture rate in 21 cancer patients with bone metastases who received intravenous pamidronate and whose baseline NTX levels were above the normal range. The bone resorption markers PYD, DPD and NTX were measured at baseline and at 1, 3 and 6 months. In 12 of the 21 patients, NTX levels were normal at 6 months and 9 of the 21 remained abnormally elevated. In the group with NTX returning to normal levels, 42% developed fractures whereas in the group which failed to normalise, the corresponding figure was 89% ($p = 0.07$). The respective figures for each group of patients who went on to disease progression in bone were 25% and 78% ($p = 0.03$). Although these data represent small numbers of patients, it was suggestive that normalisation of bone resorption should also be a goal so as to reduce the fracture rate in metastatic bone disease patients.

Very little work has been published on the possible correlation between bone markers and the occurrence of skeletal events. Despite the obvious clinical benefits of bisphosphonates, it is clear that only a proportion of events are prevented and some patients do not experience a skeletal event despite the presence of metastatic bone disease. It is currently impossible to predict whether an individual patient needs, or will benefit from, a bisphosphonate.

We have recently reported on 121 patients with metastatic bone disease treated at our own institution (Brown *et al.* 2003). These patients had monthly measurements of urinary NTX during treatment with a range of bisphosphonates. All skeletal related events, plus hospital admissions for control of bone pain, and death during the period of observation were recorded. NTX was strongly correlated with the number of skeletal related events and/or death ($p < 0.001$). Patients with NTX values above 100 nmol/mmol creatinine were many times more likely to experience a skeletal related event/death than those with NTX below this level ($p < 0.01$).

Overall, bisphosphonates reduce the frequency of skeletal events by 25–40%. However, bisphosphonates are a relatively costly additional intervention in cancer care which is now applicable to a very large proportion of patients with advanced malignancy. The cost effectiveness of routine long-term treatment has been questioned (Hillner 2001) and prioritisation of bisphosphonate use is needed. A more cost-effective use of bisphosphonates might be to reserve them until patients have an NTX levels above either 50 or 100 nmol/mmol creatinine, and adjust the dose and schedule to maintain a normal rate of bone resorption. Randomised trials to assess this approach are planned.

## Prevention of bone metastases

Bone is the most frequent site of distant relapse, accounting for around 40% of all first recurrence (Coleman & Rubens 1987). In addition to the well-recognised release of bone cell activating factors from the tumour, it is now appreciated that release of bone derived growth factors and cytokines from resorbing bone can both attract cancer cells to the bone surface and facilitate their growth and proliferation (Boissier *et al.* 2000). Inhibition of bone resorption could therefore have an effect on the development and progression of metastatic bone disease, and is an adjuvant therapeutic strategy of potential importance.

Encouraging animal studies with a variety of animal tumour models and a range of bisphosphonates have shown inhibition of bone metastasis development and a reduction in tumour burden within bone (Yoneda *et al.* 1999). More recently, several clinical trials have been reported using the relatively low potency oral bisphosphonate, clodronate (Table 20.2). In the largest study, 1079 women with primary operable breast cancer were randomised to receive either clodronate 1600 mg daily or placebo for two years in addition to standard adjuvant systemic treatment. Recent data presented with a median follow-up time of 5 years revealed a non-significant reduction in the frequency of bone metastases in the clodronate treated patients (63 (12%) versus 80 (15%) patients, $p = 0.127$) (Powles *et al.* 2002). However, during the two years on active treatment, there was a reduction in bone metastases, but this disappeared on discontinuation of the study drug, suggesting that adjuvant bisphosphonate treatment trials in the future should test a longer duration of treatment. There was no effect on non-bone recurrence (112 (21%) v 128 (24%) patients, $p = 0.26$) but, despite little effect on the primary endpoint (bone recurrence), patients randomised to the clodronate arm had a better survival (82 versus 77%, $p = 0.047$).

In a second study, Diel and colleagues studied 302 breast cancer patients randomly allocated to either oral clodronate 1600 mg daily ($n = 157$) for 3 years or a control group ($n = 145$). These women had no overt evidence of metastatic disease, but were selected for the trial on the basis of immunocytochemical detection of tumour cells in the bone marrow, a known risk factor for the subsequent development of distant metastases (Diel *et al.* 1998). Patients received appropriate adjuvant chemotherapy and endocrine treatment. There were no discernable prognostic or treatment imbalances between the two groups and the follow-up schedules were similar. The median observation period was 36 months. The incidence of osseous metastases was significantly lower in the clodronate group (11 (7%) versus 25 (17%) patients, $p < 0.002$). There was also an unexpected large reduction in the incidence of visceral metastases in the clodronate group (19 (13%) versus 42 (29%) patients,

**Table 20.2** The use of adjuvant clodronate in primary operable breast cancer trials.

| Number of patients | Period of clodronate treatment (years) | Occurrence of bone metastases (clodronate versus placebo) | Occurrence of non-bone metastases (clodronate versus placebo) | Deaths (clodronate versus placebo) | Reference |
|---|---|---|---|---|---|
| 1079 | 2 | At two years, 2% versus 5%; $p = 0.016$. At >2 years, 10% versus 10%; $p = 0.73$ | At >2 years 21% versus 24%; $p = 0.26$. | At 2 years 8% versus 8% (approx.). At 5 years 17% versus 22%; $p = .047$ | Powles *et al.* (2002) |
| 299 | 3 | 21% versus 17% $p = .27$ | 43% versus 25%; $p = 0.009$. | At 5 years 30% versus 17%; $p = 0.01$. | Saarto *et al.* (2001) |
| 302 | 2 | 14% versus 24% $p = .044$ | 16% versus 26%; $p = 0.091$. | At 5 years 10% versus 22%; $p = 0.002$. | Diel *et al.* (2000) |

In all cases 1,600 mg clodronate was given orally. Average follow-up time was 4.5–5.5 years.

$p < 0.001$). These results have subsequently been updated (Diel *et al.* 2000) and show similar results, although the striking effect on extra-skeletal visceral relapse seen in the earlier report was less and no longer statistically significant.

The exciting findings of the Diel study must, however, be viewed in the light of a further trial which produced conflicting results. Saarto *et al.* (2001) randomised 299 women with primary node-positive breast cancer to oral clodronate 1600mg daily ($n = 149$) or a control group ($n = 150$). The median follow-up was 5 years. Treatment with clodronate in this study did not lead to a reduction in the development of bone metastases (29 (19%) versus 24 (16%) patients, $p = 0.27$ for the clodronate and control groups respectively). Additionally the development of non-skeletal recurrence was significantly higher in the clodronate group (60 (40%) versus 36 (24%) patients, $p = 0.0007$) and, most importantly, the overall five year survival was significantly lower in the clodronate group (70% versus 83%, $p = 0.009$). It is possible that there were some prognostic imbalances favouring the control group but the safest assumption is to consider that the Diel and Saarto studies cancel each other out and probably reflect the usual heterogeneity of results seen in relatively small studies of adjuvant treatment.

Identifying a definite adjuvant role for bisphosphonates will require further large randomised studies. The National Surgical Adjuvant Breast Project (NSABP) have recently started a placebo controlled trial of oral clodronate ($n > 3000$) in an attempt to resolve the value or otherwise of adjuvant clodronate.

Adjuvant trials are just beginning with zoledronic acid. It is hoped that the added potency of zoledronic acid may have beneficial effects not only through the inhibition of bone resorption, but also through direct effects on tumour cells in the bone marrow. There is increasing evidence, from a range of cell line experiments, that zoledronic acid can inhibit tumour cell adhesion and invasion (Van der Pluijm *et al.* 1996). Additionally, zoledronic acid promotes apoptosis both directly and in synergy with paclitaxel (Jagdev *et al.* 2001). These effects are mediated through the mevalonate pathway using the same molecular pathway that aminobisphosphonates exploit to inhibit osteoclast function. Finally, there are experimental data from animal models that indicate that zoledronic acid can suppress angiogenesis (Wood *et al.* 2002).

## Effects of cancer treatments on skeletal health

There are now increasing numbers of long-term survivors from breast cancer who have received combination chemotherapy, radiotherapy and hormonal cancer treatment. Many of these individuals are at increased risk of osteoporosis largely because of the endocrine changes induced by treatment. There may also be clinically relevant, direct effects of cytotoxic drugs on bone. This is a particularly important long-term problem in women with breast cancer for whom there are concerns about the safety of hormone replacement therapy.

Oestrogen is known to be critical in the maintenance of normal bone mass in women. After the menopause a reduction in bone mineral density (BMD) occurs, most pronounced in the first three years where the rate can be as high as 5% per year, but then reduces to a rate of about 0.5% per annum thereafter. The aromatase inhibitor anastrozole leads to nearly complete suppression of circulating oestradiol and causes accelerated bone loss. As a consequence these women may be at greater risk of suffering a low trauma fracture. Preliminary data from the ATAC adjuvant trial indicate that fractures are increased to 5.8% in patients taking anastrozole compared with 3.7% in women taking tamoxifen (ATAC Trialists' Group 2002). Part of this difference can be attributed to the bone sparing effect of tamoxifen. However, a contribution from the direct effect of anastrozole on BMD and bone strength is also assumed.

The bisphosphonates, as potent inhibitors of bone resorption, have emerged as an important class of agents in the management of postmenopausal osteoporosis. The use of alendronate, an aminobisphosphonate, has demonstrated a significant reduction in osteoporotic fractures. A dose of 10 mg of alendronate in postmenopausal women resulted in an increase in BMD of 6% and 9% at the lumbar spine and femoral neck respectively, with a concomitant decrease in fracture rates (Black *et al.* 1996). A meta-analysis of five studies with alendronate in this population has shown a reduction a 30% reduction in the incidence of non-vertebral fractures (Karpf *et al.* 1997). However, there are only a few studies addressing the effectiveness of these compounds in the management of cancer treatment-induced bone loss, especially in populations where the use of hormone replacement therapy may be undesirable.

A few studies have evaluated women with breast cancer and treatment-induced premature menopause. In the first, Saarto *et al* studied the effect of 1600 mg clodronate in 148 pre-menopausal women receiving adjuvant chemotherapy for breast cancer and no evidence of bone metastases (Saarto *et al.* 1997). They observed that rapid bone loss occurred in the women who became amenorrhoeic after chemotherapy (6% and 2% losses at 2 years in the spine and hip respectively). However, in those receiving clodronate, the bone effects of chemotherapy induced premature menopause were attenuated (2% loss and 1% gain at 2 years in the spine and hip respectively). In a comparison of risedronate with placebo in a postmenopausal group of patients receiving tamoxifen, Delmas *et al* observed an approximately 2.5% increase in BMD at the lumbar spine and femoral neck in the risedronate group compared with placebo (Delmas *et al.* 1997).

Intravenous bisphosphonate administration is widely used in oncology in the treatment of metastatic disease. In a recent study, Reid *et al* investigated the use of 3 monthly, six monthly, and annual intravenous zoledronic acid administration, in a general population of osteoporotic, post-menopausal women (Reid *et al.* 2002). It was found that a single 4 mg intravenous dose of zoledronic acid resulted in an increase in BMD at the spine of 4.6% and the hip of 3.3%, both measured one year later. This was comparable to the increase in BMD achieved by giving the same total dose at 3- or 6-monthly intervals. In breast cancer patients, 6 monthly zoledronic acid has also been shown to reverse the bone loss induced by medical castration with the LHRH analogue goserelin (Zoladex) plus oestrogen suppression with anastrozole. In this study a 10% loss of bone in the lumbar spine occurred with this combination without bisphosphonate compared with a small 1% gain in BMD with six monthly zoledronic acid (Gnant *et al.* 2002).

## Conclusions

Bone metastases are a common and very important clinical problem in advanced breast cancer. Bisphosphonates should now be part of standard management for breast cancer patients with symptomatic bone disease. The available evidence indicates that the aminobisphosphonates, and in particular zoledronic acid, are the most effective agents to prevent skeletal complications and relieve bone pain. Further work to define the optimum schedule of treatment, and when to start and stop treatment is needed. Bone resorption markers may be useful in this regard. Current data suggest that oral clodronate may be useful in the adjuvant setting and that it reduces treatment induced bone loss. However, larger confirmatory trials are required before adjuvant bisphosphonates can be recommended for routine use.

*References*

Andersen, P. K. & Gill, R. D. (1982). Cox's regression model for counting processes: a large sample study. *Annals of Statistics* **10**, 1100–1120.

ATAC Trialists' Group (2002). Anastrozole alone or in combination with tamoxifen versus tamoxifen alone for adjuvant treatment of postmenopausal women with early breast cancer: first results of the ATAC randomised trial. *The Lancet* **359**, 2131–2139.

Berenson, J. R., Rosen, L. S., Howell, A., Porter, L., Coleman, R. E., Morley, W. *et al.* Zoledronic acid reduces skeletal-related events in patients with osteolytic metastases. *Cancer* **91**, 1191–1200.

Berenson, J. R., Vescio, R., Henick, K., Nishikubo, C., Rettig, M., Swift, R. A. *et al.* (2001). A phase I, open label, dose ranging trial of intravenous bolus zoledronic acid, a novel bisphosphonate, in cancer patients with metastatic bone disease. *Cancer* **91**, 144–154.

Black, D. M., Cummings, S. R., Karpf, D. B. *et al.* (1996). Randomised trial of the effect of alendronate on the risk of fracture in women with existing vertebral fractures. *The Lancet* **148**, 1535–1541.

Body, J. J., Bartl, R., Burckhardt, P., Delmas, P. D. *et al.* (1998). Current use of bisphosphonates in oncology. International Bone and Cancer Study Group. *Journal of Clinical Oncology* **16**, 3890–3899.

Body, J. J., Dumon J. C., Gineyts E., Delmas P. D. (1997). Comparative evaluation of markers of bone resorption in patients with breast cancer-induced osteolysis before and after bisphosphonate therapy. *British Journal of Cancer* **75**, 408–412.

Body, J.-J., Greipp, P., Coleman, R. E. *et al.* (2003). A phase I study of AMGN-0007, a recombinant osteoprotogerin construct, in patients with multiple myeloma or breast carcinoma related bone metastases. *Cancer* **97**, 887–892.

Body, J. J., Diel, I. J., Lichinitser, M. R., Kreuser, E. D., Dornoff, W., Gorbunova, V. A., Budde, M. & Bergstrom, B. (2003). MF 4265 Study Group. Intravenous ibandronate reduces the incidence of skeletal complications in patients with breast cancer and bone metastases. *Annals of Oncology* **14**, 1399–1405.

Body, J. J., Lortholary, A., Romieu, G., Vigneron, A. M., Ford, J. (1999). A dose-finding study of zoledronate in hypercalcaemic cancer patients. *Journal of Bone Mineral Research* **14**, 1557–1661.

Body, J. J., Diel, I. J., Lichinitzer, M., Lazarev, A., Pecherstorfer, M., Bell, R., Tripathy, D. & Bergstrom, B. (2004). Oral ibandronate reduces the risk of skeletal complications in breast cancer patients with metastatic bone disease: results from two randomised, placebo-controlled phase III studies. *British Journal of Cancer* **90**, 1133–1137.

Boissier, S., Ferreras, M., Peyruchaud, O. *et al.* (2000). Bisphosphonates inhibit breast and prostate carcinoma cell invasion, an early event in the formation of bone metastases. *Cancer Research* **60**, 2949–2954.

Brown, J. E. & Coleman, R. E. (2002). Assessment of the effects of breast cancer on bone and the response to therapy. *The Breast* **11**, 1–11.

Brown. J. E., Thomson, C. S., Ellis, S. P., Gutcher, S. A., Purohit, O. P. & Coleman, R. E. (2003). Bone resorption predicts for skeletal complications in metastatic bone disease *British Journal of Cancer* **89**, 2031–2037.

Coleman, R. E. (1998). Pamidronate Disodium in the treatment and management of hypercalcaemia. *Reviews in Contemporary Pharmacotherapy* **9**, 147–164.

Coleman, R. E. (2002). The clinical use of bone resorption markers in patients with malignant bone disease. *Cancer* **94**, 2521–2533.

Coleman, R. E., Purohit, O. P., Black, C. *et al.* (1999). Double-blind, randomised, placebo-controlled study of oral ibandronate in patients with metastatic bone disease. *Annals of Oncology* **10**, 311–316.

Coleman, R. E. & Rubens, R. D. (1987). The clinical course of bone metastases from breast cancer. *British Journal of Cancer* **55**, 61–66.

Conte, P. F., Mauriac, L., Calabresi, F. *et al.* (1996). Delay in progression of bone metastases treated with intravenous pamidronate: Results from a multicentre randomised controlled trial. *Journal of Clinical Oncology* **14**, 2552–2559.

Costa, L., Demers, L. M., Gouveia-Oliveira, A., Schaller, J., Costa, E. B., de Moura, M.C. & Lipton, A. (2002). Prospective evaluation of the peptide-bound collagen type I cross-links N-telopeptide and C-telopeptide in predicting bone metastases status. *Journal of Clinical Oncology* **20**, 850–856.

Delmas, P. D., Balena, R., Confravreux, E. *et al.* (1997). Bisphosphonate Risedronate prevents bone loss in women with artificial menopause due to chemotherapy of breast cancer: a double-blind, placebo-controlled study. *Journal of Clinical Oncology* **15**, 955–962.

Diel, I. J., Solomayer, E. F., Costa, S. D., Gollan, C., Goerner, R., Wallwiener, D. *et al.* (1998). Reduction in new metastases in breast cancer with adjuvant clodronate treatment. *New England Journal of Medicine* **339**, 357–363.

Diel, I. J., Solomayer, E., Gollan, C., Schutz, F., Bastert, G. (2000). Bisphosphonates in the reduction of metastases in breast cancer – results of the extended follow-up of the first study population. *Proceedings of the American Society of Clinical Oncology* **19**, 82a, (abstract 314).

Elomaa, I., Blomqvist, C., Grohn, P., Porkka, L., Kairento, A. L., Selander, K. *et al.* (1983). Long-term controlled trial of bisphosphonate in patients with osteolytic bone metastases. *The Lancet* **i**, 146–149.

Gnant, M., Hausmaninger, H., Samonigg, H. *et al.* (2002). Changes in bone mineral density caused by anastrozole or tamoxifen in combination with goserelin(+/- zoledronate) as adjuvant treatment for hormone receptor premenopausal breast cancer, results of a randomised multicentre trial. *Breast Cancer Research and Treatment* **76** (Suppl. 1), S31 (abstract 11).

Hillner, B. E. (2001). Pharmaco-economic issues in bisphosphonate treatment of metastatic bone disease. *Seminars in Oncology* **28**(4 Suppl. 11), 64–68.

Hortobagyi, G. N., Theriault, R. L., Porter, L. *et al.* (1996). Efficacy of pamidronate in reducing skeletal complications in patients with breast cancer and lytic bone metastases. *New England Journal of Medicine* **335**, 1785–1791.

Hultborn, R., Ryden, S., Gunderson, S., Holmberg, E., Wallgren, U.-B. (1996). Efficacy of pamidronate on skeletal complications from breast cancer metastases. A randomised prospective double blind placebo controlled trial. *Acta Oncologica* **35** (Suppl. 5), 73–74.

Hughes, D. E., Wright, K. R., Uy, H. L. *et al.* (1995). Bisphosphonates promote apoptosis in murine osteoclasts in vitro and in vivo. *Journal of Bone Mineral Research* **10**, 1478–1487.

Jagdev, S., Coleman, R. E., Shipman, C. M. & Croucher, P. (2001). The bisphosphonate zoledronic acid induces apoptosis of breast cancer cells: evidence for synergy with paclitaxel. *British Journal of Cancer* **84**, 1126–1134.

Jagdev, S. P., Purohit, O. P. Heatley, S. *et al.* (2001). Comparison of the effects of intravenous pamidronate and oral clodronate on symptoms and bone resorption in patients with metastatic bone disease. *Annals of Oncology* **12**, 1433–1438.

Karpf, D. B., Shapiro, D. R., Seeman, E. *et al.* (1997). Prevention of nonvertebral fractures by alendronate. *Journal of the American Medical Association* **277**, 1159–1164.

Kong, Y.-Y., Yoshida, H., Sarosi, O. *et al.* (1999). OPGL is a key regulator of osteoclastogenesis, lymphocyte development and lymph-node organogenesis. *Nature* **397**, 315–323.

Lipton, A., Demers, L., Curley, E. *et al.* (1998). Markers of bone resorption in patients treated with pamidronate. *European Journal of Cancer* **34**, 2021–2026.

Luckman, S. P., Coxon, F. P., Russell, R. G. G. & Rogers, M. J. (1998). Nitrogen-containing bisphosphonates inhibit the mevalonate pathway and prevent post-translational prenylation of GTP-binding proteins, including Ras. *Journal of Bone Mineral Research* **13**, 581–589.

Major, P. P., Lortholary, A., Hon, J. *et al.* (2001). Zoledronic acid is superior to pamidronate in the treatment of hypercalcemia of malignancy – a pooled analysis of two randomized, controlled clinical trials. *Journal of Clinical Oncology* **19**, 558–567.

Neville-Webbe, H., Holen, I. & Coleman, R. E. (2002). The anti-tumour effects and potential of bisphosphonates. *Cancer Treatments Reviews* **28**, 305–320.

Paterson, A. H. G., Powles, T. J., Kanis, J. *et al.* (1993). Double-blind controlled trial of oral clodronate in patients with bone metastases from breast cancer. *Journal of Clinical Oncology* **11**, 59–65.

Powles, T., Paterson, S., Kanis, J. A. *et al.* (2002). Randomised, placebo-controlled trial of clodronate in patients with primary operable breast cancer. *Journal of Clinical Oncology* **20**, 3219–3224.

Reid, I. R., Brown, J. P., Burckhardt, P. *et al.* (2002). Intravenous zoledronic acid in postmenopausal women with low bone mineral density. *New England Journal of Medicine* **346**, 653–661.

Rogers, M. J., Watts, D. J. & Russell, R. G. G. (1997). Overview of bisphosphonates. *Cancer* **80**, 1652–1660.

Roodman, G. D. (2003). Role of stromal-derived cytokines and growth factors in bone metastasis. *Cancer* **97**, 733–738.

Rosen, L. S, Gordon, D., Kaminski, M., Howell, A., Belch, A. *et al.* (2001). Zoledronic acid versus pamidronate in the treatment of skeletal metastases in patients with breast cancer or osteolytic lesions of multiple myeloma: a phase III, double-blind, comparative trial. *Cancer Journal* **7**, 377–387.

Rosen, L. S, Gordon, D., Kaminski, M. *et al.* (2003). Long-term efficacy and safety of zoledronic acid compared with pamidronate disodium in treatment of skeletal complications in patients with advanced multiple myeloma of breast cancer: a randomized, double-blind, multicenter, comparative trial. *Cancer* **98**, 1735–1744.

Saarto, S., Blomqvist, C., Valimaki, M., Makela, P., Sarna, S. & Elomaa, I. (1997). Chemical castration induced by adjuvant cyclophosphamide, methotrexate, and fluorouracil chemotherapy causes rapid bone loss which is reduced by clodronate: A randomised study in premenopausal patients. *Journal of Clinical Oncology* **15**, 1341–1347.

Saarto, T., Blomqvist, C., Virkkunen, P. & Elomaa, I. (2001). Adjuvant clodronate treatment does not reduce the frequency of skeletal metastases in node-positive breast cancer patients: 5 year results of randomised controlled trial. *Journal of Clinical Oncology* **19**, 10–17.

Theriault, R. L., Lipton, A., Hortobagyi, G. N. *et al.* (1999). Pamidronate reduces skeletal morbidity in women with advance breast cancer and lytic bone lesions: A randomised, placebo-controlled trial. *Journal of Clinical Oncology* **17**, 846–854.

Van Holten-Verzantvoort, A. T, Bijvoet, O. L. M., Cleton, F. J. *et al.* (1987). Reduced morbidity from skeletal metastases in breast cancer patients during long term bisphosphonate (APD) treatment. *The Lancet* **ii**, 983–985.

Van der Pluijm, G., Vloedgraven, H., van Beek, E. *et al.* (1996). Bisphosphonates inhibit adhesion of breast cancer cells to bone matrices in vitro. *Journal of Clinical Investigation* **98**, 698–701.

Vinholes, J., Coleman, R., Lacombe, D., Rose, C., Tubiana-Hulin, M., Bastit, P. *et al.* (1999). Assessment of bone response to systemic therapy in an EORTC trial: preliminary experience with the use of collagen cross-link excretion. European Organization for Research and Treatment of Cancer. *British Journal of Cancer* **80**, 221–228.

Vinholes, J. J., Guo, C.-Y., Purohit, O. P., Eastell, R., Coleman, R. E. (1996). Metabolic effects of pamidronate in patients with metastatic bone disease. *British Journal of Cancer* **73**, 1089–1095.

Vinholes, J. J., Purohit, O. P., Abbey, M. E., Eastell, R & Coleman R. E. (1997). Relationships between biochemical and symptomatic response in a double-blind trial of pamidronate for metastatic bone disease. *Annals of Oncology* **8**, 1243–1250.

Vinholes, J. J., Purohit, O. P., Abbey, M. E., Eastell, R. & Coleman, R. E. (1997). Evaluation of new bone resorption markers in a randomized comparison of pamidronate or clodronate for hypercalcaemia of malignancy. *Journal of Clinical Oncology* **15**, 131–138.

Walls, J., Assiri, A., Howell, A., Rogers, E., Ratcliffe, W. A., Eastell, R. *et al.* (1999). Measurement of urinary collagen cross-links indicate response to therapy in patients with breast cancer and bone metastases. *British Journal of Cancer* **80**, 1265–1270.

Wood, J., Schnell, C. & Green, J. (2002). Novel anti-angiogenic effects of the bisphosphonates compound zoledronic acid. *Journal of Pharmacology and Experimental Therapeutics* **302**, 1055–1061.

Yoneda, T., Michigami, T., Yi, B. *et al.* (1999). Use of bisphosphonates for the treatment of bone metastasis in experimental animal models. *Cancer Treatment Reviews* **25**, 293–299.

Zegels, B., Eastell, R., Russell, R. G., Ethgen, D., Roumagnac, I., Collette, J. *et al.* (2001). Effect of high doses of oral risedronate (20 mg/day) on serum parathyroid hormone levels and urinary collagen cross-link excretion in postmenopausal women with spinal osteoporosis. *Bone* **28**, 108–112.

# PART 5

# The menopausal patient, enhancing emotional adjustment and the role of the clinical nurse specialist

# Chapter 21

# Treatment of menopausal symptoms in women with breast cancer

*Lorraine E. Turner and Nigel J. Bundred*

## Natural menopause

> *'The term menopause simply means last menstrual bleed.'*
> Abernethy (1997)

The phase either side of this last bleed is described as the climacteric. In the UK, the mean age for the start of the menopause is 50 years and 9 months. During this time many women experience physical and psychological symptoms due to the decreasing levels of oestrogen. These include vasomotor symptoms such as hot flushes and night sweats, vaginal dryness and mood swings. Night sweats in particular interrupt sleep patterns and contribute to insomnia, which can negatively affect women's quality of life (Le Boeuf & Carter 1996). The most common reported vasomotor symptom is hot flushes, which is experienced by 68–92% of menopausal women (Harper 1990).

## Menopause for women with breast cancer

Seventy per cent of women who develop breast cancer are post-menopausal. The remaining 30% will often become prematurely post-menopausal after breast cancer treatment (McPhail & Smith 2000). Such treatments include oophorectomy, chemotherapy, hormonal drugs (including tamoxifen and aromatase inhibitors) and/or the abrupt discontinuation of hormone replacement therapy (HRT) at diagnosis. Thus many women will have climacteric symptoms (before) during and after treatment for breast cancer.

Hot flushes are experienced by approximately 65% of women after breast cancer treatment, with most describing their symptoms as severe (Carpenter *et al.* 1998). In addition, one of the main side effects of tamoxifen, the drug most widely prescribed for patients with breast cancer, is hot flushes (ATAC Trialists' Group 2002).

## Management of menopausal hot flushes
### Lifestyle interventions

Numerous lifestyle suggestions have been suggested to help post-menopausal women adopt a more preventative role. For example, maintaining lower room temperatures and better air circulation. Paced respirations and progressive muscle relaxation training have also been reported to reduce hot flushes (Freedman & Woodward 1992; Irvin *et al.* 1996). Hence, many post-menopausal women are now taking an active role in reducing the number of hot flushes by frequent exercise, weight management, wearing loose cotton fabrics, limiting the intake of spicy foods, caffeine and alcohol and increasing their daily intake of fruits, fresh vegetables and grains.

Although none of these last interventions have been clinically tested so far, it is worth acknowledging that such simple and inexpensive lifestyle interventions could be easily implemented by women.

## Randomised controlled trials

Randomised controlled trials of non-oestrogen, i.e. therapies that have improved vasomotor symptoms, are shown in Table 21.1. The problem, however, with many of these clinical trials is the high placebo response rate. The improvement of hot flushes in the placebo group reported in clinical trials has been considerable in the range of 25– 51%, despite effective blinding (Scambia *et al.* 2000; Umpalis *et al.* 2000; Patten *et al.* 2002). Regardless, a placebo effect with any therapy for hot flushes may be caused by the variability and spontaneous improvement that occurs over time. Other researchers have speculated that it may be simply a result of monitoring and expectation, particularly in highly motivated women. A randomized controlled trial, which recommended intervention such as attending lectures, reading relevant material and the use of medications, was compared with standard care. The intervention group did not particularly avail themselves of literature or attendance at lectures but had a significantly higher uptake of medications (such as progestogens) to relieve hot flushes.

## Vitamin E

Barton *et al.* (1998) performed a double blind, randomised placebo-controlled, crossover trial to investigate the efficency of Vitamin E for controlling hot flushes in breast cancer survivors. Vitamin E (800 IU/day) treatment produced a significant reduction in hot flushes compared with placebo, with low toxicity. However, this amounted to one less hot flush a day than placebo, and it required the Vitamin E to be taken for at least one month to see benefit. In response to this study, Vitamin E was recommended as an antidote for hot flushes in the initial National Surgical Adjuvant Breast and Bowel Project (NSABP).

## Clonidine

Compounds such as clonidine (an $\alpha$-adrenergic agonist) have been investigated as a potential therapy for use of tamoxifen associated hot flushes. Goldberg *et al.* (1993) found a significant decrease in hot flushes in women assigned to receive transdermal clonidine, compared with women who were allocated placebo. Similarly, Pandya *et*

**Table 21.1** Summary of effective treatments for vasomotor symptoms.

| Source | Intervention | Type of study | Response | Conclusion |
|---|---|---|---|---|
| Barton *et al.* 1998 | Vitamin E 800mg/day | Double-blind, randomised placebo-controlled, cross-over | 25% reduction in hot flushes compared to 22% placebo | One less hot flush than placebo |
| Pandya *et al.* 2000 | Oral Clonidine 0.1mg/day | Randomised, placebo-controlled trial | 37% reduction in hot flushes compared to 20% placebo | Only 1% increase in quality of life |
| Loprinzi *et al.* 2000 | Venlafaxine 37.5mg/day 75–150mg/day | Randomised, placebo-controlled trial | 40% reduction in hot flushes with 37.5mg/day, 60% reduction with 75–150mg/day compared to 27% placebo | Ongoing clinical trials |
| Loprinzi *et al.* 1994 | Megestrol acetate 40mg/day | Double-blind, randomised placebo-controlled, cross-over | 75–80% reduction in hot flushes compared to 20–25% placebo | ? long term risk of breast cancer |
| Preliminary results of Study 32930 | Tibolone 2.5mg/day | Double-blind, randomised placebo-controlled pilot study | 50–60% reduction in hot flushes compared to 10–20% placebo | Awaiting results from larger, multi-national clinical trials |
| Albertazzi *et al.* 1998 | Phytooestrogen (soy) 60g/day | Double-blind, randomised placebo-controlled | 45% reduction in hot flushes compared to 30% placebo | Similar findings with other phytooestrogen studies |

*al.* (2000) found a 37% reduction of hot flushes in the oral clonidine arm versus 20% in the placebo arm after 4 weeks' treatment with 0.1 mg/day of clonidine and 38% compared with 24% after 8 weeks' treatment. However, only a 1% increase in quality of life was experienced because of its toxicity with several unpleasant side effects such as mouth dryness, constipation, drowsiness and difficulty sleeping.

## Venlafaxine and selective serotonin reuptake inhibitors

The mechanism of action of venlafaxine and selective serotonin reuptake inhibitors (SSRIs) paroxetine and fluoxetine is not clear, although it is thought that the effects are central and related to alterations in dopamine, serotonin or norepinephrine pathways. A small dose of venlafaxine (37.5 mg/day) was shown to reduce hot flushes by approximately 50% (Loprinzi *et al.* 1998). With a higher dose of 75 mg/day, Loprinzi *et al.* (2000) found an even greater effect (60% reduction) (Figure 21.1). The only evident side effects noted of venlafaxine, a dual serotonin norepinephrine reuptake inhibitor, were mouth dryness, decreased appetite and nausea. In most cases the nausea resolved after the first week. However, venlafaxine is not licensed for the indication of relief of hot flushes, and patients have experienced problems when stopping the drug. Galactorrhoea and sexual dysfunction have been reported on rare occasions with long-term therapy.

Indeed, paroxetine (an SSRI) has been shown to have a similar effect with a 75% reduction in hot flushes as seen in Stearns *et al.* (2000) study.

Gottlieb (2000) does, however, state the importance for further research using SSRIs in reference to potential side effects and specific doses in well-designed

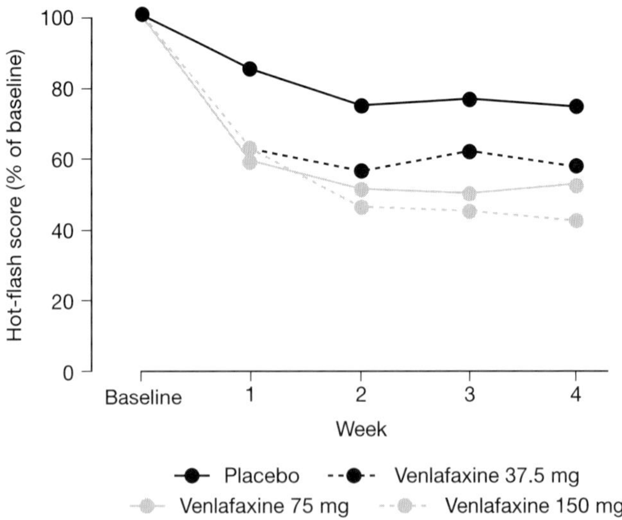


**Figure 21.1** The effect of venlafaxine on vasomotor symptoms

placebo-controlled crossover trials. Reviewing the current evidence, venlafaxine should be offered to women following breast cancer treatment as long as the dose and side effects are reviewed on a regular basis to reach optimum effectiveness.

## Progestogens

Many clinicians choose progestational agents such as megestrol acetate as a first-line treatment for hot flushes in breast cancer. Various clinical trials have found that progestogens significantly reduce vasomotor symptoms compared with placebo. A placebo-controlled, double blind, randomised crossover trial involving a 4-week period of oral megestrol acetate (40 mg/day) followed by placebo for 4 weeks, or vice versa, was performed by Loprinzi *et al.* (1994). Those receiving placebo first had a 21% reduction in hot flushes. More significantly, those receiving megestrol acetate had a 75–80% reduction. With this type of improvement the dose can then be reduced to 20 mg per day or less after one month's treatment.

It is notable that for the first 7–10 days after starting progestogens a 'flare' or increase in hot flushes occurs, and women must be encouraged to persevere beyond 10 days to get the longer-term benefits of therapy.

Reginster *et al.* (1996) found that progesterone (150 mg of depot medroxyprogesterone for 25 days/month) was better than oestrogen alone over a 3 month period in relieving vasomotor symptoms (18% of women taking oestrogen and 33% taking progesterone had no symptoms).

Unfortunately, there are long-term effects of megestrol acetate, including weight gain and carpel-tunnel syndrome (Quella *et al.* 1998). With any hormonal treatment given to women with a history of breast cancer, risks and benefits have to be scrutinized.

Pharmacological doses of progesterone used in combined hormone replacement therapy are associated with an increased risk of breast cancer. Convincing evidence from the latest randomised Women's Health Initiative Study (2002), which parallels that of the observational 'Million Women Study' (2003), has shown that combined oestrogen–progestogen use significantly increases a woman's risk of developing breast cancer (Relative Risk (RR) 2.00; 95% confidence interval (CI) 1.88–2.12), which increases with prolonged use (Million Women Study Collaborators 2003). One needs to acknowledge theoretical concerns because of some *in vitro* data that suggest that these drugs might stimulate the growth of micrometastatic breast cancer, potentiate the development of new primary breast cancers, or interfere with tamoxifen therapy.

## Phytoestrogens

Phytoestrogens are so named because they are plant-derived molecules possessing oestrogen-like activity. Their chemical structure is a steran frame and is structurally similar to 17β-oestradiol and selective oestrogen receptor modulators, although their effects are estimated to be some thousand-fold weaker compared with those of 17β-oestradiol.

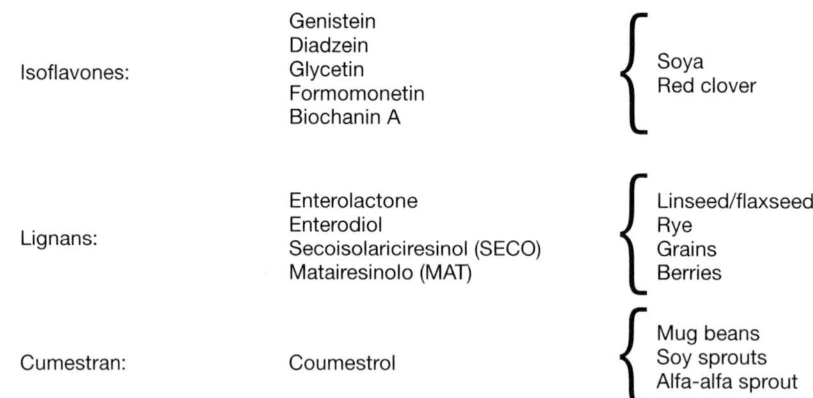


**Figure 21.2** Classification of phytooestrogen subtypes

Potentially, phytoestrogens can act as both oestrogen agonists and antagonists depending on tissue metabolites and processing (Quella *et al.* 2000). The three main types of phytoestrogen are the isoflavones found in soy (the most potent), coumestan and lignans found in flaxseed (Figure 21.2).

The incidence of menopausal vasomotor symptoms is much lower in Asian countries, where consumption of soy phytoestrogens is high. Evidence from several human studies is controversial. In randomised controlled trials there is a minimal effect of soy on hot flushes, with a prominent placebo effect. Vincent & Fitzpatrick (2000) found a 45% reduction in hot flushes using soy supplements compared with 30% on placebo. A similar trend was also mirrored in a randomised placebo controlled trial of 104 post-menopausal women (Albertazzi *et al.* 1998). Although these studies had statistically significant results, the clinical significance is unclear.

The trial by Germain *et al.* (2001) involving 69 post-menopausal women found no treatment effect on severity of hot flushes or night sweats at any point in a 24-week period using isoflavone rich (80 mg/day) protein supplements.

There is even more uncertainty about the use of phytoestrogens in reducing vasomotor symptoms for women treated for breast cancer. Recent studies show no statistical variations between soy and placebo treatments in the reduction of hot flushes. A trial involving 177 women treated for breast cancer, of whom 66% were receiving tamoxifen, established that those taking a soy pill equivalent of 150 mg/day were not observed to be any more effective than placebo in reducing hot flushes (Quella *et al.* 2000). Interestingly, 36% of women who took the placebo reported their hot flush frequency was reduced by 50%, compared with 24% of patients taking the soy pill. In addition, more patients at the end of the study preferred the placebo to the soy supplement (37% versus 33%, respectively).

Two randomised controlled trials of red clover tablets versus placebo showed that at doses of both 40 mg and 160 mg a day, no effects on hot flushes were seen over a three month period (Baber *et al.* 1999; Knight *et al.* 1999).

Many researchers have argued that concentrated soy isoflavone / high-dose plant oestrogen supplements should not be given to women who have been diagnosed with breast cancer, because theoretically and until proven otherwise, it may encourage tumour growth in a potentially low-oestrogen environment.

Recent evidence has found genistein, one of the main isoflavones in soy, to inhibit thyroid metabolism in animals and humans, potentially leading to hypothyroidism (Harding *et al.* 1996; Divi *et al.* 1997). The uses of phytoestrogens have also been linked to effects on concentrations of insulin and glucagons; they therefore have the potential to act as endocrine disrupters (Ohno *et al.* 1993).

It must also be remembered that the metabolism of phytoestrogens, in particular, is predominantly determined by gastrointestinal flora, and antibiotic use, bowel disease or gender may modify metabolism. The inter-individual diversity and complexity in dietary phytoestrogen makes the bioavailability of these compounds unpredictable. In one study, conversion by gut microflora of the isoflavone diadzein to its isoflavan metabolite equol, which is a more potent oestrogen, occurred only in some individuals (about 35% of subjects tested in the study were equol excretors) (Wiseman 1999). Therefore questions about bioavailability, absorption, compliance and dosage highlight the importance in determining clinical efficacy.

## Non-effective studies

Black cohosh (*Cimicifuga racemosa*) is an herbal agent that has been approved by the German Government's Commission for the treatment of menopausal symptoms. Several studies completed in Germany have suggested that black cohosh could have a role in reducing menopausal symptoms (Liske 1998; Pepping 1999). However, inconsistencies exist between clinical trials. Jacobson *et al.* (2001) performed a randomised, placebo-controlled study involving 69 women with a history of breast cancer. They found no difference in hot flushes between those who took black cohosh or placebo. Until further data are made available on its physiological effects, black cohosh should not be recommended for alleviating hot flushes.

Other non-traditional treatments or supplements, which include ginseng, *Angelica sinensis*, also known as dong quai, and evening primrose oil, have very little research-based evidence to support their effectiveness as a substitute for HRT. Hirata *et al.* (1997) found dong quai to have no effect on reducing hot flushes in 71 post-menopausal women compared with placebo over a 24-week period. In addition, evening primrose oil, which has been shown to have a high concentration of γ–linolenic acid (GLA; an omega-6 fatty acid), was found to be no more effective than placebo for hot flushes in several studies (Chenoy 1994; Bassey *et al.* 2000). Those studies that have been performed appear generally weak in their methodology.

## Validity and reliability of clinical evidence

One of the main problems when researching into the frequency and intensity of hot flushes is that they form part of a subjective experience. Reporting of vasomotor symptoms may fluctuate in a given individual for various reasons. The fact that many women may sleep through their night sweats makes the data unreliable.

Unfortunately, researchers cannot control such things as weather, stressful situations and the simple improvement with time, which have all been shown to influence the frequency and intensity of symptoms.

Most studies quoted throughout this chapter have clearly outlined that a placebo effect does exist. Moyad (2002) claims that it is not unusual to observe a placebo response of 20–40% from studies of dietary supplements.

## Hormone replacement therapy in breast cancer

A meta-analysis of the risk of breast cancer on the oral contraceptive pill based on approximately 150,000 women indicated an increased risk of breast cancers in heavy users (RR 1.24; 95% CI 1.15–1.33). The cancers that developed on breast cancer were in general well differentiated, oestrogen receptor positive and node negative. The Women's Health Initiative (WHI) randomised trial was stopped early in 2002 because an interim analysis suggested that risks with oestrogen plus progestin treatment exceeded benefits. The hazard ratio for breast cancer among HRT users in the WHI study was estimated at 1.26 (1.00–1.59) after a mean follow up of 5.2 years. However, women randomised to oestrogen-only HRT continued in the study and there has been no increased risk of breast cancer.

A recent meta-analysis of four randomised trials including the WHI has been published. The results of these studies when overviewed show the relative risk of breast cancer is significantly increased among women randomised to combined oestrogen and progesterone HRT use (1.27; 95% CI 1.03–1.56). The risk of coronary heart disease was not reduced by either oestrogen or combined oestrogen and progesterone in these randomised studies, and there was an excess of major, potentially fatal conditions. Thus, the use of oestrogen therapy has to be set against this background. Oestrogen therapy will relieve hot flushes irrespective of whether the hot flushes were part of a natural menopause or chemotherapy-induced menopause. HRT will lower total serum cholesterol and increase high-density lipoprotein cholesterol (Barret-Connor *et al.* 1998).

Women are prepared to consider the use of HRT under medical supervision (Couzi *et al.* 1995) and clinicians are more likely to discuss the use of HRT in the short term for relief of severe menopausal symptoms. Indeed, several authors have reported no increased recurrence of breast cancer in women using HRT preparations. These studies have, however, been non-randomised and have selected women at low risk of recurrence or other good prognostic factors (Eden *et al.* 1995).

The Italian Prevention Trial reported in women on oestrogen based HRT that tamoxifen prevented the development of breast cancer. Tamoxifen has a much greater affinity to the oestrogen receptor than oestradiol, and at a 20 mg/day dose it has been calculated that almost 200 times more 4-hydroxy tamoxifen molecules will surround a single oestrogen receptor compared with oestradiol molecules. Tamoxifen also prevents breast recurrence in pre-menopausal cancer sufferers (Early Breast Cancer Trialists' Collaborative Group 1998).

Importantly, the combination of tamoxifen- and oestrogen-based HRT appears to have an additive effect on increasing femoral bone density, but further studies will be required before such a combination becomes routine. Thus, potentially, the combination of tamoxifen and HRT may be safe, but newer drugs such as aromatase inhibitors cannot be combined with oestrogen-based HRT. However, the HABITS trial addressing whether hormone-replacement therapy (HRT) is safe for women with previous breast cancer showed an increased recurrence of breast cancer (RR 3.5, 95% CI 1.5–8.1). However, the Stockholm trial showed no increased recurrence (Holmberg & Anderson 2004). Both trials used predominantly oestrogen–progestogen-combined HRT.

### Tibolone

Tibolone is a synthetic sex hormone agent that is being evaluated in clinical trials of breast cancer patients (Moore 1999). Comparison of tibolone with oestrogen and progesterone combinations (Hammar *et al.* 1998) found that tibolone had a similar reduction in the number of hot flushes compared with combined HRT over a 48 week trial period. In addition, livial was less likely to cause increased breast density and breast pain. Tibolone had a similar effect to HRT on bone metabolism, with reduction in bone loss in post-menopausal women compared with placebo (Rymer *et al.* 2001). It is within this context that a large randomised adjuvant study of tibolone is now underway to test its value after breast cancer treatment. The main advantage of tibolone is that it has weak oestrogenic and progestogenic properties and cannot be converted to ethinyl oestradiol, unlike progestin.

A pilot study of 62 women with breast cancer taking tamoxifen compared tibolone with placebo for a year immediately after cancer surgery demonstrated an improved quality of life, and a reduction in hot flushes with no increased risk of recurrence. Importantly, endometrial biopsies revealed no increased incidence of endometrial hyperplasia on the combination therapy. Emerging evidence shows that aromatase inhibitors are more effective than tamoxifen in preventing recurrence of breast cancer, and the widespread use of aromatase inhibition may limit the potential use of oestrogen-based HRT after breast cancer except in women at low risk of recurrence such as screen-detected breast cancers.

One randomised placebo-controlled trial of tibolone after breast cancer is underway in Europe. Evidence so far suggests a combination of tamoxifen and tibolone is safe to relieve hot flushes after breast cancer treatment and low-dose vaginal oestrogen is safe to relieve vaginal symptoms after breast cancer treatment.

In general, the move away from oestrogen-based HRT after breast cancer treatment will lead to more use of progestogens or potentially tibolone to relieve hot flushes and menopausal symptoms.

For many women with screen-detected cancers and a 95%, 5 year survival, the quality of the remaining life is more important than the prevention of breast cancer recurrence for which they are at extremely low risk. In these women the use of HRT to relieve vasomotor symptoms will be efficacious and valuable. For other women whose risk of recurrence of breast cancer is high, it would be inappropriate to use HRT and other therapies after breast cancer treatment.

## Management of osteoporosis

Recent estimates have reported that 23% of women aged 50 years and over in Europe have osteoporosis. It is known that oestrogen-replacement therapy is highly effective in preventing early post-menopausal bone loss and subsequent hip fractures. Conversely, to obtain such a significant skeletal benefit, HRT should be given continuously; Lindsey *et al.* (1978) estimated at least a 10 year period. In light of recent research about the prolongation of HRT use, many clinicians and post-menopausal women are reluctant to try long-term hormonal treatment.

## Phytoestrogens

There are few data to support the claim that phytoestrogens protect against bone loss, with published studies not having controlled for confounding factors such as exercise and short-term usage.

Studies such as that by Kardinaal *et al.* (1998) found no relation between genistein or daidzein excretion and the rate of cortical bone loss. Only recently, the Menfis Trial (Chiechi 2002), consisting of 187 healthy post-menopausal women, was set up to assess the effect of a phytoestrogen (soy)-rich diet on the risk of post-menopausal cardiovascular disease and osteoporosis, compared with the outcome of HRT. The findings suggest that a phytoestrogen-rich diet is not as effective as HRT in reducing the increased post-menopausal bone turnover. With lignans, studies have shown that flaxseed does not alter biomarkers of bone metabolism in post-menopausal women (see Lucas *et al.* 2002).

### *Ipriflavone*

Ipriflavone (a synthetic isoflavone) has been reported to function in post-menopausal women by inhibiting bone resorption, thus improving bone density in these women. Halpner *et al.* (2000) found that urinary N-linked telopeptides, another marker of bone breakdown, declined by 29% in those receiving ipriflavone supplements. In some countries, it has already been marketed as a non-hormonal treatment for osteoporosis for those women who cannot receive HRT.

Despite such positive results caution must be applied. A topical large-scale trial by Alexandersen *et al.* (2001) involving 474 oesteoporotic participants found no changes between the treatment (ipriflavone) arm and placebo for bone loss or biochemical markers of bone metabolism. This group also documented the ability of ipriflavone to cause lymphocytopenia in a significant number of women ($p < 0.05$). This particular side effect could represent a significant negative factor in its long-term use. There needs to be further research to identify other long-term side effects of ipriflavone use.

## Calcium

The use of daily supplements such as calcium and vitamin D have been linked to improved bone mineral density (BMD) and the prevention of fractures. The National Institutes of Health (1994) found that post-menopausal women with a history of breast cancer consumed well below the 1500 mg recommended daily intake of calcium for women not using HRT. The usual dietary intake of calcium in this age group of women has been reported to be as low as 300–600 mg per day (Borody *et al.* 1998). However, calcium supplementation alone in the initial years of menopause does not prevent fully the loss of bone that occurs more rapidly with the loss of oestrogen. Studies involving post-menopausal women that compare the effects of calcium supplementation, placebo or control on BMD generally provide evidence of a decreased rate of bone loss in those taking calcium supplementation (Chiu 1999).

As well as increasing calcium and vitamin D intake, maintaining a well balanced diet, taking regular exercise, reducing the intake of alcohol and avoiding smoking are all important factors in the prevention of osteoporosis.

## Selective oestogen receptor modulators

Raloxifene, like tamoxifen, is a selective oestrogen receptor modulator (SERM) that has been approved for the treatment and prevention of osteoporosis. It provides somewhat less of a beneficial effect on bone density than HRT and has not been shown to help relieve flushes and sweats. In one study, a 6% increase in the occurrence of hot flushes has been observed, mostly during the first six months (Glusman *et al.* 1998).

Irrespective of this, raloxifene has been shown to increase bone density at the hip and spine and provide beneficial changes in lipids, which may help reduce the risk of coronary heart disease (Clemett 2000). Given that raloxifene is a selective oestrogen receptor modulator, it could potentially affect breast cancer recurrence, but the direction and magnitude of any effect is unknown.

Raloxifene has also been shown to increase the risk of venous thrombo-embolism to the same degree as tamoxifen. Therefore women at risk of developing deep vein thrombosis or pulmonary emboli should be steered away from SERMs or oestrogen use. Thus, raloxifene cannot be routinely recommended to prevent osteoporosis in a woman with breast cancer without further investigation.

## Bisphosphonates

More encouraging is the wide array of bisphosphonates that have been shown to inhibit bone resorption and normalise bone turnover. Such agents have been used effectively in women with breast cancer as seen in the study by Powles *et al.* (1997).

Bisphosphonates are non-hormonal drugs that induce a decrease in resorption of calcium from bone, and an increase in the intestinal absorption. Their action on the resorption is achieved by inhibition of the osteoclastic cells, thus enabling the osteoblasts to work more effectively in increasing bone density.

Currently there are three bisphosphonates used to treat osteoporosis: alendronate, etidronate and risedronate. Alendronate, however, has been the landmark in treatment. The FIT trial was the first large, well-designed trial that demonstrated a positive effect on bone mass in all the relevant skeletal areas; in particular, hip fracture risk was reduced by 63% (Figure 21.3).

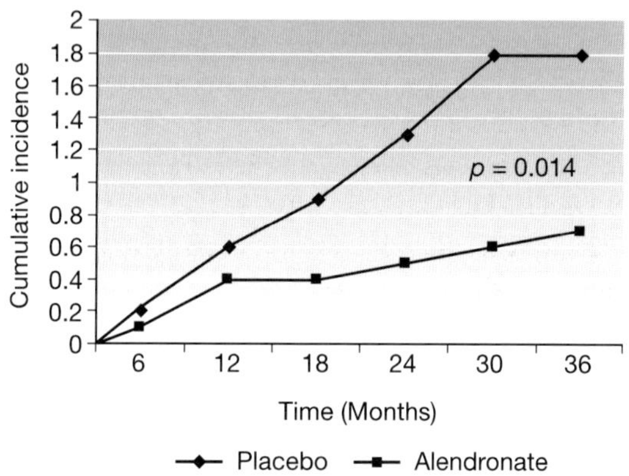


**Figure 21.3** Alendronate: efficiency on hip fractures (FIT) (Black *et al. Journal of Clinical Endocrinology & Metabolism*, **85** (11))

Risedronate has been incorporated more recently into our armamentarium. In two large clinical trials a positive effect on bone mass has been demonstrated, as well as on bone turnover markers. The risk of vertebral fracture was reduced by approximately 40–50%. In a separate study, specifically designed for demonstrating hip fracture risk, risedronate demonstrated a reduction of 30–40% (Clemmesen *et al.* 1997).

Risedronate is the bisphosphonate being used to combat bone loss in the International Breast Intervention Study II comparing anastrazole and tamoxifen in ductal carcinoma *in situ* (DCIS).

Bisphosphonates appear safe and in general well tolerated, especially when the patient follows the administration rules carefully. Unlike alendronate and etidronate, which have been shown to cause digestive disturbances, risedronate has shown few such side effects.

## Management of cardiovascular disease

It is known that the risk of mortality from of coronary heart disease (CHD) in women is approximately one in three compared with the risk of developing breast cancer, which is estimated to be one in nine. Although fear and awareness of breast cancer is high among post-menopausal women, 30% will die of heart disease compared with 4% from breast cancer.

### Phytoestrogens

Clinical studies have shown that an addition of soy protein to the diet has demonstrable effects on blood lipid levels, particularly on cholesterol, triglycerides and low-density lipoprotein (LDL).

An average daily consumption of 47 g of soy protein per day has been reported to decrease plasma triglyceride concentration by 11%, plasma LDL concentration by 13% and to increase high-density lipoprotein (HDL) by 2%.

Not all phytoestrogens have been shown to have the same effect. Studies looking at soy, red clover and flaxseed have shown little improvement in lipid profile either in normal or hypercholesterolaemic subjects (Nestel *et al.* 1999; Howes *et al.* 2000).

Other components of soya may also contribute to or be responsible for the hypocholesterolaemic effects. For example, phytosterols such as β-sitosterol in soy are structurally similar to cholesterol and, although poorly absorbed from the intestine, human studies have shown that they reduce levels of serum or plasma total cholesterol and LDL.

### Selective oestrogen receptor modulators

Tamoxifen and raloxifene both appear to have beneficial effect on lipids. Hence, significant cardiovascular benefits have been shown recently in studies of long-term tamoxifen treatment of women with breast cancer. In the study by Rutqvist & Mattsson (1993), the incidence of fatal myocardial infarctions and morbidity from cardiac disease were significantly lower in patients who received tamoxifen therapy than in those treated without. The cardiovascular benefits of this drug appear related not only to the lowering of serum cholesterol levels but also to the protection of cardiac muscle cell membranes against the damage caused by lipid peroxidation.

## Conclusion

For breast cancer patients to make an informed decision about their transition through the menopause, their educational needs must be met. Indeed, it is important that clinicians counsel women about the precipitation or exacerbation of hot flushes, especially if they are about to begin chemotherapy or tamoxifen.

Worryingly, Schneider (1997) identified that among pre- and post-menopausal women in the UK, between 40% and 60% had never discussed the menopause with their doctor. Only 4% of women aged 40–69 years in a study reported by Barlow *et al.* (1991) consulted their general practitioner in relation to their menopausal symptoms. Clinicians and breast care specialists should therefore consider the development of protocols guiding appropriate menopausal management for women with a history of breast cancer as well as women going through the 'natural' menopause. Any of the above therapies discussed in this chapter must be re-evaluated regularly to assess response, monitor side effects and, if necessary, to adjust the dose or consider an alternative agent.

In addition to making the appropriate changes in lifestyle, a reasonable strategy for women with a history of breast cancer suffering from mild hot flushes would be to commence on vitamin E (800 IU/day) given its safety and cost effectiveness. A reasonable next step for women would be to consider venlafaxine or one of the new SSRIs given their dual benefit on vasomotor symptoms and affect. An alternative would be to employ a progestational agent such as megestrol acetate. However, patients should be made aware of the potential side effects as well as informed that progestogens and venlafaxine generally do not convey long-term protection against osteoporosis and cardiovascular disease. An alternative strategy would be to reduce the tamoxifen dose to 10 mg/day or combine it with tibolone to relieve menopausal symptoms, or both.

If women with breast cancer are diagnosed as having osteoporosis or at risk of developing it, then bisphosphonates or raloxifene should be prescribed and then monitored. As for those women at risk of or suffering from cardiovascular disease, selective oestrogen receptor modulators are generally considered to represent first-line treatment.

Future treatment may also include the use of HRT. However controversial this recommendation appears, one needs to consider the most effective method of extending life expectancy against the risk of osteoporotic fracture, coronary heart disease and vasomotor symptoms, and the relative efficacy of these therapies.

## *References*

Abernethy, K. (1997). *The Menopause and HRT*. London: Bailliere Tindall.

Albertazzi, P., Pansini, F., Bonaccorsi, G., Zanotti, L., Forini, E., De Aloysio, D. (1998). The effects of soy supplementation on hot flushes. *Obstetrics and Gynecology* **91**, 6–11.

Alexandersen, P., Toussaint, A., Christiansen, C., Devogelaer, J. P., Roux, C., Fachtenbanno, J., Gennari, C. & Reginster, J. Y. Ipriflavone Multicentre European Fracture Study (2001). Ipriflavone in the treatment of postmenopausal osteoporosis: randomised controlled trial. *Journal of the American Medical Association* **286**, 1836–1837.

ATAC Trialists' Group (2002). Anastrazole alone or in combination with tamoxifen versus tamoxifen alone for adjuvant treatment of postmenopausal women with early breast cancer: first results of the ATAC randomised trial. *The Lancet* **359**, 2131–2139.

Baber, R., Templeman, C., Morton, T., Kelly, G. & West, L. (1999). Randomised placebo-controlled trial of an isoflavone supplement and menopausal symptom in women. *Climacteric* **2**, 85–92.

Barlow, D., Brockie, J. & Rees, C. (1991). Study of general practice consultations and menopausal problems. *British Medical Journal* **302**, 274–276.

Barrett-Connor, E., Wingard, D. & Criqui, M. (1998). Postmenopausal oestrogen use and heart disease factors in the 1980's. *Journal of the American Medical Association* **261**, 2095–2100.

Barton, D., Loprinzi, C. & Quella, S. (1998). Prospective evaluation of vitamin E for hot flashes in breast cancer survivors. *Journal of Clinical Oncology* **16**, 495–500.

Bassey, E., Littlewood, J. & Rothwell, M. (2000). Lack of effect of supplementation with essential fatty acids on bone mineral density in healthy pre – and postmenopausal women: two randomised controlled trials of Efacal vs calcium alone. *British Journal of Nutrition* **83**, 629–635.

Borody, W. L., Brown, T. E. & Boroditsky, R. S. (1998). Dietary fat and calcium intakes of menopausal women. *Menopause: Journal of the North American Menopause Society* **5**, 230–235.

Carpenter, J., Andrykowski, M. & Cordova, M. (1998). Hot flashes in postmenopausal women treated for breast carcinoma. *Cancer* **82**, 1682–1691.

Chenoy, R., Hussain, S., Tayob, Y., O'Brien, P., Moss, M. & Morse, P. (1994). Effect of oral gamolenic acid from evening primrose oil on menopausal flushing. *British Medical Journal* **308**, 501–503.

Chiechi, L., Secreto, G., D'Amore, M., Fanelli, E. & Venturelli, E. (2002). Efficacy of a soy rich diet in preventing postmenopausal osteoporosis: the Menfis randomised trial. *Maturitas* **42**, 295–300.

Chiu, K. M. (1999). Efficacy of calcium supplements on bone mass in postmenopausal women. *Journal of Gerontology* **54**, M275–M280.

Clemett, D. & Spencer, C. M. (2000). Raloxifene: a review of its use in postmenopausal osteoporosis. *Drugs* **60**, 379–411.

Clemmesen, B., Ravn, P., Zegels, B., Taquet, A., Christiansen, C. & Reginster, J. (1997). A 2-year phase II study with 1-year of follow-up of risedronate in postmenopausal osteoporosis. *Osteoporosis International* **7**, 488–495.

Couzi, R., Helzlsouer, K. & Fetting, J. (1995). Prevalence of menopausal symptoms among women with a history of breast cancer and attitudes toward oestrogen replacement therapy. *Journal of Clinical Oncology* **13**, 2737–2744.

Divi, R. L., Chang, H. C. & Doerge, D. R. (1997). Anti-thyroid isoflavones from soybean: isolation, characterization, and mechanisms of action. *Biochemical Pharmacology* **54**, 1087–1096.

Early Breast Cancer Trialists' Collaborative Group (1998). Tamoxifen for early breast cancer: an overview of the randomised trials. *The Lancet* **351**, 1451–1467.

Eden, J.A., Bush, T. & Nand, S. (1995). A case–control study of combined continuous oestrogen–progestin replacement therapy among women with a personal history of breast cancer. *Menopause* **2**, 67–72.

Freedman, R. & Woodward, S. (1992). Behavioural treatment of menopausal hot flashes: evaluation by ambulatory monitoring. *American Journal of Obstetrics and Gynecology* **167**, 436–438.

Germain, A., Peterson, C., Robinson, J. & Aleker, L. (2001). Isoflavone-rich or isoflavone-poor protein does not reduce menopausal symptoms during 24 weeks of treatment. *Menopause* **8**, 17–26.

Glusman, J. E., Huster, W. J. & Paul, S. (1998). Raloxifene effects on vasomotor and other climacteric symptoms in postmenopausal women. Primary care update. *Obstetrics and Gynaecology* **5**, 166.

Goldberg, R., Loprinzi, C. & O'Fallon, J. (1993). Transdermal clonidine for ameliorating tamoxifen-induced hot flushes. *Journal of Clinical Oncology* **12**, 155–158.

Gottlieb, N. (2000). Non-hormonal agents show promise against hot flushes. *Journal of the National Cancer Institute* **92**, 1118–1120.

Halpner, A. D., Kellermann, G., Ahlgrimm, M. J., Arendt, C. L., Shail, N. A., Hargrave, J. & Tallas, P. C. (2000). The effect of an ipriflavone-containing supplement on urinary linked telopeptide levels in postmenopausal women. *Journal of Women's Health and Gender Based Medicine* **9**, 995–998.

Hammar, M., Christau, S., Nathorst-Boos, J., Rud, T. & Garre, K. (1998). A double-blind, randomized trial comparing the effects of tibolone and continuous combined hormone replacement therapy in postmenopausal women with menopausal symptoms. *British Journal of Obstetrics and Gynaecology* **105**, 904–911.

Harding, C., Morton, M. & Gould, V. (1996). Dietary supplementation is oestrogenic in postmenopausal women. Abstract from the second International Symposium on the role of soy in preventing and treating chronic disease, September 15–18, Brussels, Belgium. (Abstract.)

Harper, D. C. (1990). Perimenopause and aging. In: *Gynaecology: Well-women Care* (eds. R. Lichtman & S. Papera), pp. 405–424. East Norwalk, CT: Appleton & Lange.

Hiruta, J., Swierz, L., Zell, B., Small, R. & Ettinger, B. (1997). Does Dong Quai have oestrogenic effects in postmenopausal women? A double blind placebo controlled trial. *Fertility and Sterilisation* **68**, 981–986.

Holmberg, L. & Anderson, H. (2004). HABITS (hormonal replacement therapy after breast cancer – is it safe?), a randomised comparison: trial stopped. *The Lancet* **363**, 453–455.

Howes, J. B., Sullivan, D. & Lai, N. (2000). The effects of dietary supplementation with isoflavones from red clover on the lipoprotein profiles of postmenopausal women with mild to moderate hypercholesterolaemia. *Atherosclerosis* **152**, 143–147.

Irvin, J., Domar, A., Clark, C., Zuttermeister, P. (1996). The effects of relaxation response training on menopausal symptoms. *Journal Psychological Obstetrics and Gynecology* **17**, 202–207.

Jacobson, J., Troxel, A. & Evans, J. (2001). Randomised trial of black cohosh for the treatment of hot flushes among women with a history of breast cancer. *Journal of Clinical Oncology* **19**, 2739–2745.

Kardinaal, A., Morton, M., Bruggemann-Rotgans, I. & Van Berestseijn, E. (1998). Phytooestrogen excretion and rate of bone loss in postmenopausal women. *European Journal of Clinical Nutrition* **52**, 850–855.

Knight, D., Howes, J. & Eden, J. (1999). The effects of Promensil an isoflavone extract on menopausal symptoms. *Climacteric* **2**, 79–84.

Le Boeuf, B. & Carter, S. (1996). Discomforts of the perimenopause. *Journal of Obstetrics and Gynaecology Neonatal Nursing* **25**, 173–180.

Lindsay, R., Hart, D., MacLean, A., Clarke, A., Kraszewski, A. & Garwood, J. (1978). Bone response to termination of oestrogen treatment. *The Lancet* **i**, 1325–1327.

Liske, E. (1998). Therapeutic efficacy and safety of cimicifuga racemosa for gynaecologic disorders. *Advanced Therapy* **15**, 45–53.

Loprinzi, C., Kugler, J. & Sloan, J. (2000). Phase III controlled trial of venlafaxine in the management of hot flushes. *The Lancet* **356**, 2059–2063.

Loprinzi, C., Michalak, J. & Quella, S. (1994). Megestrol acetate for the prevention of hot flushes. *New England Journal of Medicine* **331**, 347–352.

Loprinzi, C., Pisansky, T. M. & Fonseca, R. (1998). Pilot evaluation of venlafaxine hydrochloride for the therapy of hot flushes in cancer survivors. *Journal of Clinical Oncology* **16**, 2377–2381.

Lucas, E. A., Wild, R., Hammond, L., Khalil, D. A., Juma, S., Daggy, B. P., Stoecher, B. J. & Arjmandi, B. H. (2002). Flaxseed improves lipid profile without altering biomarkers of bone metabolism in postmenopausal women. *Journal of Clinical Endocrinology and Metabolism* **87**, 1527–1532.

McPhail, G. & Smith, L. (2000). Acute menopause symptoms during adjuvant systemic treatment for breast cancer. *Cancer Nursing* **23**, 430–443.

Million Women Study Collaborators (2003). Breast cancer and hormone-replacement therapy in the Million Women Study. *The Lancet* **362**, 419–427.

Moore, R. A. (1999). Livial: a review of clinical studies. *British Journal of Obstetrics & Gynaecology* **106** (Suppl. 19), 1–21.

Moyad, M. (2002). Complementary / alternative therapies for reducing hot flushes in prostate cancer patients: re-evaluating the existing indirect data from studies of breast cancer and postmenopausal women. *Urology* **59** (Suppl. 4A), 20–33.

National Institutes of Health (1994). Consensus Development Panel on Optimum Calcium Intake. NIH consensus conference, optimum calcium intake. *Journal of the American Medical Association* **272**, 1942–1948.

Nestel, P. J., Pomeroy, S. & Kay, S. (1999). Isoflavones from red clover improve systemic arterial compliance but not plasma lipids in menopausal women. *Journal of Clinical Endocrinology and Metabolism* **84**, 895–898.

Ohno, T., Kato, N. & Ishii, C. (1993). Genistein augments cyclic adenosine 3'5'-monophosphate accumulation and insulin release in MIN6 cells. *Endocrine Research* **10**, 273–285.

Pandya, K., Raubertas, R. & Flynn, P. (2000). Oral clonidine in postmenopausal patients with breast cancer experiencing tamoxifen-induced hot flushes. A University of Rochester Cancer Centre CCOP Program Study. *Annals of International Medicine* **132**, 788–793.

Patten, C. L., Olivotto, I. A., Chambers, K., Gelmon, K. A., Hislop, G., Templeton, E., Wattie, A. & Prior, J. (2002). Effect of soy phytooestrogens on hot flushes in postmenopausal women with breast cancer: A randomized, controlled clinical trial. *Journal of Clinical Oncology* **20**, 1449–1455.

Pepping, J. (1999). Black cohosh: *Cimicifuga racemosa. American Journal of Health-System Pharmacy* **56**, 1400–1402.

Powles, T., McCloskey, E., Paterson, A., Ashley, S., Tidy, A. & Kanis, J. (1997). Oral clodronate will reduce the loss of bone mineral density in women with a primary breast cancer. *Proceedings of the American Society of Clinical Oncology* **16**, 130a.

Quella, S., Loprinzi, C. & Barton, D. (2000). Evaluation of soy phytooestrogens for the treatment of hot flushes in breast cancer survivors: an NCCTG trial. *Journal of Clinical Oncology* **18**, 1068–1074.

Quella, S., Loprinzi, C. & Sloan, J. (1998). Long-term use of megestrol acetate for treatment of hot flushes in cancer survivors. *Cancer* **82**, 1784–1788.

Reginster, J. Y., Zartarian, M. & Colau, J. C. (1996). Influence of nomogestrel acetate on the improvement of the quality of life induced by oestrogen therapy in menopausal women. *Contraception, Fertility, Sexuality* **24**, 847–851.

Rutqvist, L. & Mattsson, A. (1993). The Stockholm Breast Cancer Study Group. Cardiac and thromboembolic morbidity among postmenopausal women with early stage breast cancer in a randomised trial of adjuvant tamoxifen. *Journal of the National Cancer Institute* **85**, 1398–1406.

Rymer, J., Robinson, J. & Fogerman, I. (2001). Effects of 8 years of treatment with tibolone 2.5mg daily on postmenopausal bone loss. *Osteoporosis International* **12**, 478–483.

Scambia, G., Mango, D. & Signorile, P. (2000). Clinical effects of a standardized soy extract in postmenopausal women: a pilot study. *Menopause* **7**, 105–111.

Schneider, H. (1997). Cross-national study: women's use of HRT in Europe. *International Journal of Fertility* **42**, 365–375.

Stearns, V., Isaacs, C. & Rowland, J. (2000). A pilot trial assessing the efficiency of paroxetine hydrochloride in controlling hot flashes in breast cancer survivors. *Annals of Oncology* **11**, 17–22.

Upmalis, D., Rogerio, L. & Bradley, L. (2000). Vasomotor symptom relief by soy isoflavone extract tablets in postmenopausal women: a multicentre, double-blind, randomised, placebo-controlled study. *Menopause* **7**, 236–242.

Vincent, A. & Fitzpatrick, L. A. (2000). Soy isoflavones: are they useful in menopause? *Mayo Clinic Proceedings* **75**, 1174–1184.

Wiseman, H. (1999). The bioavailability of non-nutrient plant factors: dietary flavonoids and phytooestrogens. *Proceedings of the Nutrition Society* **58**, 139–146.

Writing Group of the Women's Health Initiative Investigations (2002). Risks and benefits of oestrogen plus progestin in healthy postmenopausal women. *Journal of the American Medical Association* **288**, 321–333.

# Chapter 22

# A novel intervention aimed at increasing the emotional adjustment of breast cancer patients

*Ann McPherson, Suman Prinjha and Julie Evans*

## Introduction

Imagine being told you have a life-threatening illness. Imagine that you are at home preparing supper for your family, the telephone rings: it's your doctor. The doctor says that, unfortunately, the lump you found is indeed cancer. Or imagine being told that the cancer has spread and the treatment available will not necessarily be a cure, will cause your hair to fall out, make you sick, may cause diarrhoea and has other possible nasty side effects. The diagnosis of breast cancer will be given to 36,000 women each year in the UK, all of whom have to deal with unfamiliar and unexpected issues and feelings.

To be diagnosed as suffering from a serious illness such as breast cancer can be bewildering and frightening. Despite the fact that breast cancer is now a high-profile disease, many people receiving the diagnosis have little or no previous knowledge of the condition. They suddenly need all sorts of information about the disease itself, its treatment and how it might affect the rest of their lives.

DIPEx – experiences of health and illness (www.dipex.org) – is a unique website that shows what the experience of illness is really like for patients. It links a video and audio database of patients' experiences with evidence-based information about the illness and treatment options. DIPEx acknowledges and accommodates the overlapping nature of many lay and professional information needs. The same database is available for patients, carers, professionals and students, policy makers and researchers. It has been developed for UK users, but we envisage international collaborations that would make it possible to compare different cultures and health systems and that would promote solidarity between patients internationally.

## Background

The revolution in communication and information technology has changed people's ability to gain information about their health. Increased access to the Internet has the potential to change the consultation radically. Some patients already arrive with computer printouts about the disease. Patients with rare conditions are particularly likely to be at least as well informed as their GP. Often professionals respond with caution and suspicion, and worry about the partiality and quality of the information.

It is increasingly recognised that a well-informed patient is likely to be less anxious and better prepared for a consultation with a doctor than one who knows little. Patients who share in decision making may have improved health outcomes and those patients who do not want an active role in decision-making may also benefit from good-quality information. An understanding of treatment choices can improve psychological status and treatment outcome, independent of participation in the decision-making process.

Patients rarely have a previous experience on which to draw and therefore may be anxious or apprehensive. Many people with a new diagnosis seek information from formal and informal sources, including self-help groups; through the Internet or literature; from casual conversations with friends or acqaintances; or from meeting someone with a similar diagnosis.

Self-help groups provide a forum for patients to exchange information about experiences of illness. They are usually formed by people who share a common problem or condition, who get together for mutual support and to find new ways of coping. Many of these groups lack the resources to assess the quality of information before responding to enquiries. Some people with a new diagnosis may not feel ready to engage in the two-way exchange of experiences that often occurs in a group.

Discussion lists and self-help groups on the Internet help patients to exchange experiences. They are valuable and demonstrate the appeal of narrative. Electronic narratives allow patients to describe their personal interpretation of illness, often in great detail, which can be read and added to by others. However, the truth of many of the details cannot be checked, and if the story being told is that of another person then consent becomes a concern. Furthermore, access is limited, the experiences of the participants are unlikely to be representative, and the quality of information being exchanged in these forums is uncertain. These are reasons why people worry about health information gleaned from 'anecdotal' accounts or from the Internet.

Personal accounts of the experience of illness are particularly powerful when the reader shares a diagnosis with the author. In recent years, several autobiographical accounts of experience of illness have become best sellers. Ruth Picardie, for example, published a powerful description of her own breast cancer. The impact of the illness experience on partners has also inspired moving written accounts such as that by Ruth Picardie's sister. Many doctors have admitted that they realised how little they understood about what it was like to be ill only when they became ill themselves. Readers of the 'personal view' column of the *British Medical Journal* will be aware of accounts of doctors' responses to their own illness. Such accounts provide important insights into illness and caring. But although these sources of information are arresting and perceptive, none can represent the wide variation and the commonality of individual patient experiences. Nor can they be expected to include rigorous and detailed information about the disease, the effects of different treatments or the range of support materials that are available.

## What is the DIPEx breast cancer site?

The DIPEx breast cancer site combines a systematic collection and analysis of interviews with 44 women and one man with breast cancer. The patients talk about their diagnosis, their interaction with health professionals, the tests involved, the different treatments and side-effects and many other issues. There is also information about the illness, treatments and side effects, questions and answers, an index and search facility, links to other websites and details of support groups. Users are invited to forward their comments, suggestions and their own experience to the DIPEx team.

## How the DIPEx breast cancer site is compiled

### Interviews

The 45 interviews with breast cancer patients were systematically collected and analysed using the same qualitative research methods as all DIPEx projects. The qualitative method of maximum variation, or purposive, sampling was used to ensure the widest practical range of experiences of patients rather than to replicate the frequency of occurrence in the population, as would be intended in a quantitative survey. Participants are sought from a variety of sources including GPs, consultants and self-help groups. DIPEx qualitative interviews use a combination of an illness narrative approach and a semi-structured section where we ask about issues that have been discussed in the literature or have arisen in earlier interviews. DIPEx interviews are all collected by experienced qualitative researchers from a variety of social science backgrounds. Respondents are interviewed in their homes and are asked to describe in their own words what has happened to them since the health problem first began, structuring the narrative in whatever way they prefer. These methods yield an 'oral history' of the illness experience, analysis of which identifies the concerns, meanings and priorities of the respondents rather than the agenda of the health researcher. Supplementary questions, guided by the systematic search of the field, explore areas of particular interest, such as what they knew about the condition before they became ill, how treatment decisions were made, and how information has been sought. Interviews are recorded on audio or videotape with the patients' written consent. Interviews continue until it is judged that no new themes are emerging from the data analysis (this stage is known as 'data saturation'). The site presents summaries of the main themes from the interviews (including symptoms, diagnosis, treatments, complementary approaches, talking to children, ideas about causes, support groups and information seeking), each containing an overview of the prevalence of the range of experiences, as far as it is known from the literature. This helps to put the experiences of the participants into context.

An advisory panel of lay and professional experts is asked to guide the sampling, assist the researcher, co-author the topic summaries and identify and approve the information and links that are included on the site. Panels include patients, clinicians, members of voluntary and support groups, representatives of the relevant Cochrane consumer groups, academics and researchers. Information is reviewed regularly and the sites updated as new treatments become available.

## Links and other resources

The resources section of the database includes a wide range of material, with links to the Cochrane Library, the National Electronic Library for Health, and to other information websites that have been critically appraised and found to be of value. Other resources, many of them specific to the condition, include contact details for existing support agencies, derived from a national register, and details of biographical accounts and other forms of literature that include illuminating descriptions of the condition. Information in DIPEx is reviewed using the methods developed by the Discern Project.

## The DIPEx breast cancer interviews

The DIPEx breast cancer interviews on the site can be accessed in three ways: by topic, person by person or through the index. If the interviews are looked at by topic, there is a list of topic summaries to choose from. These summaries are based on the whole collection of interviews and provide an analysis of the broad range of experiences identified in the interviews. Clips are chosen to illustrate the written summary. It is intended, for example, that someone who has found out that they have breast cancer should be able to find that an experience akin to their own is included in the topic summary. An example is given here, with illustrative clips from the interviews.

### Example: a summary of breast cancer patients' experiences of the impact of the diagnosis

Most women described feeling shocked and upset on hearing their diagnosis. Some interviewees described how they 'switched off' and dissociated themselves from the news:

> *It was a very strange experience, I felt as though I was sitting in the corner by the window, it was rather like an out of body experience and when I came back, you know, I came back to reality, I kept trying to put myself back in the seat I was in but I kept going back to the window again. I think everybody thought I was taking it very well, I was very controlled…And fortunately I had a friend with me again because at that point I switched off completely. I heard, I've always heard that people seeing a doctor can switch off from bad news, I actually didn't realise I'd done it but I heard one sentence come out of him and I completely blanked.*

One woman described her sense of disbelief and denial, as she already had other illnesses to cope with:

*Er when they said to me that I have cancer, in fact I wept like a child. But I thought why me, why me, why, why, what person er, I'm having arthritis, this blood pressure and this too, why? So I wept. And the doctor said 'Don't weep, I'll save your life.' It was my consultant you know. He said 'I'll save your life,' he said 'I'll cut the whole breast,' I said 'What!' So in fact that day I wept. So I told them I'm doubting, I don't think what they are saying is true so they should do another examination. So it was three, three days, I had the injection, then the second one and third one and then they said 'you have to accept that it's cancer.' So what else can I do, there's nothing I can do. And so I accepted it.*

Another interviewee recalled the feelings and questions she had at the time:

*But the fact is I was so shocked because I wasn't expecting it that I didn't do anything. I just sat deadly still and I didn't know what to do. It was terrible because no one was there and then they went out of the room and they went into the office and they left me on my own in that little room, and that's when I burst into tears. That's when, that's when the reality hit me. And you get all these things going through your mind you know, how long have I got, that was the first question you know, is it terminal, am I going to die you know, what are my chances, you get all these thoughts. I think everybody must, you know, it's just, and you just, it was so much of a shock to me and I'm so young, I'd been so fit for so long you know, and I'm not the one in the family that's the smoker. I do drink at the weekend but I don't drink excessively you know. I eat fairly healthily, I keep fit, so why me, what have I done, you know. So I thought, well I must've been a bit of a bad 'un in my past life. I must you know, I must've done something wrong and I just, I wanted someone to blame really. And it's, you can't find anybody because no one's given you it, you know.*

Some women described feeling angry at the diagnosis and the timing of it. One of these women, who was interviewed two weeks after being diagnosed, recalled feeling anger as well as a sense of bereavement:

*Well here I am at nearly 74, much wiser after the event as usual. If you'd have asked me a fortnight ago to try and explain just how I felt I wouldn't have been able to do it. I'm very angry at myself because I feel I should have known better…I think if I reflect now back on that fortnight it's, I suppose, a similar thing to a bereavement, where you're going through all the normal things and yet you, as if you're behaving differently. I have been really cross at myself and then I think I got from that stage to disbelief where I felt if I'd just kept on pushing myself, just to do the ordinary everyday things, it would probably go away anyway. I was even stupid enough to put my hand and think maybe it's gone, when you know very well it hasn't, but you do it. I'm relieved now that I've got to the stage where I know exactly what is happening. I know that this is only the first stage. I'm quite confident in my mind that although there are so many people with it, you're not on your own, but I'm quite confident that everything that can be done will be done for me, and that is really reassuring.*

Other women reported feeling alone, isolated or lonely. Some of these women noted that they did not want to talk to other people at the time. One interviewee, who was diagnosed at the age of 30, described how she attempted to contain her feelings and anxieties about her young children:

*I was just in a daze the whole time. I was quite bottled up at the time, I didn't talk to people about my feelings, I coped...And everybody thought I was coping fine, which I was on the surface, but underneath I was in agony. I was lying awake in the nights thinking I would not see my children grow up. Because the daughter who'd I'd just been weaning was, she'd been born in 1981, so she was just over 1 year old when I found the lump. And my son was 2 1/2 coming up to 3 when I was having the treatment. ...Er when I say I bottled everything up, I bottled up my feelings. I didn't ask for help, I didn't talk to people about how upset I was, I didn't even tell my husband much, that I was lying awake in the night... And I was frightened that my children would lose their mother at an age when they wouldn't remember me. And having been on the receiving end of losing a parent I didn't want that for them.*

Concern for children was mentioned by several women, as well as concern for other family members. Two women described coping very much alone, and one related how she told few people:

*And I was really quite matter of fact with it I think, it hadn't sort of, I think it hadn't sort of hit me at that stage. Er I didn't cry or anything, you know, when he said it was malignant and needed to be done...Then I had to go home and it was beginning to sink in at that stage, you know, and I had to tell my husband. But I obviously didn't tell him very well because about, long after the operation, he asked me whether I had got cancer [laughs], so I obviously hadn't, I think I was trying not to worry him...My way of sort of doing it was not to tell very many people you know and people were surprised that I'd had breast cancer and so on, and I've always been like that. I don't like people to know I was ill or anything you know, but then everybody is different. The cost of not telling people is that you don't get the sort of sensitiveness and so on, kindness and so on, but I would like somebody to say 'Oh I'm so glad you're well,' not 'Oh you poor thing, you've got breast cancer,' you know* [laughs].

A few patients reported feeling 'left behind' while other people were progressing with their lives. Other women discussed dealing with the reactions of others, including pity, distance and unease:

*And people's reactions to it were, cancer sort of ugh, you know, they don't like, I mean a lot of people just don't like mentioning the word. Er like I say the oncologist didn't, and sometimes I felt some people avoided me because they didn't know what to say, and so that was, that was hard to bear really I think. Er I mean some people were great but some people, and I mean it wasn't that people didn't want to help, they just didn't know what to say, and so they just avoided it and avoided me, which was difficult... Er so I think it is more difficult when you're younger, probably. And certainly people's reactions to it are probably more marked.*

Fear was another common feeling that women discussed:

*I think the trouble is it is a very isolating thing having cancer, you, at the end of the day, have to go through it on your own...But it does, I think, also make you face up to the idea that we will all eventually die one day, and you imagine you're going to die sooner rather than later when you're first told this...I was quite surprised in a way that I dealt with it myself as well as I did. I think it's very much easier if you think you're going to get better...The fear is the overriding problem, I mean the fear of the unknown, the fear of what you've got to have done, the fear of how much is it going to hurt or make you feel ill. If you could just take all that away it would be pretty easy to deal with at the level at which I've had to deal with it.*

and several reported feeling depressed:

*I was fine I think at the beginning, I was very, I was really kind of being positive for everybody else because everybody else thought I was dying, you know, from the cancer...And it was only then, probably a couple of months ago, that I realised I wasn't fine, I was, well I mean I'm taking antidepressants now, I was really, I got really depressed, I was just really flat and irritable and not sleeping and I stopped talking to [my husband] and everything was just too much effort really...Whereas I was always somebody who would shrug off any illness, you know, I was never sick, never ever sick, and just being confronted with your own mortality I think is a scary business. And it does change how you feel about life really, because you can't forget about it and every morning*

> *I have to take this pill and I just want it all to go away and pretend it's never happened, but it has, so I have to deal with it as best I can really.*

One woman described feeling empty, and another recalled switching off from her feelings completely and relying on her faith:

> *I didn't feel at all. I didn't feel at all. I left everything in the hands of God. That was it. He's the only one who gives out suffering and He's the only one who takes it away. That's all. And even to this day I continue with life in this way. It's my philosophy, whatever the situation, that's what's written in destiny can't be erased, whatever God's written for you. There's no use in worrying. Just have faith in God. That's enough.*

Several women reported that they did not feel shock at the news of their diagnosis. One interviewee explained how she wanted to talk about her illness with all her friends, and commented that she did not feel the shock that she had been led to expect at the news of her diagnosis:

> *I came home and just phoned everybody, I just wanted, I just wanted to tell everybody, I don't know why, there was no sort of, oh dear poor me, there was nothing like that, I just wanted everybody to know. And that's when I had to deal with everybody else's emotions, and I think I thought once everybody knows I can actually be myself, I can actually then start coping with it myself, I've got to cope with everybody else for the next six weeks, it will be much more difficult…Er talking of books they've produced a book at the Breast Cancer Unit of women's experiences of breast cancer, and somebody loaned me a copy and I started reading it and I couldn't relate to it at all because every single woman who had written in it, well, it was all shock and horror and, I just, in the end, I thought, am I abnormal? Because I wasn't in that shock horror, you know, never once was I like on the floor, devastated or anything like that…But I realised that it was real but I just wasn't reacting in this shock horror way that most people anticipated.*

Some patients said that they expected the news of their diagnosis, and treated their illness, as it were, philosophically:

> *I wasn't surprised. I did say to the surgeon 'That's exactly what I expected you to say, now what are we going to do?' I don't think at the time I actually realised how severe cancer can be, not having had any close relatives suffer from cancer or you know anybody…but as you go through the treatment so you learn more. But I mean I never cried, I'm too matter of fact I think for that. I just sort of thought well you've got it girl, let's just get on with it. Let's get this

*sorted, get the next 12 months over with and then get back on with your life really...You just have to get on with it. You haven't got any option. It's happened but there's no point in asking why because nobody knows the answer to that, so you've got to just go through it and get on with it.*

A few patients mentioned continuing 'on autopilot', as it were, as things happened quickly from diagnosis to treatment, describing how it was peculiar to know that they had cancer but not to feel unwell while some patients mentioned that maintaining a positive attitude helped them cope, and others talked about fighting their illness without allowing it to control their lives. Several interviewees discussed the unfounded fears and myths associated with cancer, and one woman, aged 70, described how she saw her illness as a minor interruption that, these days, is much easier to deal with than many other conditions:

*So when he said 'Yes I'm sorry I'm afraid it is a cancer,' I thought ugh, it is a slight you know. Not because it was cancer, I will not join in this great myth that it's the most terrible diagnosis in the world, it is not. Believe me there are some nastier illnesses than cancer. I wouldn't like to have Parkinson's, I don't want to have a stroke, I don't want to have multiple sclerosis, cancer at 70, I'm 70, is like you know not such a terrible thing. It's a slow growing thing, it's easier to treat...At the moment of being told I had cancer I remember thinking frankly I thought oh bugger because it was a nuisance, because it was tiresome but I wasn't, it wasn't, I wasn't overwhelmed. I knew enough about the disease to know that I was not a candidate for immediate death and I don't think a diagnosis of cancer is a death sentence anyway. I think this is one of the great myths. Too many people have done very, very well and are doing very well.*

## Who uses DIPEx?

### Patients, their families and friends

DIPEx sites are designed to be easily used by patients, either in their own homes or in settings where there is additional support such as Cancer Information Centres and libraries. Being able to read or hear people's experiences of their illness, both good and bad, and the associated investigations and treatments they have to go through, may help patients and their families and friends to cope. Our recent evaluation of the DIPEx breast cancer sites included focus groups with women who highlighted the patchy and inconsistent nature of much information provided elsewhere. Even when information is fairly comprehensive, it can be difficult to take in:

*...you get a lot of information verbally and you remember most of it, which I did, but when I went home I realised I didn't fully understand the implications...it was just a lot of information and a lot of words and I didn't*

*really know what it meant. For example they say 'We found abnormal cells but we don't know if its invasive, come back on Tuesday' and you go away...and you think I don't really know what that means...You get a lot of verbal information but it's very hard to take in at the time, especially if you are on your own.* (breast cancer patient, Scotland)

Access to DIPEx should help patients to formulate questions for their doctors and nurses, and encourage them to identify and communicate their own anxieties.

## Education of doctors and nurses

Integrated teaching of medical students has highlighted the need to listen to what patients are saying, but in practice students may have few opportunities to spend time with patients, especially those with unusual conditions. History taking still often focuses on the narrower requirements of identifying a diagnosis rather than finding out what it is like to have the disease. The DIPEx database provides a systematic analysis of patients' experiences that is likely to improve communication and facilitate shared decision making. Medical textbooks currently make little use of patients' perspectives on their illness, and this deficiency could be enhanced by incorporating topic summaries and illustrative clips from the DIPEx database. Time is at a premium for most doctors; DIPEx could be used as part of postgraduate education and as a recommended resource for patients.

DIPEx will eventually also help GPs and other professionals faced with a disorder or disease that they may see only once or twice in their career. As the range of conditions covered extends, they will be able to use DIPEx to make up for their unavoidable lack of experience, and help newly diagnosed patients who are anxious to know what lies ahead.

## Policy makers and researchers

DIPEx can provide an additional field within systematic reviews of the effects of healthcare interventions, and help policy makers and researchers to identify the issues and outcome measures that reflect patients' concerns. It should facilitate the integration of the research agendas of investigators and funding bodies with those of patients.

## Discussion

Despite the increase in access to the worldwide web and the acknowledgement that patients need better information, too often the information provided to deal with patients' concerns is only an occasional short meeting with a doctor or nurse, perhaps supplemented with a leaflet. Although leaflets are widely used, many are of poor quality.

DIPEx is available not only to the growing number of people with their own access to the Internet, but is also being developed as a DVD for use in GPs' surgeries, public libraries, support groups and cancer information centres. The Internet is becoming increasingly available everywhere, and with it new opportunities for accessing DIPEx. Some of these settings offer opportunities for DIPEx to be used with help for those who might be unfamiliar with the technology. A key component of improving standards of care and patient choice is access to good quality information, in a range of formats to suit the differing preferences of the users. The information should of course be accurate and based on the most up-to-date scientific evidence, but also compiled to reflect the information needs of those with the condition. Even if the quality of consumer health information can be assured, patients may want material that is not usually covered by the more traditional information sources.

Advances in information and communication technologies and the explosion in access to the Internet will inevitably change what happens in consultations. People who invest time and energy gathering information about their condition do not deserve to be met with suspicion (or despair) by their health advisers. Health professionals need reassurance that there are sources on the Internet which have achieved agreed quality criteria. Patients, carers, doctors and nurses all need information that they can use to improve their understanding of illness and guide their decisions about treatments. Although there will always be individuals who prefer minimal information or who do not wish to participate in decision making, it is no longer appropriate to assume that information for doctor and patient should be prepared at different levels. Neither is it desirable nor possible to separate patients' experiences from other evidence about the effects of treatment. We need to recognise that the experience of illness is an integral part of the evidence about treatment, and an aspect that becomes particularly important when facing one's own treatment choices. The DIPEx site has clear signposts to ensure that users can access the type and level of information that interests them, which may differ according to the stage of their illness.

## Conclusions

DIPEx allows support 24 hours a day for women who have been diagnosed with breast cancer and their families, and also has great potential for educating health professionals about the patient's perspective of what it is like to have an illness. DIPEx offers a patient-centred perspective to researchers, managers and those who commission health services. At DIPEx we aim to identify the areas that matter most to people when they are ill, share their experience of illness, provide support and accessible evidence-based information, to answer the questions that are important to patients, and to be an educational resource for health professionals.

# Chapter 23

# The clinical nurse specialist and breast cancer patient: defining the *modus operandi* of the nurse and evaluating the outcome of nursing intervention

*Carmel Sheppard*

## Introduction

Although we can never truly understand the unique personal experience of any woman following a diagnosis of breast cancer, a great deal of research over the past 20 years has enabled us to understand in more detail some of the complexities of the psychological response and the effects of the disease on quality of life (Dean & Surtess 1989; Watson *et al.* 1999; Gallagher *et al.* 2002). Numerous studies have suggested that the prevalence of anxiety and depression ranges between 25% and 50% (Maguire *et al.* 1978; Sellick & Crooks 1999). Despite this knowledge, there is evidence that psychological morbidity repeatedly goes unrecognised, with the primary focus of care remaining firmly fixed on the biomedical agenda (Fallowfield *et al.* 2001, Newell *et al.* 1998). There are several reasons why the effects of cancer are often underestimated or sometimes minimised, including include poor communication skills among clinicians, time limitations, lack of experience in dealing with the emotional aspects of care, as well as 'self-protective avoidance' (Fallowfield & Hall 1994; Ramirez *et al.* 1995; Fallowfield *et al.* 2001). Clearly, there is an obvious danger that unless opportunities are grasped to explore patient concerns, with facilitated discussion around the personal effects of individual diagnosis and subsequent treatments, the emotional turbulence that many patients endure will continue to go unrecognised and patients may be denied opportunities for psychological support. The role of the breast cancer nurse has developed in response to a recognition of the need for both improved patient information and support.

## Evaluation of the role of the breast cancer nurse

The role of the breast care nurse was first described and evaluated in the early 1980s (Maguire *et al.* 1980; Watson *et al.* 1988). Watson *et al.* (1998) examined the differences in outcome for women who had received specialist nurse intervention compared with standard care (no specialist nurse access) through a randomised study of 40 newly diagnosed women. Although this study was small in numbers, the results demonstrated that the specialist nurse intervention group showed less depression at 3 months, with more beliefs in personal control over health. At 12 months there were no significant differences reported in anxiety and depression scores; however, adjustment occurred more rapidly in the specialist nurse intervention group. This study identified the importance of early intervention, particularly during the initial diagnosis period but did not support sustained long-term effects. However, a larger study undertaken by Maguire *et al.* (1980) reported the results of 172 patients randomised to either specialist nurse intervention or routine care demonstrating longer-term effects with less psychiatric morbidity in the specialist nurse intervention group (12%) versus the group receiving routine care (39%) at 12 months. The authors suggest that regular monitoring during the women's progress led the nurse to recognise and refer 76% of those requiring specialist psychiatric help. In the control group (routine care) only 15% of women requiring specialist help were referred.

The benefits of intervention by the breast care nurse are further supported in a study by McArdle *et al.* (1996), who reported the outcomes of 272 women. They compared specialist breast care nurse support versus voluntary counselling support, or routine care with ward nurse support. Although there are some methodological issues because changes from baseline were not reported, this study did compare mean scores of psychological morbidity using the General Health Questionnaire (Goldberg & Williams 1988) and Hospital Anxiety and Depression Scale (Zigmond & Snaith 1983) post-operatively and at 3, 6 and 12 month intervals. The results demonstrated that for each scale, scores were consistently lower in patients offered support from the breast care nurse compared with other groups. In addition, the authors report that in times of perceived crisis, the patient would turn to the breast care nurse, bypassing their GP, suggesting that patients may also value the breast care nurse as an integral member of the specialist team. A limitation reported within the voluntary counselling group was the lack of specialist knowledge relating to the disease process and treatment.

Although some breast care nurses have traditionally focused their roles at the diagnostic end of care, both these studies highlight the need to monitor patients beyond initial diagnosis through a follow-up mechanism whereby they can observe and identify those patients needing more advanced psychological interventions.

Nationally, some breast care nurses have begun to consider extending their role to include the long-term clinical follow up of patients, previously undertaken by doctors. Although there is considerable literature refuting the benefits of follow up from the perspective of identification of recurrence and improving survival (Schapira & Urban 1991; Rosselli Del Turco *et al.* 1994) there is less evidence about the benefits in terms of psychological outcomes of either continued or reduced follow up. In a recent study comparing doctor-led follow up versus breast care nurse follow up, the breast care nurse was reported to have recognised psychological distress in 53% of women during their follow up visit compared with only 8% recognition by the doctor (Baildam *et al.* 2001). An important point to note from this study is that the nurse did spend significantly more time with the patients and therefore the ability of the doctor to recognise psychological distress may have been limited as a function of time. Time itself is perhaps one of the most important aspects of care through which patients are given opportunities to express themselves. In addition to increased time, both the nurses involved in this study were trained in counselling, which may be considered to have contributed to their ability to undertake psychological assessment and more readily detect psychological distress.

Despite the study by Baildam *et al.* (2001), other investigators have suggested that nurses can also demonstrate little evidence of screening effectively for psychological morbidity (Heaven and Maguire, 1997; Fallowfield *et al.* 2001). It is, the present author contends, important to recognise the context in which these studies have been performed and that such studies have not necessarily considered the issues of specialist knowledge and expertise that the specialist nurse may be anticipated to develop over time. In particular, the study by Heaven & Maguire (1997) reported on the communication skills of hospice nurses, who could have been relatively newly qualified with little specialist knowledge and training in communication, and indeed this is not considered within the paper. Although advanced training in communication or counselling has not previously been an essential requirement for the role of breast care nurse, one might argue that if nurses claim advanced communication skills and counselling to be their main area of expertise then training in this area should be a prerequisite to the role.

## General framework for practice

Any long-term relationship evolves, and its development is often dependent on certain core conditions, i.e. unconditional positive regard, empathy and congruence (Mearns & Thorne 1988). To facilitate the development of this relationship through which the patient can feel respected, free to express their intimate concerns in a trusting environment and feel genuinely supported, the nurse must seek opportunities through which the relationship can begin to develop. Many breast care nurse specialists offer a planned programme of care (Table 23.1).

### Diagnosis

Normally the relationship begins at diagnosis. Weisman & Worden (1997) have highlighted the strong relationship between the number and severity of patients' concerns during the first 4–8 weeks after diagnosis, and the later development of clinical anxiety and depression. It would therefore appear particularly important to ensure that the concerns of patients are understood early on. Watson *et al.* (1988) suggest that 'counselling during the early period particularly pre operative seemed crucial in establishing a trusting and knowledgeable relationship between the counsellor and her client and provided the foundation for their continuing relationship'. It is usual practice for the breast care nurse to be present at diagnosis. Although many patients may feel unable to ask questions at this time, the breast care

**Table 23.1** Minimal points of contact and potential areas of exploration

Diagnosis: beginning the relationship, exploring family or social support, assessing the need for information and support, discussing treatment options, facilitating decision making.

Pre-treatment: assessing initial impact, clarifying treatments, supporting decision, assessing informational needs, exploring difficulties and concerns since diagnosis.

Mid-treatment: assessing psychological state, effects of treatment and body image. Giving practical advice about treatments, side effects, clothing, etc.

Post-treatment: enabling discussions about rehabilitation, psychological issues, concerns and fears. Fitting of prosthesis.

4 months: providing an opportunity to check how treatment is progressing, exploring difficulties or blocks in social and psychological rehabilitation. Identification of patients requiring specialist psychological help and referral. Offering practical advice and advice about ongoing treatment and side effects, e.g. tamoxifen.

1 year/18 months: as for 4 months.

nurse should be able to offer further consultation to support the initial information given by the surgeon or oncologist. Many patients at this time focus on the word 'cancer' with its often linked associations of pain, death, etc. (Fallowfield 1990) and are unable to assimilate much of the information given to them about treatment. During in-depth interviews women confirmed their inability to take much in at the time of diagnosis (Bottomley and Jones 1997), indicating a need for the breast care nurse to offer further opportunities for consultation prior to commencement of treatment. Whilst some patients may use this opportunity to express thoughts and fears relating to their diagnosis, the needs of others may focus on gaining more information about treatments and the options available. Patients can be encouraged to record their questions and should be given ample opportunity to express their fears. It is particularly important at this point and at all contacts that the breast care nurse is seen to have a genuine interest in the patient's feelings. It must be remembered that there is evidence that it is rare for patients to be asked about how they are feeling or reacting; consequently, this may imply to patients that clinicians are not interested in these facets of care. (Wilkinson 1991; Heaven & Maguire 1997). Most healthcare professionals focus far more on the symptomatic and treatment issues, and some healthcare professionals may even behave in such a way that positively discourages a dialogue with the patient in this context. There are often many reasons for this, including lack of time, lack of personal support (Ramirez *et al.* 1995), lack of training in communication skills and lack of experience (Maguire 1999). However, unless invited to do so, patients rarely openly offer this information for fear of being seen as ungrateful, and not wanting to overburden those caring for them (Heaven & Maguire 1997). Some patients may well believe that they should not complain about their problems and instead should 'be grateful' for the care they are receiving. It must also be remembered that many patients are reticent to disclose details of the side-effects of treatment, fearing that treatment may be withdrawn. The opportunity for more time and the nurse's specific remit to provide psychological support enables the breast care nurse to pose questions and encourage answers specific to the patient's feelings. Using key behaviours such as eye contact, clarifying, responding to verbal cues suggestive of emotional distress, enquiring about the home situation, making supportive comments, handling interruptions, being empathetic, etc., are all skills that the breast care nurse should ideally possess, emphasizing the need for training in communication and counselling skills. An initial assessment of the patient should include information about past experiences of cancer, previous psychiatric illness, recent stressful life events, spiritual support and relevance, family and social support, general hobbies and lifestyle preferences (Burton & Watson 1998).

Written information should be offered according to the patients assessed need, remembering that different coping strategies may be adopted by individual patients. Some patients may use denial as their primary strategy for coping, whereas others will have greater informational needs. Generally speaking, we know that nurses and doctors tend to underestimate the level of information required by the patient (Fallowfield *et al.* 1994). Bottomley & Jones (1997) have shown some correlation at 12 months post-treatment between information giving and reduced anxiety and depression. At this point many patients may still be struggling with decision making about their treatment options. With specialist knowledge relating to breast cancer treatments, the breast care nurse can facilitate this process.

## Pre- and post-treatment

Throughout the patients treatment it is usual for the breast care nurse to arrange to see the patient at several junctures. This will usually include both pre- and post-surgical visits on the ward at which time the breast cancer nurse will not only be assessing the patients emotional state and reactions, but also giving practical advice about bras, prostheses, arm exercises, wound care, etc.

Post-operatively, patients will generally return to the outpatient clinic for histological results and further discussion of adjuvant treatment. At this point the specialist nurse will ideally provide further support to the patients to assist decision making about further adjuvant treatments and will assess the need for further information. Degner (1997) suggests that fewer than 50% of patients achieve their preferred level of control about treatment choices, although Fallowfield & Hall (1994) suggest that it is not necessarily being given choice that is important to patients so much as the feeling that they have been given adequate information.

Interestingly, Jenkins *et al.* (2001) suggest that certain aspects of the specialist nurses role such as discussion of prognosis, discussion of investigations and treatment options are often not realised and go unseen by other members of the specialist team, yet this is widely considered to form a fairly major part of the specialist nurse role. Carroll (1998) identified up to 40% of the breast care nurse's time as being spent in facilitating the patient in decision making. Discussions about prognosis and treatments commonly occur as the relationship with the patient develops, enabling them to feel more able to discuss fears, and share intimate concerns such as perceptions of altered body image, fear of death and difficulties with their physical relationships.

At this time the nurse will generally explore the manner in which the patient has coped since discharge from hospital, and provide adequate time to encourage patients to share their concerns and fears about further treatment.

## Ongoing care

As the patient continues with her treatment, the breast care nurse will generally continue to provide on-going care. This may include practical advice and giving information about side effects from treatment, i.e. advice about hair loss from chemotherapy, lethargy, weight gain, hot flushes, vaginal dryness, and information about protheses and clothing, etc. In addition, many patients may seek on-going psychological support as there are several issues that patients may encounter as part of their illness. (Table 23.2).

**Table 23.2** Psychological issues faced by patients

Fear of recurrence.

Loss of confidence.

Difficulties getting back to work.

Blocks to future planning, e.g. organising future holidays.

Tiredness or lethargy, which may result from treatment but which might also be a sign of psychological disturbance.

Feeling low and tearful.

Feelings of anxiety.

Concerns about sexual relationships.

Low self esteem from altered body image.

Feelings of loss, anger, guilt, etc.

Fertility issues resulting from treatment.

Menopausal issues resulting from treatment.

Difficulties in regaining normal life style.

To facilitate the detection of some of the difficulties patients encounter, some breast care nurses have mechanisms in place to undertake psychological assessments at specific points in time, e.g. at 4, 12 and 18 months. Although establishing a good trusting relationship early on throughout the patient's disease will hopefully encourage the patient to feel able to access the breast care nurse at any point in time, a structured approach also gives 'permission' to those patients feeling unable to contact the breast care nurse for fear of being a burden or wasting valuable nursing time, to do so as required.

During the past 5 years the number of women receiving adjuvant chemotherapy has increased, and for many women the length of continued treatment may extend over a year from their original diagnosis. It is therefore not surprising that some women have difficulty in emotional and lifestyle re-adjustment. This follow-up mechanism also provides opportunities for the breast care nurse to identify those patients who may require additional specialist support, and who may require referral to a psychologist or psychiatrist. It has been suggested that the identification of patients with emotional distress may be better facilitated with the use of psychological screening tools (Ibbotson *et al.* 1994; Fallowfield *et al.* 2001) such as the Hospital Anxiety and Depression Scale (Zigmond & Snaith 1983), or General Health Questionnaire (Golderberg & Williams 1988).

During the follow-up visit the breast care nurse has the opportunity to explore various aspects of the patient's recovery. This will include asking the patient specific questions about any obstacles to regaining 'normality', that is to say checking whether or not the patient has returned to work or normal activity, asking how they feel about the future, and how they feel about their altered body image, etc. Some patients may also require additional information about delayed breast reconstruction, and information about dealing with side effects from ongoing endocrine treatment, e.g. coping with hot flushes, weight gain and other side-effects.

Most breast care nurses are also available to provide information and support to the partners and families of those suffering from breast cancer. It is important to remember that the effects of the diagnosis can have equally devastating effects on others close to the patient. During in-depth interviews with patients' partners, carers and relatives, Sheppard & Markby (1997) reported feelings of helplessness and fear as the most commonly described emotions.

It is also important to acknowledge that some patients may value support from other patients. Hence, some breast care nurses have become involved in either setting up support groups, facilitating them, or developing some form of 'buddy' system where patients can communicate with others in similar circumstances.

## Preparation for practice

### Specialist knowledge

It is not only the development of communication skills that influences the effectiveness of the specialist breast care nurse role but also the extent of knowledge and expertise held in relation to the disease; its investigation, diagnosis, treatment, and ongoing care and rehabilitation (which will include issues relating to body image and sexuality and the support of patients in their attempt to return to normal activities such as work, hobbies, etc.). Hence, there should be specific and adequate education about the disease to assist and enable the function of the breast care nurse. Essential for this role is a qualification in advanced breast care nursing or cancer care. In addition, it is generally accepted that nurses practising at specialist nurse level should be educated to Master's degree level (RCN 2002).

## Communication skills

As considered earlier, if the breast care nurse specialist claims expertise relating to advanced communication and counselling skills, then training in this area must be considered essential. Indeed, Maguire *et al.* (1980) states that training specialist nurses in relevant assessment skills much improves the recognition and psychiatric referral of patients who develop affective disorders. Because of this, the National Guidelines for Nurses in Screening (2002) recommend a minimum 100 hours of training in counselling or communication skills. Parle *et al.* (2001) also highlight the importance of clinical supervision, and links to psychology or psychiatry services.

## Future roles

Stepping outside the traditional breast care nursing role, some nurses have begun to expand their role to develop additional skills more traditionally associated with medical roles; for example, undertaking clinical follow up of patients, receiving new patients referrals, and advising on family history. These roles are developing in response to gaps in patient services. However, it is important to maintain good quality patient care, and also not to set aside or lessen the importance of the previously described psychological aspects of the role. Nurses undertaking extended roles should pay significant attention to the medico-legal aspects of these roles, evidencing their skills, knowledge and experience to demonstrate competence, both through audit of individual practice and reflective practice.

## Conclusion

During the past decade the breast care nurse specialist has become a core member of the multidisciplinary breast cancer team and has a pivotal role in offering emotional and psychological support as well as specialist information about treatments to women with breast cancer and their families. Whereas most nurses work with patients at a single point in time, the longitudinal relationship working with the patient throughout the cancer journey enables the development of a greater understanding of the effects on individuals over a period of time. Although Jenkins *et al.* (2001) highlight the fact that this role frequently goes unrecognised, it is not uncommon to read documentations from patients of their encounters with nurses and the significance that they have attached to the nursing function in treatment and care (Oakley 1993; Corner 2002). As well as evaluating the outcome of the specialist nurse interventions in terms of measurable outcomes, one should not forget the more subtle effects of nursing: for example, the nurse as someone to talk to, someone who has the time to sit and listen, and someone who can offer hope in times of despair which relate to individual experience and are therefore more difficult to capture or measure in large-scale quantitative studies. Although there are numerous studies that consider the value of psychological intervention for improved well being and survival outcomes (Ross *et al.* 2002), the findings of which are often inconsistent, there is a dearth of studies that explore the core value of the nurse–patient relationship and further research would usefully investigate and describe this central facet of effective clinical care.

## *References*

Baildam, A., Keeling, F., Noblet, M., Thompson, L., Bundred, N. & Hopwood, P. (2001). Nurse led follow-up for women treated for breast cancer: a randomised controlled trial. *European Journal of Cancer* **27**, 792.

Bottomley, A. & Jones, L. (1997). Breast cancer care: women's experience. *European Journal of Cancer Care* **6**,124–132.

Burton, M. & Watson, M. (1998). *Counselling People with Cancer*. Chichester: John Wiley.

Carrol, S. (1998). Role of the breast care clinical nurse specialist in facilitating decision making for treatment choice: a practice profile. *European Journal of Oncology Nursing* **2**, 34–42.

Corner, J. (2002). Nurses' experiences of cancer. *European Journal of Cancer Care* **11**, 193–199.

Dean, C. & Surtees, P. (1989). Do psychological factors predict survival in breast cancer? *Journal of Psychosomatic Research* **33**, 561–569.

Degner, L., Kristjanson, L., Bowman, D. *et al.* (1997). Information needs and decisional preferences in women with breast cancer. *Journal of the American Medical Association* **277**, 1485–1492.

Fallowfield, L. (1990). *The Quality of Life: The Missing Measurement in Health Care*. London: Souvenir Press.

Fallowfield, L., Ratcliffe, D., Jenkins, V. & Saul, J. (2001). Psychiatric morbidity and its recognition by doctors in patients with cancer. *British Journal of Cancer* **84**, 1011–1015.

Fallowfield, L., Hall, A., Maguire, G. P. & Baum, M. (1990). Psychological outcomes of different treatment policies in women with early breast cancer outside a clinical trial. *British Medical Journal* **301**, 575–580.

Fallowfield, L., Ford, S. & Lewis, S. (1994). No news is good news: information preferences of patients with cancer. *Psycho-oncology* **4**, 197–202.

Fallowfield, L. & Hall, A. (1994). Psychological effects of being offered choice of surgery for breast cancer. *British Medical Journal* **309**, 448.

Gallagher, J., Parle, M. & Cairns, D. (2002). Appraisals and psychological distress six months after diagnosis of breast cancer *British Journal of Health Psychology* **7**, 365–376.

Goldberg, D. & Williams, P. (1988). *A User's Guide to the General Health Questionnaire*. Windsor: NFER-Nelson.

Jenkins, V., Fallowfield, L. & Poole, K. (2001). Are members of multidisciplinary teams in breast cancer aware of each other's informational roles? *Quality in Health Care* **10** (2), 70–75.

Heaven, C. & Maguire, P. (1997). Disclosure of concerns by hospice patients and their identification by nurses. *Palliative Medicine* **11**, 283–290.

Ibbotson, T., Maguire, P., Selby, P., Priestman, T. & Wallace, L. (1994). Screening for Anxiety and Depression in Cancer Patients: the effects of disease and treatment. *European Journal of Cancer* **30a**, 37–40.

Maguire, P. (1999). Improving Communication with Cancer Patients. *European Journal of Cancer* **35**, 2058–2065.

Maguire, G. P., Lee, E., Bevington, D., Kuchemann, C., Crabtree, R. & Cornell, C. (1978). Psychiatric problems in the first year after mastectomy. *British Medical Journal* **1**, 963–965.

Maguire, P., Tait, A., Brooke, M., Thomas, C. & Sellwood, R. (1980). Effect of counselling on the psychiatric morbidity associated with mastectomy. *British Medical Journal* **281**, 1454–1456.

McArdle, J., George, W., McArdle, C., Smith, D., Moodie, A., Hughson, A. & Murray, G. (1996). Psychological support for patients undergoing breast cancer surgery: a randomised study. *British Medical Journal* **312**, 813–816.

Mearns, D. & Thorne, B. (1988). *Person Centred Counselling in Action.* London: Sage.

Newell, S., Sanson Fisher, R., Girgis, A. & Bonaventura, A. (1998). How well do medical oncologists' perceptions reflect their patients' reported physical and psychosocial problems? Data from a survey of five oncologists. *Cancer* **83**, 1640–1651.

NHS Cancer Screening Programmes (2002). *Quality Assurance Guidelines for Nurses in Breast Cancer Screening.* NHSBSP Publication No 29. Sheffield: NHS Cancer Screening Programmes.

Oakley, A. (1993). *Essays on Women, Medicine and Health.* Edinburgh University Press.

Parle, M., Gallagher, J., Gray, C., Akers, G. & Liebert, B. (2001). From evidence to practice : Factors affecting the specialist breast nurse's detection of psychological morbidity in women with breast cancer. *Psycho-oncology* **10**, 503–510.

Ramirez, A., Graham, J., Richards, M., Cull, A., Gregory, W. *et al.* (1995). Burnout and psychiatric disorder among cancer clinicians. *British Journal of Cancer* **71**, 1263–1269.

RCN (2002). *Advanced Nursing Practice in Breast Cancer Care.* London: Royal College of Nursing.

Royal College of Nursing (2002). *Advanced Nursing Practice in Breast Cancer Care.* London: Royal College of Nursing.

Ross, L., Boesen, E., Dalton, S. & Johansen, C. (2002). Mind and cancer: does psychological intervention improve survival and psychological well-being. *European Journal of Cancer* **38**, 1447–1457.

Rosselli Del Turco, M., Palli, D., Cariddi, A., Ciatto, S., Pacinic, P. & Distante, V. (1994). Intensive diagnostic follow-up after treatment of primary breast cancer. A randomised trial. *Journal of the American Medical Association* **271**, 1583–1597.

Schapira, D. & Urban, N. (1991). A minimalist policy for breast cancer surveillance. *Journal of the American Medical Association* **265**, 380–382.

Sellick, S. & Crooks, D. (1999). Depression and cancer: an appraisal of the literature for prevalence, detection, and practice guideline development for psychological interventions. *Psycho-oncology* **8**, 315–333.

Sheppard, C. & Markby, R. (1997). The partner's experience of breast cancer: a phenomenological approach. *International Journal of Palliative Nursing* **3**, 134–140.

Spiegel, D., Bloom, J., Kraemer, H. & Gottheil, E. (1989). Effect of psychosocial treatment on survival of patients with metastatic breast cancer. *The Lancet* **ii**, 888–891.

Watson, M., Haviland, J., Greer, S., Davidson, J. & Bliss, J. (1999). Influence of psychological response on survival in breast cancer: a population-based cohort study. *The Lancet* **354**, 1331–1336.

Watson, M., Denton, S., Baum, M. & Greer, S. (1988). Counselling Breast Cancer Patients: a specialist nurse service. *Counselling Psychology Quarterly* **1**, 25–34.

Weisman, A. D. & Worden, J. W. (1997). The existential plight in cancer: significance of the first 100 days. *International Journal of Psychological Medicine* **7**, 1–15.

Wilkinson, S. (1991). Factors which influence how nurses communication with cancer patients. *Journal of Advanced Nursing* **16**, 677–88.

Zigmond, A. & Snaith, R. (1983). The Hospital Anxiety and Depression Scale. *Acta Psychiatrica Scandinavica* **67**, 361–370.

PART 6

# Clinical governance

# Chapter 24

# Two-week wait: political versus biological reasoning on the clinical significance of pre- and postoperative delays in the treatment of breast cancer

*Timothy J. Archer*

This chapter reviews the history of political directives and whether government targets are likely to make a significant difference to the health of patients with breast cancer or continue to be merely politically expedient. It also reviews the times to treatment using performance audits conducted during 1997–2000, the period leading up to the publication of the currently operative NHS Cancer Plan.

The treatment of breast cancer is accompanied by much anxiety and fear. A delay in treatment increases the anxiety (Risberg *et al.* 1996). How much of this is the result of the perception that even a small delay causes a significantly worse outcome is uncertain. The Government's NHS Cancer Plan (2000) devoted a chapter to cutting waiting times for diagnosis and treatment and discussed in considerable depth the targets in the patient care pathway ('patient journey') (Figure 24.1). The targets set down were:

- a maximum 1-month wait from diagnosis to treatment for breast cancer from 2001
- a maximum 2-month wait from urgent general practitioner referral to treatment for breast cancer from 2002.

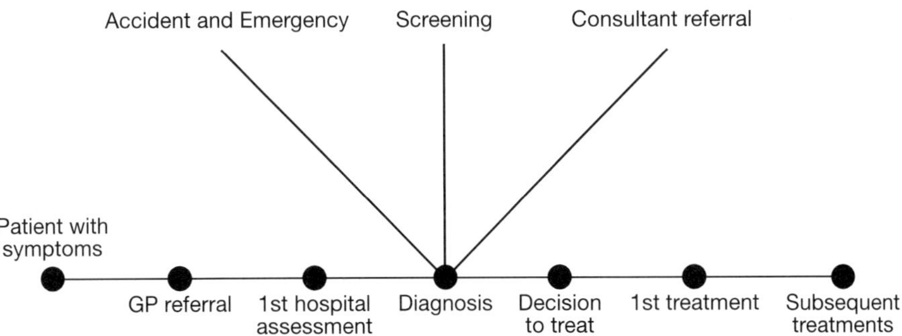


**Figure 24.1** NHS Cancer Plan (September 2000): care pathways.

## UK directives for the treatment of breast cancer

Professor Sir Patrick Forrest's report on breast cancer screening (Forrest 1986) established the NHS Breast Screening Programme (NHSBSP) with the aim of reducing breast cancer mortality. The report was specific about how screening units should be set up and made certain recommendations. Following this, triennial screening of women between the ages of 50 and 64 has been successfully implemented by the NHSBSP. In the Forrest report, there was a small section that dealt with quality assurance. This initially concerned only the radiology units, but it rapidly became apparent that all other aspects of the screening programme should be included. The Quality Assurance Guidelines for surgeons in breast cancer were produced in conjunction with the BASO (British Association of Surgical Oncologists) Breast Group and a revised edition was published in 1996 (NHSBSP 1996). This specified that 90% of all women should be admitted to hospital for therapeutic surgery within 3 weeks of being informed of the decision.

## BASO Breast Group symptomatic guidelines.

As only a quarter of breast cancer patients fall within the screening age group, the BASO Breast Group devised similar guidelines for surgeons in the management of symptomatic breast disease (Breast Surgeons Group of the British Association of Surgical Oncology 1995). These recommended that more than 80% of urgent referrals should be seen within 5 working days of receipt of the referral (the surgeon decided the priority) and 70% of all other referrals should be seen within 15 working days. In 1998 this was revised and the standard became that more than 80% of patients who subsequently proved to have breast cancer should be seen within 14 days of receipt of the referral. The recommendations for the time between diagnosis and surgery were the same as for screening. Both screening and symptomatic guidelines have undergone revision.

## Survey of waiting times for all cancers

Spurgeon *et al.* (2000) reviewed waiting times to first outpatient appointment for a month some eight years ago during October 1997. This information was collected from most of the Trusts in England, which presumably extracted the data from their own information systems. How these data were verified remains unclear. The median time for an urgent breast referral to be seen was 9 days and 90% of patients had been seen within 22. The time to first definitive treatment was 27 days and 90% were treated within 62. This contrasted favourably with colorectal disease where the median time to first appointment was 13 days, with 90% being seen in 35 and the median time to first definitive treatment 39 days, 90% of patients being treated within 95. It was not clear whether time to first definitive treatment is from GP referral to treatment or from time-definitive diagnosis to treatment. If the latter is true, the times to treatment fall considerably outside the breast-screening targets. The authors also suggest that to end the waiting times for cancer surgery would help thousands of women waiting for breast cancer treatment, with the assumption that reduced waiting times would lead to more rapid diagnosis, earlier instigation of care and reduced psychological morbidity.

## The 2-week wait rule

Health Service Circular 1998/242 introduced the 2-week target. This stated that 'everyone with suspected cancer will be able to see a specialist within two weeks of their general practitioner deciding they need to be seen urgently and requesting an appointment'. This was started in April 1999 for breast with the aim of being in place for all other cancers by 2000. The directive set up machinery in every hospital to monitor waiting times for cancers. These were recorded and returned for central review. All patients suspected of having breast cancer were expected to be seen in the time limit, suggesting a lack of realism and ignorance of biological statistics on behalf of the directive makers. The decision about the urgency of the referral was shifted from the doctors receiving the letters to the GP. This led to the justifiable fear that anxiety and an inability to rule out cancer in low-risk patients would lead to a flood of urgent referrals. Patients with non-urgent referrals, some of whom would have breast cancer, might thus be disenfranchised (Jones *et al.* 2001). GPs had already been circulated with guidelines for the referral of breast disease in 1995 and a revised edition was produced in 1999 by the NHSNSP (Austoker *et al.* 1999). These guidelines emphasized the importance of using only the classification 'urgent' for those patients whose symptoms were highly suggestive of breast cancer. This has often been ignored. It was hoped that the guidelines would minimise inappropriate referrals. This hope has not been realised.

## The Cancer Services Collaborative

The Cancer Services Collaborative was set up as part of the National Cancer Plan late in 1999. The nine first phase cancer networks tried out many small-scale re-engineering projects for the patient journey. For the second phase, all 34 networks in England were targeted and the key standards required related to:

- time to first definitive treatment
- patient's appointments being booked at three key stages
- all patients being reviewed by a multidisciplinary team
- continuing analysis of patient and carer experience and satisfaction.

With this is the requirement that the Cancer Services Collaborative staff shall measure and fully document the patient care pathway.

## Biological significance of delays in treatment

### Adverse survival outcomes

The theoretical concepts of whether delay in the diagnosis of breast cancer leads to adverse outcomes concern cell doubling times and are discussed in detail by Andrews and Bates (2000). It is unlikely that a delay of 10 months for a tumour with a 90-day doubling time causes more metastases than will already have arisen during the tumour's 90-month life time, although the size will increase from 10 to 21.5 mm. The majority of metastases in lymph nodes, which have occurred at the time of surgery, are likely to have occurred long before the tumour was detected.

Two observational surveys were published in 1999. Richards *et al.* (1999) performed a meta-analysis of 89 studies and reached the conclusion that a delay of 3–6 months produced a reduction in survival of 7%. Sainsbury *et al.* (1999) analysed the Yorkshire Breast Cancer Registry with 36,222 patients, suggesting that delays by providers in diagnosis of 3 months or more did not seem to be associated with decreasing survival in patients presenting with breast cancer. There is likely to be a very small adverse effect from any delay (Bentzen *et al.* 1999); however, the statistical power of studies makes it unlikely that this will be demonstrated in practice.

Sainsbury *et al.* (1999) confirmed earlier work by Afzelius *et al.* (1994) that patients who presented with longstanding symptoms had unfavourable outcomes. Patients who were treated rapidly after presentation also faired poorly. This is presumably because patients who ignore their symptoms have more advanced disease when they are first seen and patients with more alarming disease are treated more rapidly than those with fewer physical signs.

### Psychological effects

Most patients who delay reporting symptoms of breast cancer to GPs regard the condition as definitely not serious (Greer 1974). On the other hand, the principal reason for such a delay was the fear of diagnosis, suggesting a combination of denial strategies to defend against perceived stressful events. These observations have been confirmed more recently (Nosarti *et al.* 2000).

Risburg *et al.* (1996) studied 252 patients with different types of cancer showing that psychological distress correlated positively with the total length of delay for both men and women and that the distress was worse between treatment at the local hospital and being seen in the department of oncology. Women were more distressed than men, however long the delay. This study can be criticised because only a quarter of the patients had breast cancer.

A study of patients with metastatic breast cancer (Spiegel 1996) showed that patients randomly allocated to psychotherapeutic intervention survived on average 18 months longer than control patients. This study has not been definitively verified and there are no studies of this type of intervention in patients with early breast cancer.

## Surveys of waiting times

### BASO Breast Group prospective audit of referrals.

The historical example is given of 15 breast units who studied their referrals for 3 months during 1999 and 2000. Three of these units studied their referrals for a further 3 months after the introduction of a new referral proforma. This was designed to support the NHSBSP guidelines (Austoker *et al.* 1999) for the referral of patients with breast problems. The units observed 12,358 referrals which produced 1121 breast cancers. Seven units assessed whether the GP referrals were outside the guidelines. The median figure was 18.5% (range 8–51%). Fourteen units recorded percentage of cancers referred non-urgently. The median was 31% (range 6–60%). Of the three units that studied their results again after the introduction of the proforma, the percentage of referrals outside the guidelines had risen from 19% to 26%. The percentage of non-urgent referrals with cancer fell from 32% to 30% and the percentage of urgent referrals with cancer remained at 30%.

### BASO UK Symptomatic Breast Audit

Between 1 April 2000 and 30 September, 2000 symptomatic breast referrals were audited; 34 breast units reported all referrals and 56 units reported cancers only. This produced a total of 23,596 referrals with 4049 cancers. The percentage of referrals seen within 2 weeks varied between 20% and 80%. Some units defined all referrals as urgent and some defined all referrals as routine. At both extremes units were seeing 80% of the referrals within 2 weeks. The median for urgent referrals, where they were subdivided, was 32% seen within 2 weeks. The percentage of cancers referred non-urgently varied between 0 and 95%, with a median of 15. The extremes of range probably reflect the way in which urgency is defined in some units. The number of cancers seen within 2 weeks varied from 40% to 100% with a median of 75%. Several units were not seeing some of the cancers referred to them for 3 months. The number of patients with and without cancer was stratified for age (Figure 24.2), confirming the large preponderance of younger patients without cancer who are referred to breast clinics.

### Eastern Region Referral Pattern (urgent referrals per cancer)

Between April 1999 and September 2000, the total number of urgent referrals to all 14 breast units was recorded. This was divided by the maximum number of cancers found in that unit per year at any time in the past 10 years in order to judge the activity. The subsequent ratio was multiplied by 100. The range of ratios was 1.1–7.3 with a median of 2.35. Even discounting the two outlying units, there is a threefold disparity in the number of urgent referrals per cancer found across the region.

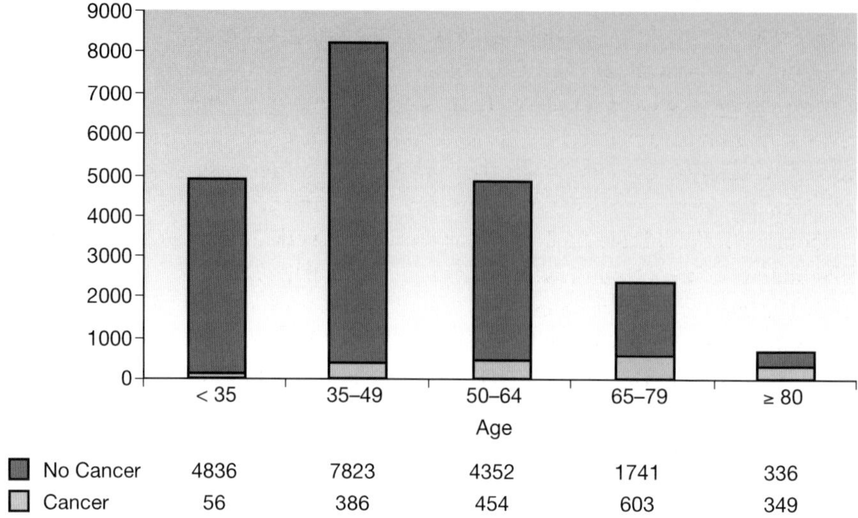



| | | < 35 | 35–49 | 50–64 | 65–79 | ≥ 80 |
|---|---|---|---|---|---|---|
| ■ | No Cancer | 4836 | 7823 | 4352 | 1741 | 336 |
| □ | Cancer | 56 | 386 | 454 | 603 | 349 |

**Figure 24.2** Numbers of breast cancers diagnosed compared with number of referrals, stratified by age.

## BASO Audit of Screen Detected Breast Cancers

As part of the Quality Assurance mechanism for breast cancer screening, there is an annual audit of waiting times for surgery. The cumulative table for the 4 years between 1997 and 2000 of the historical period examined is reproduced in Table 24.1. There has been a steady fall in the number of patients admitted for surgery within the BASO Guidelines (see NHSBSP and BASO Breast Group 2001 for the initial discussion of these results).

**Table 24.1** Four-year comparison: waiting times for therapeutic surgery

| Year of data collection | Number of cases in sample | Percentage admitted within 21 days allowing for clinical decision and patient choice |
|---|---|---|
| 1997 | 1245 | 82 |
| 1998 | 1516 | 81 |
| 1999 | 1748 | 80 |
| 2000 | 2092 | 77 |

## Discussion

The UK has devised a successful national breast screening programme, set targets and produced reliable data. This has typically been fed back to the surgeons responsible annually at the BASO Breast Group teaching day (see NHSBSP and BASO Breast

Group 2001 for earlier discussion). Only a quarter of the breast cancers are found by the Breast Screening Programme, and audit for the rest of the breast cancers is poorly funded but is undertaken by the BASO Breast Group. To improve the processes in the patient journey (referral time to first appointment, etc.) the Cancer Services Collaborative set up a mechanism for and organised meetings and workshops for all involved to catalyse change in working practice. This met with some success and many changes were reported in the Service Improvement Guide (Cancer Services Collaborative 2001) (Table 24.2). In every cancer network there is a Cancer Services Collaborative office charged with recording the patient journeys for breast, lung, prostate, ovary and gastrointestinal cancers. This rudimentary audit could be harnessed to a more sophisticated symptomatic audit of breast cancer, which had been the aim of the BASO Breast Group. None of the examples in Table 24.2 did anything other than improve the use of existing resources. Not all were successful, but many have improved the quality of patient care and the morale of staff.

**Table 24.2** Cancer Services Collaborative Service Guide Improvements

---

**Charing Cross Hospital**
Patients arriving for chemotherapy had to wait for drugs to be made up: 40 minutes taken off the total time from patient's arrival at the unit to completion of treatment by making up the drugs beforehand and storing them in the ward refrigerator

**Tunbridge Wells**
Time pressures precluded oncologist attending multidisciplinary meeting. He or she now only sees patients once and further follow-up is by the surgeon

**Mid-Anglia (Ipswich)**
Mammographic follow-up alone for breast cancers after 2 years. Difficulty appointing a suitable administrator to help breast screening maintain database and process general health questionnaire

---

## Audit data

The three surveys of waiting times from referral to consultation discussed as part of this historical review show a wide variation in both referral practice and breast unit performance. In many units the number of inappropriate urgent referrals was high. As extra provision had to be made for these referrals to be seen within 14 days, there were fewer outpatient spaces for non-urgent referrals that contain a third of symptomatic breast cancers (Jones *et al.* 2001). The National Cancer Plan's response to this disparity was to produce the target that all cancer patients shall have a wait of less than a month from referral to first treatment by 2002. This implied that all breast referrals should be seen within a fortnight. This aim remains laudable but requires the diversion of some major resource in addition to the efforts of the Cancer Services Collaborative. The problem is exacerbated by the large number of referrals, particularly of younger patients, who are at low risk of breast cancer.

Transferring the classification of urgency from secondary care to primary care physician under the 14-day rule has not improved referral patterns and some patients have had a further delay in their treatment. Although there are no biological reasons for the 14-day rule, prompt diagnosis and treatment are desirable, for both patients and providers. There is still very little information available about time from diagnosis to treatment; however, the BASO breast screening audit reviewed in this retrospective showed a deterioration, most of which was caused by a lack of beds and surgical time. Continuing audits conducted by the breast group, now developed into the British Association for Breast Surgery, will address many of these issues.

## Conclusions

- There is no evidence that political imperatives about the cancer journey have any biological justification; however, the psychological effects of delay in cancer and failure for patients to have the phases of their treatment booked in advance are very real.
- Attempts to measure the patient journey are laudable, because without this information there is no hope for objective demonstration of change.
- The Cancer Services Collaborative approach aims to ensure that the current resources are used to their best advantage.
- The evidence from the BASO Breast Group suggested that real shortages in personnel and equipment in the treatment of breast cancer remain a major problem and this remains true at the time of publication in 2005.

## Acknowledgements

The BASO Breast Group referral audit discussed here was undertaken by Paul Sauven with information from the following breast units: Kidderminster, Chelmsford, RVI Newcastle, RVI Glasgow, Kingston, City Hospital Birmingham, Ipswich, Wolverhamptom, Plymouth, Portsmouth, Chertsey, Rotherham, Gateshead, Southend and Ashford, Kent. The BASO Breast Group Symptomatic Audit was undertaken by Ian Monypenny.


*References*

Afzelius, P., Zedeler, K., Sommer, H., Mouridsen, H., Blichert-Toft, M. *et al.* (1994). Patient's and doctor's delay in primary breast cancer – prognostic implications. *Acta Oncologica* **33**, 345–351.

Andrews, B. T., Bates, T. (2000). Delay in the diagnosis of breast cancer: medico-legal implications. *The Breast* **9**, 223–237.

Austoker, J., Mansel, R., Baum, M., Sainsbury, R., Hobbs, R. *et al.* (1995). *Guidelines for referral of patients with breast problems.* NHS Breast Screening Programme.

Austoker, J., Mansel, R., Baum, M., Sainsbury, R., Hobbs, R. *et al.* (1999). *Guidelines for referral of patients with breast problems.* NHS Breast Screening Programme.

Bentzen, S., Dische, S., Bond, S. *et al.* (1999). Delay in diagnosis in breast cancer. *The Lancet* **353**, 2155.

Breast Surgeons Group of the British Association of Surgical Oncology (1995). Guidelines for surgeons in the management of symptomatic breast disease in the United Kingdom. *European Journal of Surgical Oncology* **21** (suppl A), 1–13.

Cancer Services Collaborative (2001). *Breast Cancer Service Improvement Guide.* NHS Modernisation Agency. Hayward Medical Communications. London.

Forrest, P. (1986). *Breast Cancer Screening, Report to the Health Ministers of England, Wales, Scotland and Northern Ireland.* London: HMSO.

Greer, S. (1974). Psychological aspects: delay in the treatment of breast cancer. *Proceedings of the Royal Society of Medicine* **67**, 470–473.

HSC (1998). 242. Two Week Waiting Time for Breast Cancer Referrals from 1st April 1999. Department of Health Circular.

Jones, R. *et al.* (2001). Is the two week rule for cancer referrals working? Not too well. *British Medical Journal* **322**, 155–156.

NHS Breast Screening Programme (1996). *Quality Assurance Guidelines for Surgeons in Breast Cancer Screening.* NHSBSP Publication No 20. NHS Breast Screening Publications.

NHS Cancer Plan (2000). Cutting waiting for diagnosis and treatment. London: Department of Health.

NHSBSP and BASO Breast Group (2001). An Audit of Screen Detected Breast Cancers for the year of screening April 1999 to March 2000. NHS Breast Screening Programme 2001 – NHS Breast Screening Programme. Sheffield.

Nosarti, C., Crayford, T., Roberts, J., Elias, E., McKenzie, K., David, A. *et al.* (2000). Delay in presentation of symptomatic referrals to a breast clinic: patient and system factors. *British Journal of Cancer* **82**, 742–748.

Richards, M., Westcombe, A., Love, S., Littlejohns, P., Ramirez, A. *et al.* (1999). Influence of delay on survival in patients with breast cancer: a systematic review. *The Lancet* **353**, 1119–1126.

Risberg, T., Sorbye, S., Norum, J., Wist, E. *et al.* (1996). Diagnostic delay causes more psychological distress in female than in male cancer patients. *Anticancer Research* **16**, 995–1000.

Sainsbury, R., Johnston, C., Haward, B. *et al.* (1999). Effect on survival of delays in referral of patients with breast cancer symptoms: a retrospective analysis. *The Lancet* **353**, 1132–1135.

Spiegel, D. (1996). Cancer and depression. *British Journal of Psychiatry* **168** (suppl.30), 109–116.

Spurgeon, P., Barwell, F., Kerr, D. *et al.* (2000). Waiting times for cancer patients in England after General Practitioner's referrals: retrospective national survey. *British Medical Journal* **320**, 838–839.

# Chapter 25

# NICE: a clinician's view

*Paul Ellis*

## Introduction

It is currently an exciting time for those working in breast cancer medicine. Further advances in our understanding of the molecular genetics of the disease, improved diagnostic technologies, the ability of pharmaceutical companies to fast track development of new agents, and the trend for increasing collaboration in large-scale clinical trials has meant an increase in potential treatment options available to breast cancer clinicians. What has not kept pace with these developments is the ability of a cash-strapped and understaffed NHS to assess and assimilate these often costly new therapies into everyday practice. The result has been the development of areas of regional inequality around the UK and a perception by many that the UK lags behind western Europe and the USA in the delivery of state-of-the-art cancer care. It is this type of inequality, not just in cancer care but across the health spectrum, that led to the establishment of the National Institute for Clinical Excellence (NICE).

## What is NICE and how does it work?

### The NICE organizational structure

NICE was launched as a Special Health Authority (SHA) in April 1999 and has a remit covering England and Wales. Its role is (1) to appraise new technologies and provide guidance to the NHS on clinical effectiveness and cost-effectiveness and (2) to develop new clinical guidelines outlining best practice.

It consists of a board of executive and non-executive directors (NICE Board), the secretariat and a technology appraisals committee (Figure 25.1). Representatives of relevant stakeholder groups are appointed by the Secretary of State as appropriate.

### The appraisal process

The technology appraisal committee is likely to ask two questions of the new technology or treatment to be considered: Is it likely to result in a significant health benefit taken across the NHS as a whole? What is the likely impact on NHS resources?

The appraisal process for the consideration of existing and new cancer therapies involves a series of steps over approximately a 10-month period (Figure 25.2). NICE initially commissions an independent assessment of the published literature (Assessment Report). It also receives a written submission from the manufacturer as well as additional submissions from interested parties such as professional organisations

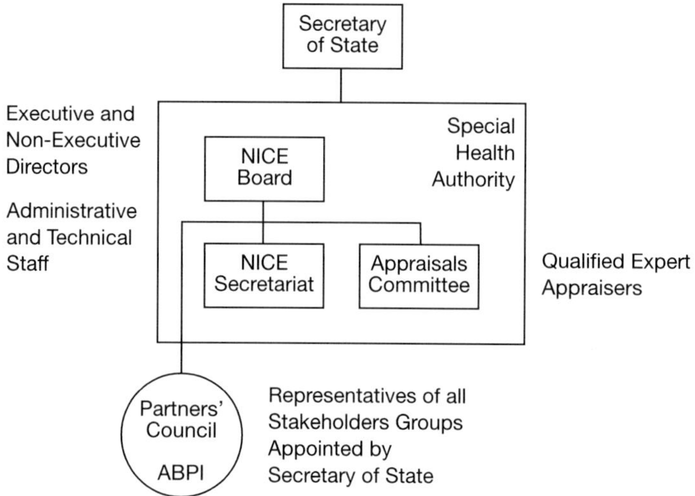



**Figure 25.1** Schematic representation of the NICE organisation.

(e.g. National Cancer Research Institute – NCRI) and patient advocacy groups. These are combined into an Evaluation Report which is considered by the appraisal committee and results in the release of a Provisional Appraisal Determination (PAD). After a 4-week consultation period, the committee meets for a second time to reconsider the PAD in the light of feedback received. This is then released as a Final Appraisal Determination (FAD). An appeals process is available, with appeals heard by an independent panel and if upheld referred back to the technology appraisal committee. If no appeal is forthcoming or the appeal is not upheld, the FAD becomes NICE Guidance and is released directly to the NHS and public. The guidance is released in a standard format and makes a recommendation on use in the NHS (Figure 25.3).

## Breast cancer guidance to date

A growing number of therapeutic areas in cancer medicine have been assessed and released as guidance. These have included the use of taxane therapy in advanced breast cancer and ovarian cancer, gemcitabine in pancreatic cancer, temozolomide in cerebral tumours, and vinorelbine, gemcitabine and taxanes in non-small cell lung cancer. Other areas include fludarabine, rituximab and imatinib in haematological malignancies with new therapies for colorectal cancer also investigated. The use of trastuzumab and vinorelbine in advanced breast cancer has also been assessed.

The guidance for taxanes in breast cancer suggested that these agents had a role in the management of advanced disease but should not be used in the adjuvant or neoadjuvant setting outside a clinical trial. It was predicted that approximately 4000

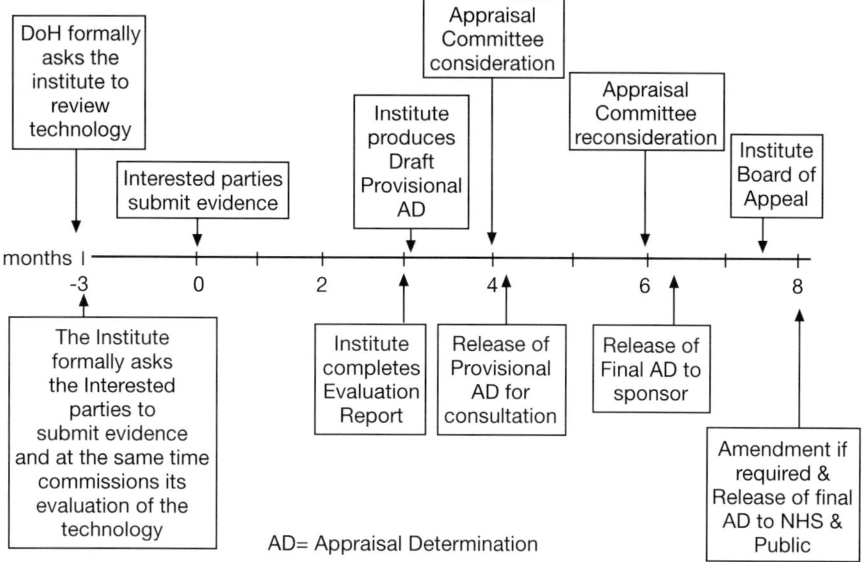



**Figure 25.2**  Summary of technology appraisal process



**Figure 25.3**  Example of guidance format when released

women annually would benefit from this treatment at a cost to the NHS of around £16 million.

## Is it working?

## What impact is NICE having?

1.  The issue of assessing new innovative therapies has been thrust into the political

spotlight with implementation of NICE Guidance and the resources available to do this becoming a major political issue.

2. Global awareness of the NICE process is generating interest in other countries (e.g. USA, Australia, Canada) with some of these looking at putting similar systems in place.

3. NICE is impacting on the resource planning of the UK pharmaceutical industry.

4. It is apparent that there are major variations in rate of uptake of new therapies around the UK both before and after the emergence of NICE Guidance. In-house research from Aventis (Figure 25.4a) suggests a trend in rising use of the agent docetaxel well before the release of the associated guidance in the second quarter of 2000. It is also clear that there were very significant regional variations in the use of this drug around the UK (Figure 25.4b, c). Disappointingly this appeared to continue in some parts of the UK for a significant period after the guidance and such geographical disparities in treatment availability across the UK remain in evidence in 2005.

## What is working well?

The selection of drugs/technologies for referral to NICE has by necessity led to the development of constructive interactions between often separate interest groups (e.g. industry, patient advocacy groups, clinicians). Dissemination of the guidance once released has also been impressively speedy and comprehensive with appropriate use made of the media and the internet.

## What could be improved?

There are a number of areas within the appraisal process where, from the point of view of the clinician, uncertainty and frustration remain, including the following:

- The appraisal process at times appears inflexible. The 'one size fits all' methodology is not always appropriate in oncology. Although the use of randomised clinical trial (RCT) evidence is rightly considered the gold standard, there are times when too much reliance seems to be placed on RCTs of varying quality, with other seemingly robust clinical non-randomised evidence appearing to be side-lined. Non-randomised evidence may often need to be taken into account, given the limitations of phase III clinical trials on likely clinical effectiveness and cost-effectiveness in routine clinical practice. At times, suggestions are made for RCT to be performed in disease settings where such trials may, from the point of view of the treating clinician, be unfeasible, impractical or even unethical.
- Related to this point there is a paucity of involvement of clinical experts with specialist knowledge in the field being assessed often until the appeals process.
- There is an increasing feeling by patient groups, professional organisations and

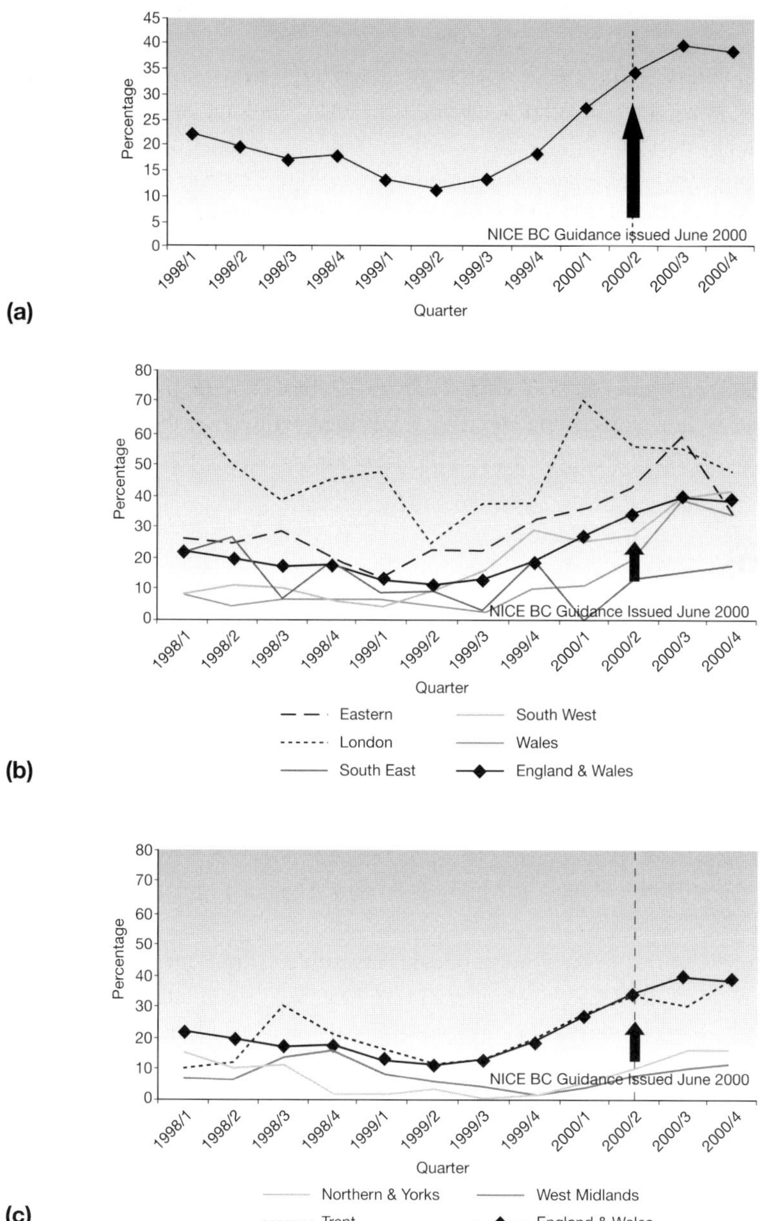



**Figure 25.4** Impact of NICE guidance on docetaxel usage in advanced breast cancer: (a) percentage of eligible patients treated with docetaxel in England and Wales overall; (b) percentage of eligible patients treated with docetaxel – Southern Region and Wales only; (c) percentage of eligible patients treated with docetaxel – Northern Region only. For explanation and commentary see text.

pharmaceutical companies that much of the evidence submitted and subsequent feedback provided are unacknowledged or ignored.
- One of the major purposes of the NICE process is to rid the UK of obvious inequalities in patient access to health care, and this is certainly to be applauded. Nevertheless, NICE Guidance has resulted in downgrading of often sophisticated local assessment mechanisms such that there may be little local autonomy in decision-making and priority setting with regard to new therapies.
- Most importantly there is a lack of clarity as to how affordability is addressed. A treatment may be cost-effective, but whether it can then be 'afforded' by the NHS is still not an issue that NICE as an independent body is able to address.

## Conclusion

The regional inequality in cancer care across the UK and the increasing development of a two-tiered system whereby patients with wealth or health insurance have access to treatments that the rest of the world considers standard, whereas NHS patients do not, is nothing short of a national disgrace. The author's hope is that the increasing prominence and influence of NICE will eradicate such inequality.

The NICE concept was necessary and timely, and the aims in the view of this author, laudable. It potentially allows the UK to 'catch up' with the rest of the world in the ability to offer state-of-the-art therapy to cancer patients. There are a number of issues that will need to be addressed to allow the process to work more efficiently in 2005 than it has to date, and definitive improvements in its methodologies may have the potential to lead to large-scale investment for proven effective existing and new cancer therapies for all UK residents. Many sceptical clinicians wait with interest to see if ring-fenced resources will automatically become available following 'positive' NICE guidance. NICE has much to address in cancer medicine in 2005.

*Further reading*

www.nice.org.uk. Official website of the UK National Institute for Clinical Excellence.

# Chapter 26

# Monitoring the performance of breast cancer teams: experience in Wales

*Fergus Macbeth, Jane Hanson and Andrew Champion*

Clinical governance has made it explicit that all health professionals are now accountable individually and collectively for the quality of the care that they give to patients. At the same time there has been an increasingly sharp focus on cancer services throughout the UK following the publication of the NHS National Cancer Plan for England some four years ago (Department of Health 2000). The quality and performance of cancer teams are increasingly being questioned and failures are attracting unwelcome public attention. Ultimately this need for more open scrutiny must be a good thing, but there are real problems in measuring how 'good' a clinician or a team is.

## Assessing clinical quality

Assessing clinical quality is tricky. First what should we measure? We should be measuring the effectiveness of the clinical service, the clinical outcomes; however, for breast cancer this might mean 5- or 10-year survival. Clearly we cannot wait for that information, even if we could be certain of the accuracy of the data and could allow for all the case-mix factors. So we instead have to use surrogate measures of structure or process. Unless we have very good research results that clearly relate certain components of the breast cancer team or of the clinical process to improved outcomes, we cannot really be certain how valid and relevant these measures are.

Once we have decided what to measure, we then need to define standards and to assess current performance against those standards – the familiar mechanics of clinical audit. There are a number of important questions about standards, however. First, who sets them? Until relatively recently, standards have been set by key professional groups such as Royal Colleges or specialist societies, but now we are having to get used to standards being set by managers or politicians. Second, what evidence is there to support the published standards as being reasonable and appropriate? Third, what kind of standards should they be – minimum, average or ideal? These will be different and have different effects. Setting minimum standards should discourage unacceptably poor performance but may have little effect on most of the adequate performers. Conversely, setting very high or aspirational, ideal standards, which only a few can currently achieve, may stimulate improvement, but may equally generate cynicism or despair if there are real or perceived resource constraints. Setting average standards may have little effect other than fossilising the status quo.

Measurement of performance is often difficult. Retrospective collection of data from case records is time-consuming and often incomplete. Prospective data collection requires agreement on what should be collected, as well as the resources and the commitment to do it routinely. Finally there may be difficulties in deciding who analyses the data and has access to the results, and whether traditional anonymity should be preserved.

In this chapter we reflect on some of these difficulties with particular reference to our experience with breast cancer teams in Wales.

## Implementing Calman–Hine in Wales

After the publication of the Calman–Hine Report in 1995 (Expert Advisory Group on Cancer 1995), the Welsh Office commissioned work to describe how cancer services should be taken forward in Wales. This high level backing and the active involvement of clinicians throughout were key to the success of the resulting Cameron Report, which was published in 1996 (Cancer Services Expert Group 1996). Implementation of the Report's recommendations was ensured by establishing the Cancer Services Co-ordinating Group (CSCG) in 1997.

The CSCG is composed of representatives of trusts, health authorities, general practitioners, community health councils, patients, specific professional groups and academia. This group was the only example of a focused, service-specific, multidisciplinary advisory body to the Welsh Office, now the National Assembly for Wales (NAW), and to the health authorities. Subgroups were also set up, one of which is the Minimum Standards Working Group (MSWG). Advice on breast cancer services in Wales is provided by a Breast Cancer Steering Group. These and other tumour site-specific groups were recommended by the Cameron Report in 1996 with terms of reference that focused on:

- Assessment of clinical guidelines and their implementation in Wales.
- Development of an All Wales clinical minimum data set.
- Identification of tumour site priorities, e.g. workforce and training, equipment, clinical information, organisation.
- Involvement with clinical audit and research
- Collaboration with the CSCG and its working groups in an advisory capacity.

Membership had to reflect the disciplines and professions in the breast cancer multidisciplinary teams with the addition of a patient representative and general practitioner. Before the CSCG was set up, a considerable amount of important work had already been done by breast care professionals in Wales. Much of this work laid the foundations for the rapid development of breast teams and locally agreed clinical guidelines. The newly created Breast Cancer Steering Group subsequently carried this work forward.

## Setting standards

Between 1997 and 1999 the CSCG, in consultation with its cancer expert advisory groups, issued minimum standards and monitoring tools for the major tumour sites and specialist palliative care. All the standards and monitoring tools originated from the cancer site expert groups, after consultation with clinical teams across Wales, but were finally assessed by the MSWG to ensure consistency and a generic 'core' set of standards. Once completed, the draft standards required agreement of the CSCG Board before they were issued to the commissioners, who had to make sure that they were implemented.

At the outset, the MSWG had to decide how comprehensive and how detailed the standards should be. It seemed pointless to reiterate existing national or Royal College standards. Emphasis was therefore placed on communication between primary and secondary care and information to patients. For many cancers, time targets were set, not only for the initial consultation, but also for a management plan to be agreed (Table 26.1). In 1999 this was a novel approach to national cancer service standards. They were also quite deliberately *minimum* standards and the intention was gradually to increase their scope year on year. From the outset, the MSWG decided it wanted to foster a culture of continuous improvement. It was not, nor did it wish to be, a policing agency.

The Breast Cancer Steering Group was central to the initial standard setting process in 1997 and subsequent revisions in 1998 and 2000 (Table 26.2). It refined the monitoring tool and assessed the national perspective from the data collected. It also advised on the allocation of funding ear-marked for breast cancer and updated the CSCG on continuing gaps in the service.

The first standards issued in 1997 (see Table 26.1) took the British Association of Surgical Oncologists (BASO) standard of all urgent referrals being seen within 5 working days. The findings of a CSCG national survey on waiting times and the move to the generic 2-week wait resulted in revision of this standard. Also, although everyone was prepared to accept, in principle, the 2-week waiting time standard for urgent cases, the CSCG decided, on advice from the steering groups, that the 'urgency' of individual cases should be defined by the hospital clinicians rather than by the GPs.

## Monitoring the standards

Clearly, there is no point in setting national standards for clinical care unless there is some mechanism for measuring how well teams are performing against them. In Wales there have been three separate pieces of work which have aimed to obtain information about this:

- Reports from the five health authority cancer teams.
- A national retrospective audit for 1997.

**Table 26.1** All Wales breast cancer minimum standards (first published 1997)

**Standards**
***Organisational standards***
There should be a named lead clinician in each Trust with overall responsibility for cancer services

There should be a named lead clinician for the breast cancer specialist team

Cancer care should be provided by a specialist multi-professional/disciplinary team as detailed in the CSEG report

**Communication**
All local GPs should know of the existence of the specialist breast team and the person to contact

The breast team should ensure that results for women with a diagnosis of cancer should reach the GP within 24 hours after the outpatient clinic

There should be effective communication with the patient and their carers

Information should be provided for the patient

**Rapid diagnosis**
There should be a mechanism to provide GPs rapid access to the specialist team. At least 80% of urgent referrals with a possible diagnosis of breast cancer should be seen within 5 working days of receipt by the hospital of the referral

Diagnosis of primary disease should be carried out using 'triple assessment' for each new patient at a single visit. Results should be given to the patient within 5 working days and, if necessary, an appointment for treatment within 14 working days

**Treatment**
Breast teams should work within written evidence-based clinical guidelines

Chemotherapy must be given according to the Joint Council for Clinical Oncology criteria

Radiotherapy centres should have Quality Assurance in Radiotherapy accreditation

**Clinical Information**
The team should recognise the importance of cancer registration and ensure that the items in the minimum dataset required for high quality cancer registration are correctly recorded and transmitted to the Welsh Cancer Intelligence and Surveillance Unit

The team should regularly carry out multidisciplinary audit of its services. Data should be collected using the BASO database

**Table 26.2** Revisions to the 1997 breast cancer minimum standards (published September 2000)

---

**Organisational**

[a]Cancer services in Wales should be integrated at cancer centre level

[a]A cancer centre and its associated units must provide an integrated network for cancer care

**Rapid diagnosis**

There should be a mechanism, e.g. by telephone, secure fax or email, to provide GPs rapid access to the appropriate specialist in the multidisciplinary team (MDT). Urgent referrals with a suspected diagnosis of breast cancer must be seen within 10 working days of receipt by the hospital of the referral

All diagnostic tests that are needed should be carried out in one visit. Results should be given to the patient within 5 working days and, if necessary and taking account of patient choice, an appointment for treatment within 15 working days

**Treatment**

[a]Patients should be given the opportunity to enter approved clinical trials for which they fulfil the entry criteria

[a]All services caring for cancer patients, in particular those with progressive life-threatening disease, have a responsibility to provide care with a palliative approach. All patients should have access to specialist palliative care services as described in the CSCG Minimum Standards for Specialist Palliative Care

**Follow-up**

[a]There should be an agreed means for patients and GPs to have rapid access to the MDT if recurrent breast cancer is suspected

---

[a]Indicates a new standard added for 2000.

- Snapshot audits of breast referral waiting times (including the '2-week wait'). Each of these approaches has given some information but none is complete or necessarily reliable.

## Health authority reports

The guiding principle for monitoring these standards is that individual teams monitor their own performance, using a centrally provided tool, through their own audit mechanisms. A uniform monitoring tool, drawn up by the CSCG and its All Wales Cancer Steering Groups, is important because data are collated by CSCG to provide a national perspective. The tool offsets the variation in approach and 'culture' in the different health authorities, and ensures the same core questions are asked of all multidisciplinary teams (MDTs). Information and data provided by MDTs are 'signed off' by Trust Chief Executives and the health authority cancer lead, and verified and used by the health authority cancer teams to focus on gaps in service provision and priority areas.

The strength of this approach has been that it has brought commissioners and MDTs together to run a locally owned rather than a central process. There is a completed circle between commissioner and provider, which informs local Health Improvement Plans. The down side has been uncertainty about the quality of some of the data provided and the time required for health authorities to visit MDTs and verify what has been provided before detailing action plans. The time to publication of the national picture is inevitably also unacceptably long. The solution to this must be the move to prospective data collection with information of high quality at source used by MDTs to audit their performance.

One prominent report of the national compliance to breast, colorectal and lung cancer standards was published some four years ago (Cancer Services Co-ordinating Group 2000a). The key findings were a lack of data and the need for more robust audit with regard to written policies. The final stage was to supplement this self-assessment with independent peer review.

The monitoring process for 1998/1999, for example, indicated that 12 of 16 teams (75%) were using the BASO database to enter data on new referrals. Of those 12, only 4 (25%) reported complete data entry. This resulted partially from lack of staff to input data. During the first few months of 1999, CSCG-funded information staff were appointed. Smaller trusts were allocated a part- or full-time data entry clerk with larger trusts being allocated in addition a cancer information coordinator. The three cancer centres were also allocated a cancer information specialist. Looking back, this use of resources only just begun to meet the need and has emphasised the importance of supporting MDTs with a coordinator who is able to access all the necessary information. As a result of this support, the monitoring process unpublished data for 1999/2000 showed a clear improvement with all teams using BASO and 64% reporting complete data entry.

## Retrospective audit (1997)

It became increasingly clear that some kind of comprehensive baseline assessment of breast cancer services was needed. By chance, audits of colorectal cancer and lung cancer in Wales had already been carried out. Information from these had been important in identifying shortfalls in the service and problem areas, and had influenced the work of the CSCG. So a retrospective audit of breast cancer services was commissioned in 1999 to include all patients diagnosed during 1997, a time period before the CSCG had started work. A report was subsequently published in February 2001 (Cancer Services Co-ordinating Group 2001).

This audit was carried out by staff from the breast cancer screening service, Breast Test Wales. They were supervised by an advisory steering group of relevant clinicians, and the anonymity of the hospitals and individual clinicians was scrupulously maintained. Patients were identified from a number of sources including the Breast Test Wales database and the Welsh Cancer Registry. Case notes were found and data extracted from them by trained clerks using a standardised proforma.

The strengths of this method are that it is an external, impartial scrutiny using consistent methodology and, provided that the clerks are properly trained and supervised, the data should be accurate. The weaknesses are the difficulties of obtaining complete data retrospectively, when case notes may be missing or incomplete or data items not clearly documented. It is also a costly and time-consuming exercise with an inevitable time lag between the events and the report.

The key findings from this report were that in 1997:

- Of the records, 96% were available.
- The caseload of the 49 surgical consultants ranged from 1 to 200 new cases per year, with a mean of 40; however, 85% of patients were seen by 16 consultants, who saw more than 50 new cases per year.
- The waiting time from referral to first being seen was an average of 9 working days, but only 28% were seen within 5 and 65% within 10 working days (note that there was no retrospective identification of 'urgency'); the results varied significantly between hospitals and health authorities and there was no clear relationship between workload and efficiency.
- The processes of care were generally adequate and consistent; the results in Wales for variables, such as the diagnostic tests before surgery, the completeness of pathological information and axillary node biopsy, were generally as good if not better than those from comparable audits carried out in other parts of the UK.
- Things were not perfect and there was room for improvement, especially in meeting the minimum standards that were being set.

## Snapshot audits

With the publication of the minimum standards for breast cancer services in 1997 (with revisions published in 1998 and 2000) (Cancer Services Co-ordinating Group 1997, 2000b) and the publication three years ago of the document *Improving Health in Wales* (NHS Wales, 2001), there is now a need to monitor waiting times for access to cancer teams and to treatment. To do this properly would mean continuous data collection on all individuals as they move along the care pathway. Appropriate information systems are slowly being put in place to be able to collect such data routinely and to analyse it centrally. So, without the appropriate information infrastructure, any alternative mechanism would inevitably be time-consuming and expensive.

An interim strategy was developed, based on a survey of all new breast clinic attendees run over a 4-week period during October 1999. This time-span was chosen to allow enough referrals to access the clinic and ensure that the data would be meaningful. This approach provided a 'snapshot' of the performance of the breast teams against waiting time targets, which could be fed back quickly to the NAW and the individual breast teams.

This meant that the CSCG had to work closely with the Breast Cancer Steering Group and Trust breast cancer teams to develop a simple and reliable way of collecting data. A standard proforma was produced to collect all waiting-time data and the priority status of the patient (urgent, non-urgent or family history). Data were provided by the teams themselves. This ensured that, as far as possible, accurate information was obtained that reflected the running of each breast clinic. All breast clinics in Wales participated in the survey, with the agreement of the clinicians. In most cases data collection was carried out by CSCG-funded information staff and was returned to the CSCG for central analysis. On completion, a summary of the data was returned to individual breast cancer teams for verification and an All Wales report published (Cancer Services Co-ordinating Group 2000c).

One of the most striking features of the data was the apparent lack of consistency across Wales in the interpretation of 'urgency' as deemed by the surgeon. Categorisation of urgency varied considerably between teams (11.6–83.0% of all referrals). Of the total patients subsequently categorised as urgent across Wales, 88.1% were seen within 10 working days of receipt by the hospital of the GP referral. In addition 99.2% of all referrals had all their diagnostic tests within two hospital visits and 94.3% were given their results within 5 working days from the date of their last diagnostic test. Of those patients subsequently diagnosed with breast cancer, 79.1% were offered an appointment for surgical treatment within 15 working days from the time that they were informed of the diagnosis.

The findings of the October 1999 'snapshot' survey have resulted in:

- guideline development (including guidance on criteria for 'urgent' referrals)
- the re-definition of an NAW guarantee on the waiting time for access of urgent referrals to breast teams
- additional CSCG funding to support GP referral processes.

One inherent weakness of this type of audit is that it provides only a short-term overview of the service. There may be particular local problems before or during the audit period (e.g. absence of key staff or cancellation of clinics) that affect performance. All teams were asked to provide full details of such difficulties. Conversely a 'Hawthorne effect' may operate and a team may perform better than usual when it knows that it is being scrutinised.

However, the strength of this approach has been its relative simplicity, with accurate results available to the service quickly enough to be meaningful. Furthermore, both the survey itself and associated data are 'owned' by the participating clinicians.

## The future

We have already described the potential hazards of snapshot audits and the difficulties of large-scale retrospective audits. Clearly, if there is thought to be a need to monitor continuously standards of clinical care, this can be done only by routine, prospective data collection and analysis. At the moment we cannot obtain data on all patients all of the time, but this may have to change in light of a more formal performance management approach.

This of course will in turn need robust data collection and information systems. The information can subsequently be used in three ways:

* to engage trust senior management
* to enable the breast cancer teams to assess their service
* to enable the CSCG to advise the NAW.

This is the long-term vision of the CSCG and of the Cancer Information Framework (Cancer Services Co-ordinating Group 2000d). But three important things are needed:

* Agreed data sets that capture the key data items.
* The infrastructure (data staff, computer hardware, uniform software) to support prospective, real time data collection and analysis.
* Willingness of the clinical staff to ensure that data collection is complete, accurate and up to date.

Consultation on data sets for key sites began in Wales in 2001 and the breast cancer dataset set was based on the BASO one, with additional fields to monitor the Welsh minimum standards. This project was separate from, but parallel to, a similar, more ambitious project in England. The philosophy underpinning the Welsh approach is different. We are trying to keep the number of data items to a minimum by concentrating on the outputs – the things we need to know to monitor quality, rather than the things it would be nice to know. Pragmatism and the knowledge that there is unlikely to be the same investment of resources as in England have determined this.

The intention is that the data will 'belong' to the clinical teams and the responsibility for primary analysis and local reporting will be theirs. However, reports on data relating to the minimum standards will be analysed centrally from regular returns. This will be fed back not only to the individual teams but also to the Breast Cancer Steering Group, who will take responsibility for interpreting the data and assessing its significance. They will compare performance with the published standards and make recommendations for action. The data will be owned throughout by the clinicians and analysed by their peers. In this way, we hope that the process will seem to be fair and believable, the quality of the data will be maintained and genuine improvements made.

Huge uncertainties still remain. There is no good evidence that this elaborate process of standard setting and performance monitoring across a national service will either reassure the public or politicians or, more importantly, actually improve clinical care. There are at the moment no clear mechanisms for dealing with non-compliance, although perhaps clinical governance provides a framework and the Healthcare Commission (CHAI) may represent the ultimate judge. Finally, it is not clear that the clinical time and effort to make this process reliable and effective will be supported by real investment in staff and resources. Inaccurate information is as unhelpful as no information, and good information is not cheap.

## Conclusions

NHS Wales has, for better or worse, embarked on a course of setting and monitoring the standards of breast cancer care. As far as possible the process has been carried out in close consultation with the health professionals actually involved in clinical care and not imposed from above without wide consultation. A retrospective audit has been largely reassuring about important clinical aspects of care but raised questions about workload and times to diagnosis and treatment, which were confirmed by the snapshot audits. The routine monitoring of standards has also highlighted problems about the availability and reliability of relevant information.

There is now an ambitious plan to monitor the standards by collecting data prospectively and routine analysis. Time will tell whether this is possible and effective.

## Acknowledgements

We are grateful to Dr Peter Barrett-Lee for valuable comments on an early draft of this manuscript.

*References*

Cancer Services Co-ordinating Group (1997). *Breast Cancer Services. All Wales Minimum Standards.* Cardiff: CSCG.

Cancer Services Co-ordinating Group (2000a). *Minimum Standards for Cancer Services in Wales 1998-1999. Breast, Colorectal and Lung Cancer Summary Report.* Cardiff: CSCG.

Cancer Services Co-ordinating Group (2000b). *Breast Cancer Services. All Wales Minimum Standards.* Cardiff: CSCG.

Cancer Services Co-ordinating Group (2000c). *All Wales Survey of Primary Breast Referral Waiting Times.* Cardiff: CSCG.

Cancer Services Co-ordinating Group (2000d). *Cancer Services Information Framework.* Cardiff: NHS Wales.

Cancer Services Co-ordinating Group (2001). *The Management of Breast Cancer in Wales.* A retrospective audit carried out on behalf of the CSCG. Cardiff: CSCG.

Cancer Services Expert Group (1996). *Cancer Services in Wales.* A Report by the Cancer Services Expert Group (Chairman, Professor Ian Cameron). Cardiff: NHS Wales.

Department of Health (2000). *The NHS Cancer Plan. A plan for investment. A plan for reform.* London: Department of Health.

Expert Advisory Group on Cancer (1995). *A Policy Framework for Commissioning Cancer Services. Improving the Quality of Cancer Services*. A Report by The Expert Advisory Group on Cancer to the Chief Medical Officers of England and Wales.

NHS Wales (2001). *Improving Health in Wales. A Plan for the NHS with its partners*. Cardiff: National Assembly for Wales.

# Index